Evidence-Based CBT for Anxiety and Depression in Children and Adolescents

Evidence-Based CBT for Anxiety and Depression in Children and Adolescents

A Competencies-Based Approach

Edited by

Elizabeth S. Sburlati, Heidi J. Lyneham,
Carolyn A. Schniering, and
Ronald M. Rapee

WILEY Blackwell

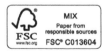

To Melba: your strength, resilience, commitment, warmth and playfulness continue to inspire
Liz

To my Mum, who inspires people to strive for competence every day
Heidi

To Mark, Nicola, and Henry
Carolyn

To Wendy, Alice, and Lucy
Ron

Contents

Part III   Specific CBT Techniques   **157**

Notes on Editors

Elizabeth S. Sburlati, PhD MClinPsych, is involved in research at Macquarie University's Centre for Emotional Health. Elizabeth is also a clinical psychologist. Her research interests are in the dissemination and implementation of evidence-based practice in "real-world" settings, as well as in the treatment of child and adolescent anxiety and depression. She has published journal articles in peer-reviewed journals, has presented research at conferences, has peer-reviewed articles for numerous journals, and has peer-reviewed presentation proposals for the 1st and 2nd biennial Global Implementation Conferences.

Heidi J. Lyneham, PhD MClinPsych, is the Clinic Director at the Emotional Health Clinic, Centre for Emotional Health, Macquarie University, Australia. Heidi's research interests include improving assessment and treatment methods for emotional problems experienced by children and adolescents. With a specific focus on improving access to services, Heidi has published a number of papers that investigate the use of supported bibliotherapy in treating anxiety, particularly for those from rural areas. She is an author of the well-known Cool Kids Anxiety Treatment Program.

Carolyn A. Schniering, PhD MClinPsych, is a senior lecturer and child psychologist at the Centre for Emotional Health, Department of Psychology, Macquarie University, Australia. Carolyn has first-hand experience in the treatment of adolescents with emotional difficulties and recently developed and evaluated a new transdiagnostic treatment that targets both anxiety and depression in youth. She also developed the Children's Automatic Thoughts Scale (CATS), which has been used on a national and international scale to identify thinking styles associated with emotional syndromes in children and adolescents.

Ronald M. Rapee, AM PhD MSc (Psych), is currently Distinguished Professor in the Department of Psychology, Macquarie University, Sydney and Director of the Centre for Emotional Health. He has published extensively on the understanding and management of emotional difficulties across the lifespan and has written and edited books for professionals and for the general public. Ron has received several awards for his scientific contributions, and in 2012 he was made a Member of the Order of Australia for his contributions to clinical psychology in Australia.

Notes on Contributors

Rinad S. Beidas, PhD, conducts research centered on the dissemination and implementation of evidence-based practices (EBPs) for youth in community settings. Previous work includes an NIMH-funded F31 MH 083333 randomized controlled trial investigating the efficacy of three training methods and ongoing support of therapist fidelity. Current work involves an NIMH funded K23 MH099179 project that prospectively investigates the impact of a policy on implementation of EBPs in outpatient mental health services for youth.

James Bennett-Levy is an associate professor at the University of Sydney's University Centre for Rural Health (North Coast). He has been one of the leading writers and researchers on CBT therapist training over the past decade. He has also co-authored the *Oxford Guide to Imagery in Cognitive Therapy* (2011) and co-edited the *Oxford Guide to Behavioural Experiments in Cognitive Therapy* (2004) and the *Oxford Guide to Low Intensity CBT Interventions* (2010).

Gemma Bowers works as a clinical psychologist with children and young people in Norfolk, UK. She has a particular interest in working with families who have a child with a chronic health problem, such as diabetes. She has also worked with children in mental health services and has an interest in the treatment of anxiety disorders in children.

Ruth C. Brown, PhD, is a postdoctoral fellow at the Virginia Institute for Psychiatric and Behavioral Genetics at Virginia Commonwealth University. Her primary research interest is the assessment of etiological factors and treatment mechanisms among youth and emerging adults with anxiety disorders. She is also interested in the adaptation and evaluation of evidence-based practices for anxiety disorders among youth with intellectual disabilities.

Sarah Clark works as a clinical psychologist in the NHS in Suffolk, UK and as a clinical tutor on the clinical psychology doctoral training programme at the University of East Anglia in Norwich. In her clinical work she has an interest in anxiety disorders and in obsessive compulsive disorder in children and adolescents.

Jonathan S. Comer, PhD, is Associate Professor of Psychology at Florida International University and the Center for Children and Families. Before this he was director of the Early Childhood Interventions Program at Boston University, an interdisciplinary clinical research laboratory devoted to expanding the quality and accessibility of mental health care for young children. His research examines anxiety and disruptive behavior disorders, with particular focus on the innovative use of new technologies for extending the availability of care.

Cathy Creswell, PhD, is a principal research fellow, MRC clinician scientist fellow, and honorary consultant clinical psychologist at the Winnicott Research Unit, School of Psychology and Clinical Language Sciences, University of Reading, UK. Cathy's research interests are the development and treatment of childhood anxiety disorders. Key recent publications are "Cognitive, Affective, and Behavioral Characteristics of Mothers with Anxiety Disorders in the Context of Child Anxiety Disorder" (co-authored with A. Apetroaia, L. Murray, and P. Cooper), published in 2012 in the *Journal of Abnormal Psychology*, and "Interpretation and Expectation in Childhood Anxiety Disorders: Age Effects and Social Specificity" (co-authored with L. Murray and P. Cooper), awaiting publication in the *Journal of Abnormal Child Psychology*.

Colleen M. Cummings, PhD, is a postdoctoral fellow at the Child and Adolescent Anxiety Disorders Clinic at Temple University, under the mentorship of Dr Philip C. Kendall. Her dissertation in graduate school at Ohio State University focused on anxiety comorbidity within mood disorders, resulting in a publication with Dr Mary Fristad ("Anxiety in Children with Mood Disorders: A Treatment Help or Hindrance?"). Other research interests include interventions for childhood anxiety disorders and dissemination of evidence-based treatments.

Matthew Ditty is a lecturer at the University of Pennsylvania School of Social Policy and Practice. As a psychotherapist in the Philadelphia area, he has applied evidence-based treatments with children, adults, and families in the Hospital of the University of Pennsylvania, in the United States Navy, and in private practice. His current research focus is the dissemination and implementation of dialectical behavior therapy, cognitive behavioral therapy, and other evidence-based treatments.

Caroline L. Donovan, PhD, is a lecturer and clinical psychologist at Griffith University in Brisbane, Australia. Her research focuses on youth psychopathology, with a particular focus on online delivery of treatment interventions for youth anxiety disorders.

Margaret Mary Downey is a research specialist at the University of Pennsylvania's Center for Mental Health Policy and Services Research. She supports several NIH-funded projects that focus on dissemination and implementation (DI) of evidence-based practices, in partnership with the Philadelphia School District and Department of Behavioral Health. To combine her additional interests in reproductive justice, task shifting, and DI, she will pursue an MSW/PhD in Social Welfare.

Julie Edmunds is a recent graduate of Temple University's clinical psychology doctoral program. She is currently a postdoctoral fellow at the Center for Effective Child Therapy at Judge Baker Children's Center in Boston, MA. Dr Edmunds' primary interests include providing evidence-based mental health care to youth and families and training others in evidence-based practices. Recent research conducted by Dr Edmunds examined the role of behavioral rehearsals during consultation sessions on training outcomes.

Christina Hardway, PhD, is an assistant professor in the Department of Psychology at Merrimack College. She received her PhD from the University of Michigan, and prior to joining the faculty at Merrimack College she was a postdoctoral fellow in Harvard University's Judge Baker Children's Center Clinical Research Training Program. Her research has largely investigated the factors that promote circumstances and interventions that allow an individual to approach the world in an intellectually engaged manner.

Jennifer L. Hudson, MClinPsych, PhD, is professor at the Centre for Emotional Health, Department of Psychology, Macquarie University. Her research endeavors to improve understanding of the genetic and environmental factors that contribute to anxiety disorders in children. Her work also focuses on evaluating and disseminating programs to improve outcomes for children's emotional health.

Emily Jones, BSc, is a student in the Master's of Medical Science program at the University of Toronto and a research student at the Hospital for Sick Children in Toronto. She completed her BSc in Psychology at Trent University. Emily is an experienced child and youth therapist and director of the Summer Youth Camp at Dr Fountain's in Oshawa, a day treatment camp for children with mental health issues.

Nikolaos Kazantzis, PhD, is founder of the Cognitive Behaviour Therapy Research Unit at La Trobe University, editor-in-chief of *Australian Psychologist*, and his collaborative research has resulted in over 100 publications, including the practitioner book *Using Homework Assignments in Cognitive Behavior Therapy*. He developed training programs for over 4,000 professionals in 11 countries worldwide, and he is the recipient of the Beck Institute for Cognitive Behavior Therapy's 2012 Scholar Award for "significant contributions to the field of cognitive therapy."

Philip C. Kendall, PhD, ABPP, is Laura H. Carnell Distinguished University Professor at Temple University. He has been a fellow at the Center for Advanced Study in the Behavioral Sciences, won the Outstanding Contribution for Educational/Training Activities from ABCT, the Distinguished Career Research Award (Division 53) and the Distinguished Scientific Contribution Award (Division 12) from the APA, the Research Recognition Award from the Anxiety Disorders Association of America, and was identified as a "top therapist" by Philadelphia Magazine. Philip's contributions include the treatment of anxiety disorders in youth, research methodology, and cognitive behavioral theory, assessment, and treatment.

Caroline E. Kerns, MA, is a doctoral student at the Center for Anxiety and Related Disorders at Boston University. Her research interests include difficulties with emotion regulation and distress intolerance in children with anxiety disorders and their families. Her clinical interests include using evidence-based cognitive behavioral treatments and parent training programs to treat children and families with psychopathology.

Lauren S. Krumholz, PhD, is a postdoctoral fellow in the Department of Psychology at Harvard University. Her research interests include the treatment and prevention of mental illness among diverse children and adolescents through the design, evaluation, and dissemination of community-based, multi-system interventions targeting the individual, family, and school.

Maria Loades is a clinical psychologist working at the University of Bath's Clinical Psychology Doctorate Programme as a clinical tutor. This role includes clinical time spent working in child and adolescent mental health. Her special interests include developing and delivering cognitive behavioural treatments for children and young people with internalizing disorders in clinical settings and refining methods and tools for evaluating therapist competence in delivering CBT.

Ryan J. Madigan, PsyD, is an instructor of psychology at Harvard Medical School, a clinical psychologist in the Dialectical Behavior Therapy Program at McLean Hospital, and a research fellow at Boston University's Center for Anxiety and Related Disorders. He also serves on the Treatment Adaptations Taskforce Advisory Board of PCIT International. His clinical and research interests include the development and dissemination of evidence-based primary and tertiary interventions targeting child and adolescent behavior and emotion regulation.

Katharina Manassis, MD, FRCP (C), is a psychiatrist and senior associate scientist, Hospital for Sick Children, Toronto. She is a professor in the Department of Psychiatry, University of Toronto, and in the Applied Psychology & Human Development Department, Ontario Institute for Studies in Education. She leads several funded research studies to better understand and treat childhood anxiety disorders. She has published over 70 peer-reviewed papers in this field, and books for both parents and mental health professionals.

Sonja March, PhD, is a psychologist and lecturer at the University of Southern Queensland in Ipswich, Australia. Her research focuses on internalizing disorders of youth, with particular interests in youth PTSD and online program delivery.

Sandra L. Mendlowitz, PhD, is a psychologist at SickKids Hospital in Toronto, Canada and an assistant professor in the Department of Child Psychiatry, Faculty of Medicine, at the University of Toronto. Her research has focused on the development and evaluation of effective treatment interventions for children and adolescents. She has presented these findings both locally and at international conferences. She has also developed several intervention programs aimed at treating anxiety, mood disorders, and obsessive–compulsive disorder.

Bryce D. McLeod, PhD, is Associate Professor of Psychology at Virginia Commonwealth University. He is the author or co-author of numerous scientific articles and book chapters, along with a book entitled *Child Anxiety Disorders: A Family-Based Treatment Manual for Practitioners* (co-authored with Jeffrey Woods). He is the recipient of NIMH grant awards and his clinical and research interests include youth diagnostic and behavioral assessment, child anxiety disorders, therapy process research, and the implementation of evidence-based practices in practice settings.

Talia Morris is a PhD candidate at the Centre for Emotional Health, Department of Psychology, Macquarie University. Her research focuses on the development of emotional health problems such as anxiety and depression in children.

Carol Newall, MClinPsych, PhD, is a postdoctoral fellow at the Centre for Emotional Health, Department of Psychology, Macquarie University. Her research focuses on advancing knowledge on the learning and unlearning of fears, particularly in children.

Thomas H. Ollendick is University Distinguished Professor of Psychology and director of the Child Study Center at Virginia Tech. He is the author or co-author of several research articles, book chapters, and books and the recipient of several National Institute of Mental Health grant awards. His clinical and research interests range from the study of diverse forms of child psychopathology to the assessment, treatment, and prevention of these child disorders from a social learning or social cognitive theory perspective.

Monika Parkinson, DClinPsy, is a clinical psychologist at the Winnicott Research Unit, School of Psychology and Clinical Language Sciences, University of Reading, UK. Monika has particular interests in the role of family factors in the transmission and maintenance of youth internalizing disorders. Key recent publications are "Feasibility of Guided Cognitive Behaviour Therapy (CBT) Self-Help for Childhood Anxiety Disorders in Primary Care" (co-authored by Cathy Creswell, Frances Hentges, Monika Parkinson, Paul Sheffield, Lucy Willetts, and Peter Cooper), published in 2010 in *Mental Health in Family Medicine*, and "Worry and Problem-Solving Skills and Beliefs in Primary School Children" (co-authored with Cathy Creswell), published in 2011 in the *British Journal of Clinical Psychology*.

Kimberly M. Parker, MS, is a clinical psychology doctoral student at Virginia Commonwealth University. She is the author of several presentations on child therapeutic alliance, including on the role of competence in youth alliance. Overlapping clinical and research interests include youth measure development, parental factors impacting child functioning, and therapeutic alliance.

Sarah J. Perini, MA, is a clinical psychologist in private practice. Her research and clinical interests include modes of treatment delivery for anxious and depressed clients and mechanisms of change in social phobia.

Jeremy S. Peterman is a doctoral candidate in clinical psychology at Temple University. He received his BA in international relations and MA in psychology from Boston University. His research examines psychosocial predictors of sleep problems in youth with anxiety disorders, as well as the effects of cognitive behavioral treatment for anxiety on sleep problems. Jeremy has also written several publications on cognitive behavioral therapy for youth.

Donna B. Pincus, PhD, is Associate Professor of Psychology at Boston University and director of the Child and Adolescent Fear and Anxiety Treatment Program at the Center for Anxiety and Related Disorders at Boston University. She has focused her clinical research on the development and testing of new treatments for anxiety disorders in youth as well as on the integration of evidence-based psychological treatments into schools and primary-care settings.

Shirley Reynolds is Professor of Evidence-Based Psychological Therapy at the University of Reading, UK. She is a clinical psychologist by profession and has served as president of the British Association of Behavioural and Cognitive Psychotherapy. Shirley works mainly with children and young people who have problems with anxiety or depression and has been involved in a number of randomized controlled trials of CBT for young people. Shirley is co-editor of *Cognitive Behaviour Therapy for Children and Fa*milies (2013).

Lauren C. Santucci, PhD, is a postdoctoral fellow in the Department of Psychology at Harvard University. Lauren's research interests include the development, testing, and dissemination of cognitive behavioral interventions for youth with anxiety disorders, with an emphasis on employing innovative treatment formats and delivery contexts, such as summer camp, to reach a greater number of children in need of services.

Sophie C. Schneider is a PhD candidate at the Centre for Emotional Health, Department of Psychology, Macquarie University. Her research focuses on emotional health disorders in children and adolescents, in particular anxiety disorders and body dysmorphic disorder.

Cara A. Settipani is a doctoral candidate in clinical psychology at Temple University. She received her BA in psychology from Northwestern University and her MA in psychology from Temple University. Cara's current research interests include the relationship between parenting behaviors and cognitive and affective processes associated with anxiety in youth, as well as implications for cognitive behavioral therapy. She has also published on social functioning in anxious youth and on anxiety symptomatology associated with autism spectrum traits.

Michael A. Southam-Gerow, PhD, is Associate Professor of Psychology and Pediatrics at Virginia Commonwealth University (VCU). His research focuses on the dissemination of evidence-based treatments (EBTs) for mental health problems in children and adolescents. Michael's other research interests include the study of emotion processes (e.g., emotion regulation) in children and adolescents and treatment integrity research. He is associate editor of the *Journal of Clinical Child & Adolescent Psychology* and author of dozens of scholarly papers.

Ana M. Ugueto, PhD, is a research associate in the Department of Psychology at Harvard University. Ana's interests include the treatment and prevention of anxiety, depression, trauma, and behavior problems as well as the dissemination and implementation of evidence-based treatments for youths and adults in the US and in developing countries. She has trained over 300 clinicians in the US and over 100 community workers in Colombia, Ethiopia, and Thailand in cognitive behavioral therapy.

Polly Waite, DClinPsy, is an MRC clinical research training fellow and clinical psychologist at the Winnicott Research Unit, School of Psychology and Clinical Language Sciences, University of Reading, UK. Her primary clinical and research interest is anxiety in adolescence, specifically the role of parents in the development and maintenance of anxiety disorders and in the development of treatment. Key recent publications are "Cognitive Behavior Therapy for Low Self-Esteem: A Preliminary Randomized Controlled Trial in a Primary Care Setting" (co-authored with Freda McManus and Roz Shafran), published in 2012 in the *Journal of Behavior Therapy and Experimental Psychiatry*, and *CBT with Children, Adolescents and Families: Cognitive Behavioral Approaches and Interventions for Obsessive Compulsive Disorder* (co-edited with Tim Williams), published in 2009.

John R. Weisz, PhD, ABPP, is Professor of Psychology in the Harvard University Department of Psychology, Faculty of Arts and Sciences, and also in the Harvard Medical School. His research involves developing and testing interventions for youth mental health problems, complemented by meta-analyses and systematic reviews characterizing the state of the science of youth mental health care. In 2013 he received the highest honor awarded by the Association for Psychological Science: the James McKeen Cattell Lifetime Achievement Award.

Stephen P. Whiteside, PhD, ABPP, is Associate Professor of Psychology and director of the Child Anxiety Disorders Program at Mayo Clinic in Rochester, Minnesota. He conducts research on the assessment and treatment of childhood anxiety disorders, including the use of neuroimaging to examine the effects of cognitive behavioral therapy. He has received research funding from the International OCD Foundation as well as from Mayo Clinic and has published over 40 articles and book chapters.

Lucy Willetts, PhD, is a consultant clinical psychologist at the Winnicott Research Unit, School of Psychology and Clinical Language Sciences, University of Reading, UK. Her research interests include the intergenerational transmission of childhood anxiety and the treatment of childhood anxiety disorders. Key recent publications are "Feasibility of Guided Cognitive Behaviour Therapy (CBT) Self-Help for Childhood Anxiety Disorders in Primary Care" (co-authored with Cathy Creswell, Frances Hentges, Monica Parkinson, Paul Sheffield, Lucy Willetts, and Peter Cooper), published in 2010 in *Mental Health in Family Medicine*; and *Overcoming Your Child's*

Fears and Worries: A Guide for Parents Using Cognitive Behavioral Techniques, together with *Overcoming Your Child's Shyness and Social Anxiety: A Guide for Parents Using Cognitive Behavioral Techniques* (both co-authored with Cathey Creswell), both published in 2007.

Brennan J. Young received his PhD in child clinical psychology from the University of Denver and is completing a postdoctoral fellowship in pediatric medical psychology at Mayo Clinic. Brennan has a longstanding clinical and research interest in assessing and treating childhood anxiety disorders, particularly in the identification of mechanisms of treatment. In addition, his research has focused on the development of romantic relationships from an attachment perspective and on the influence of dating violence on psychopathology.

1

An Introduction to the Competencies-Based Approach

Elizabeth S. Sburlati, Heidi J. Lyneham, and Carolyn A. Schniering

The Genesis of This Book

Empirically supported treatment, evidence-based practice, and the real world

There are a number of cognitive behavioral empirically supported treatments (ESTs) available for treating child and adolescent anxiety and depressive disorders that therapists practicing in routine clinical practice (RCP) can use when delivering evidence-based practice (EBP). However, interventions for children and adolescents may not be as effective when implemented in real world RCP settings as they are when implemented in research settings (Weisz, Ugueto, Cheron, and Herren 2013). Research is now indicating that poor real-world implementation of ESTs could be partly due to inadequate training of the therapists who work in RCP (Beidas, Barmish, and Kendall 2009; Herschell, Kolko, Baumann, and Davis 2010). As a result, there has been a call to examine and improve the quality of therapist EST training (Rakovshik and McManus 2010). However, until recently, the specific competencies that are required for the effective implementation of ESTs that target anxious and depressed children and adolescents were unknown, which made the development of more effective EST training difficult.

The competencies-based approach

The field of psychology is moving away from the traditional training approach, which focused on the trainee's satisfying training activities (e.g., courses, client contact hours, supervision hours) to a competencies-based approach to training that aims to

Evidence-Based CBT for Anxiety and Depression in Children and Adolescents: A Competencies-Based Approach,
First Edition. Edited by Elizabeth S. Sburlati, Heidi J. Lyneham, Carolyn A. Schniering, and Ronald M. Rapee.
© 2014 John Wiley & Sons, Ltd. Published 2014 by John Wiley & Sons, Ltd.

conceptualize, systematically train, and effectively assess the competence of trainees in performing as independent professionals (e.g., Hunsley and Barker 2011; Kaslow 2004; Kaslow et al. 2004; Knight 2011; Laidlaw and Gillanders 2011; Pachana, Sofronoff, Scott, and Helmes 2011; Roberts, Borden, Christiansen, and Lopez 2005). Competence is defined within the competencies-based approach as "the habitual and judicious use of communication, knowledge, technical skills, clinical reasoning, emotions, values, and reflection in daily practice for the benefit of the individual and community being served" (Epstein and Hundert 2002, p. 227). The competencies-based approach suggests that competence is comprised of competencies, which are the important component parts of competence (Kaslow 2004; Kaslow et al. 2004). According to the competencies-based approach, these competencies include a therapist's knowledge, attitudes, and skills that are related to his or her area of practice (Kaslow 2004; Kaslow et al. 2004).

A model of therapist competencies for the evidence-based treatment of child and adolescent anxiety and depressive disorders

As a part of a large-scale initiative in the United Kingdom, the dissemination project Improving Access to Psychological Therapies (IAPT), Roth and Pilling (2008) developed a model of therapist competencies for the evidence-based cognitive behavioral treatment of adult anxiety and depression. This model was designed to be used so as to develop a training curriculum aimed at teaching therapists in RCP to implement evidence-based practice in real-world settings. Drawing on the work of Roth and Pilling (2008) and acknowledging the vast array of different competencies required when treating children and adolescents (as opposed to adults), Sburlati, Schniering, Lyneham, and Rapee (2011) developed a therapist competence model targeting the empirically supported cognitive behavioral treatment of child and adolescent anxiety and depressive disorders. This model drew on all empirically supported treatment manuals that had been published prior to January 2010 and utilized the knowledge and feedback of experts from all around the world (for a complete description of the manuals, experts, and methods used in the model development, see Sburlati et al. 2011). The outcome was a model that provides a comprehensive listing of the individual competencies needed to conduct evidence-based practice with youth experiencing internalizing disorders in real-world clinical practice. The individual competencies in the model are grouped together by similarity, into competency categories, and these competency categories are placed under the three domains of competence (Sburlati et al. 2011). These three domains of competence are described below, in the part devoted to the subject. In the model, competencies were shaded gray if they were specific to the treatment of children and adolescents (but not adults) or require considerable adaptation when working with children and adolescents. (To view the model in its original format, see Sburlati et al. 2011, p. 94).

Sburlati et al. (2011) domains of competence

Generic therapeutic competencies

Generic therapeutic competencies, first identified by Roth and Pilling (2008), are those competencies that a therapist needs in order to interact with people within a therapeutic context, irrespective of therapeutic orientation. These competencies are not seen in cognitive behavioral therapy (CBT) only, but rather are used across all therapeutic models (Roth and Pilling 2008). The generic therapeutic competencies were reviewed, adapted, and expanded by Sburlati and colleagues (2011) to account for the needs of children and adolescents. The competency categories and individual competencies included in the generic therapeutic competencies domain can be seen in Table 1.1. These competencies are discussed across Chapters 3 to 7 of this book.

Table 1.1 Generic therapeutic competencies.

Category		*Individual competencies*
1. Practicing professionally:	(a)	knowledge of and ability to operate within professional, ethical, and legal codes of conduct relevant to working with children and adolescents, and their families (e.g., providing a duty of care);
	(b)	ability to actively participate in supervision;
	(c)	possession of an open attitude toward psychotherapy research, and the ability to access, critically evaluate and utilize this research to inform practice;
	(d)	ability to self assess current level of competence, and to seek relevant professional development.
2. Understanding relevant child and adolescent characteristics:	(a)	knowledge of developmental issues including cognitive, social, and emotional maturation from childhood to adolescence and how these can impact on therapy;
	(b)	knowledge of child or adolescent relevant individual differences (e.g., learning disorders, familial culture) and how these can impact on therapy;
	(c)	knowledge of other environmental factors (e.g., socioeconomic status, family structure, education) and life events (e.g., bullying, trauma, health issues, life transitions) and how these can impact on therapy;
	(d)	knowledge of child and adolescent psychopathology and comorbid presentations and how these can impact on therapy.
3. Building a positive relationship:	(a)	ability to engage the child or adolescent through age appropriate methods (e.g., games, activities, humour, technology, language), and appropriate session pacing;
	(b)	ability to foster and maintain a good therapeutic alliance with the child or adolescent;
	(c)	ability to foster and maintain a good therapeutic alliance with the parent;
	(d)	ability to instil hope, and optimism for change.

(Continued)

Table 1.1   (*cont'd*)

Category	Individual competencies
4. Conducting a thorough assessment:	(a) ability to undertake an evidence-based, multi method (e.g., self-report, observational), multi informant (e.g., child, parent, teacher, allied health professional) psychological assessment of the disorder presentation;
	(b) ability to integrate assessment reports from both the child or adolescent, parent and other parties;
	(c) ability to determine clinical diagnoses with consideration of differential diagnosis;
	(d) ability to undertake a generic assessment of the child or adolescent's current functioning, family functioning, peer relationships, developmental history and stage, and their suitability for the intervention;
	(e) ability to assess and manage risk of self-harm and suicide.

Source: Sburlati, Schniering, Lyneham, and Rapee (2011, p. 94).

CBT competencies
CBT competencies are those competencies required to plan, administer, and flexibly tailor specific CBT techniques to the individual needs of the child or adolescent and his or her family (Sburlati et al. 2011). The CBT competencies domain in Sburlati and colleagues (2011) is not to be found in the Roth and Pilling (2008) model; it was derived from combining two separate Roth and Pilling (2008) competence domains – basic CBT competencies and metacompetencies. The competency categories and the individual competencies included in the CBT competencies domain can be seen in Table 1.2. These competencies are discussed across Chapters 8 to 11 of this book.

Specific CBT techniques
Specific CBT techniques are techniques that target the theoretical factors that maintain anxiety and depression and that are included within empirically supported cognitive behavioral treatments for child and adolescent anxiety and depressive disorders (Roth and Pilling 2008; Sburlati et al. 2011). The competency categories and the individual techniques included in the specific CBT techniques domain can be seen in Table 1.3. These competencies are discussed across Chapters 12 to 19 of this book.

About This Book

Aims

The present book calls on the expertise of many leaders in the field to explore in detail each of the competencies in Sburlati and colleagues' (2011) model. This book is aimed at two main audiences. First, it is aimed at clinical supervisors who are

Table 1.2 CBT competencies.

Category		Individual competencies
5. Understanding relevant CBT theory and research:	(a)	knowledge of theoretical underpinnings of CBT, and the ability to implement CBT in line with these;
	(b)	knowledge of cognitions relevant to the maintenance of anxiety disorders and depression;
	(c)	knowledge of behaviors relevant to the maintenance of anxiety disorders and depression;
	(d)	knowledge of family and other environment factors relevant to the maintenance of anxiety disorders and depression in children and adolescents.
6. Devising, implementing, and revising a CBT case formulation and treatment plan:	(a)	ability to devise and revise a CBT case formulation that appropriately accounts for child or adolescent disorder presentation, developmental level, individual differences, family factors, and the presence of comorbidity;
	(b)	ability to devise, implement, and flexibly revise an evidence-based CBT treatment plan by selecting, sequencing, and applying the most appropriate specific CBT techniques, at the appropriate dosage, for the case formulation;
	(c)	ability to communicate appropriate psychoeducation about the nature of the disorder, the case formulation, and the treatment plan to both the parent and the child or adolescent;
	(d)	ability to collaboratively negotiate and agree on treatment goals;
	(e)	ability to use measures and self-monitoring to guide therapy and to monitor outcome;
	(f)	ability to manage obstacles to CBT;
	(g)	ability to plan for the end of therapy and for long-term maintenance of gains after treatment.
7. Collaboratively conducting CBT sessions:	(a)	ability to collaboratively set and adhere to session goals/agenda;
	(b)	ability to communicate rationale for each specific CBT technique;
	(c)	ability to elicit and respond to feedback;
	(d)	ability to implement specific CBT techniques flexibly for the client disorder presentation, needs or preferences, cultural background, and current mood;
	(e)	ability to make use of experiential strategies to implement specific CBT techniques (e.g., role play, modeling, corrective feedback and reinforcement);
	(f)	ability to conduct sessions with developmental sensitivity (e.g., using age-appropriate worksheets, instruction, play-based activities, token economies);
	(g)	ability to facilitate an appropriate level of *in session* collaboration between child or adolescent, parent and therapist;
	(h)	ability to facilitate parents to take an appropriate role *between sessions* (e.g., as coach);
	(i)	ability to collaboratively set, plan and review personally meaningful homework;
	(j)	ability to end sessions in a planned manner.

Source: Sburlati, Schniering, Lyneham, and Rapee (2011, p. 94).

Table 1.3 Specific CBT techniques.

Category	Individual techniques
8. Managing negative thoughts:	(a) cognitive restructuring; (b) behavioral experiments; (c) thought substitution/self-talk; (d) positive imagery; (e) thought stopping/interruption; (f) thought acceptance.
9. Changing maladaptive behaviors:	(a) interoceptive exposure; (b) *in vivo* exposure; (c) imaginal/narrative exposure; (d) response prevention; (e) behavioral activation; (f) pleasant events scheduling; (g) self-evaluation and self-rewards.
10. Managing maladaptive mood and arousal:	(a) emotion identification, expression, and regulation; (b) progressive muscle relaxation; (c) applied tension; (d) breathing retraining.
11. General skills training:	(a) problem-solving skills; (b) interpersonal engagement skills; (c) friendship skills; (d) communication and negotiation skills; (e) assertiveness skills; (f) dealing with bullying skills.
12. Modifying the family environment:	(a) family communication and conflict resolution; (b) parental expectations management; (c) parent intrusiveness and overprotection management; (d) parent contingency management; (e) parent emotion management; (f) parent modeling of adaptive behavior.

Source: Sburlati, Schniering, Lyneham, and Rapee (2011, p. 94).

mentoring therapists who will be (or are) treating children and adolescents with anxiety and depression, and at trainers who are developing and/or delivering training programs in university or college settings and continuing professional development programs. The book will assist this audience with the development of comprehensive and effective training curricula, will guide trainers and supervisors on relevant competencies that should be assessed throughout training, and can be used as a resource to support training or supervision programs leading to trainee therapists gaining a wide range of empirically based competencies. Second, given the current push for therapists to assess their own level of competence and to govern their own professional development (e.g., Bellande, Winicur, and Cox 2010), this book is aimed at therapists who wish to gain an understanding of the competencies they need to acquire in order to effectively work with the targeted population and to come to know what competent practice looks like for each individual competency; and the competency descriptions will provide a benchmark against which they can assess themselves. Third and finally, the aim of this book is to improve the quality of the treatment provided to children and adolescents as a result of the enhancement of individual therapists' abilities.

Book structure

This book is divided into three parts that reflect the three-domain structure of the competencies model described earlier. Further, chapters within these three parts broadly map onto the competency categories of each domain. For example, Part I covers the generic therapeutic competencies domain of the model and includes five chapters that focus on the four competency categories within this domain, namely "Practicing Professionally," (which is covered over two chapters) "Understanding Relevant Child and Adolescent Characteristics," "Building a Positive Relationship," and "Conducting a Thorough Assessment."

Chapter structure

In order to ensure comprehensive coverage of each of the Sburlati and colleagues (2011) competencies as well as consistency throughout the volume, most chapters in this book contain a number of recurrent sections. The headings below give a general description of these sections; the exact wording may have been adapted within each chapter. Chapters 5, 8, and 9 do not follow this structure, as their content does not fit with this manner of organizing (e.g., the chapter is knowledge-based).

Key features of competencies
The first section of each chapter describes each competency in detail, highlighting the behavioral markers of each of the individual competencies. Illustrations or examples of the competent use of therapeutic techniques and processes are also included, so as to increase the clinical utility of the book.

Competence in treating the anxiety disorders and depression
Considerable differences exist among the different anxiety disorders (e.g., between panic disorder and social phobia) and also between anxiety disorders in general and depression. Therefore all chapters include a section focused on how the competencies covered in the chapter might be uniquely tailored when treating these different disorders.

Competence in treating both children and adolescents
Since this book spans competent practice across a large age range (from early childhood to late adolescence), the third section in each chapter highlights important developmental differences in treating children from different age groups. Specifically, unique competencies required for adapting evidence-based CBT for cognitive, emotional, and social maturation are considered.

Common obstacles to competent practice and methods to overcome them
Given that there are inevitably obstacles to the competent implementation of evidence-based CBT, the final section of each chapter covers typical obstacles to competent practice and provides strategies for overcoming them. These strategies come from the literature and clinical expertise.

Conclusion

It is the editors' hope that this book will become the cornerstone of the development of a generation of therapists competent in treating children and adolescents with anxiety and depressive disorders. We believe that, by raising the standard of practice, the quality of the treatment provided to youth seeking a way out of these common and debilitating conditions in real-world RCP settings can be enhanced.

References

Beidas, Rinad S., Andrea J. Barmish, and Philip C. Kendall. 2009. "Training as Usual: Can Therapist Behavior Change after Reading a Manual and Attending a Brief Workshop on Cognitive Behavioral Therapy for Youth Anxiety?" *The Behavior Therapist*, 32: 97–101.

Bellande, Bruce J., Zev M. Winicur, and Kathleen M. Cox. 2010. "Urgently Needed: A Safe Place for Self-Assessment on the Path to Maintaining Competence and Improving Performance." *Academic Medicine*, 85: 16–18. DOI: 10.1097/ACM.0b013e3181c41b6f

Epstein, Ronald M., and Edward M. Hundert. 2002. "Defining and Assessing Professional Competence." *The Journal of the American Medical Association*, 287: 226–35. DOI: 10.1001/jama.287.2.226

Herschell, Amy D., David J. Kolko, Barbara L. Baumann, and Abigail C. Davis. 2010. "The Role of Therapist Training in the Implementation of Psychosocial Treatments: A Review and Critique with Recommendations." *Clinical Psychology Review*, 30: 448–66. DOI: 10.1016/j.cpr.2010.02.005

Hunsley, John, and Keegan K. Barker. 2011. "Training for Competency in Professional Psychology: A Canadian Perspective." *Australian Psychologist*, 46: 142–5. DOI: 10.1111/j.1742-9544.2011.00027.x

Kaslow, Nadine J. 2004. "Competencies in Professional Psychology." *American Psychologist*, 59: 774–81. DOI: 10.1037/0003-066X.59.8.774

Kaslow, Nadine J., Kathi A. Borden, Frank L. Collins, Jr., Linda Forrest, Joyce Illfelder-Kaye, Paul D. Nelson, ... Mary E. Willmuth. 2004. "Competencies Conference: Future Directions in Education and Credentialing in Professional Psychology." *Journal of Clinical Psychology*, 60: 699–712. DOI: 10.1002/jclp.20016

Knight, Bob G. 2011. "Training in Professional Psychology in the US: An Increased Focus on Competency Attainment." *Australian Psychologist*, 46: 140–1. DOI: 10.1111/j.1742-9544.2011.00026.x

Laidlaw, Ken., and David Gillanders. 2011. "Clinical Psychology Training in the UK: Towards the Attainment of Competence." *Australian Psychologist*, 46: 146–50. DOI: 10.1111/j.1742-9544.2011.00035.x

Pachana, Nancy A., Kate Sofronoff, Theresa Scott, and Edward Helmes. 2011. "Attainment of Competencies in Clinical Psychology Training: Ways Forward in the Australian Context." *Australian Psychologist*, 46: 67–76. DOI: 10.1111/j.1742-9544.2011.00029.x

Rakovshik, Sarah G., and Freda McManus. 2010. "Establishing Evidence-Based Training in Cognitive Behavioral Therapy: A Review of Current Empirical Findings and Theoretical Guidance." *Clinical Psychology Review*, 30: 496–516. DOI: 10.1016/j.cpr.2010.03.004

Roberts, Michael C., Kathi A. Borden, Martha Dennis Christiansen, and Shane J. Lopez. 2005. "Fostering a Culture Shift: Assessment of Competence in the Education and Careers of Professional Psychologists." *Professional Psychology: Research and Practice*, 36: 355–61. DOI: 10.1037/0735-7028.36.4.355

Roth, Anthony D., and Stephen Pilling. 2008. "Using an Evidence-Based Methodology to Identify the Competences Required to Deliver Effective Cognitive and Behavioural Therapy for Depression and Anxiety Disorders." *Behavioural and Cognitive Psychotherapy*, 36: 129–47. DOI: 10.1017/S1352465808004141

Sburlati, Elizabeth S., Carolyn A. Schniering, Heidi J. Lyneham, and Ronald M. Rapee. 2011. "A Model of Therapist Competencies for the Empirically Supported Cognitive Behavioral Treatment of Child and Adolescent Anxiety and Depressive Disorders." *Clinical Child and Family Psychology Review*, 14: 89–109. DOI: 10.1007/s10567-011-0083-6

Weisz, John R., Ana M. Ugueto, Daniel M. Cheron, and Jenny Herren. 2013. "Evidence-Based Youth Psychotherapy in the Mental Health Ecosystem." *Journal of Clinical Child and Adolescent Psychology*, 42: 274–86. DOI: 10.1080/15374416.2013.764824

2

Effective Training Methods

Emily Jones and Katharina Manassis

Introduction

Outcomes for cognitive behavioral therapy (CBT) and other evidence-based psycho-therapies have been evaluated extensively, but the research literature on methods of training in these therapies and on disseminating them is relatively sparse. Recent changes in the mandates of governments, mental health agencies, and research associations have, however, sharpened the focus on knowledge translation and evidence-based practices. Therefore research has started to examine what constitutes effective training for CBT and how to best help trainees implement CBT in real-world conditions of practice when working with clients of various ages who suffer from internalizing disorders. This chapter examines training methods generally, then more specifically in relation to the treatment of anxiety disorders, depression, children and adolescents. It concludes with a review of obstacles to effective training.

Key Features of Training: Presenting Training Material Using Effective Strategies

Effective strategies for presenting training material have been derived from learning models. Three different but complementary models are reviewed and then linked to specific training methods. Beidas and Kendall (2010) seek to understand how training models affect the translation of evidence-based practices (EBP) through a systems-contextual perspective. Theirs is considered a broad, holistic approach that emphasizes that an individual works within a system and thus quality of training, organizational supports, therapist variables, and client variables interact to effectively

Evidence-Based CBT for Anxiety and Depression in Children and Adolescents: A Competencies-Based Approach, First Edition. Edited by Elizabeth S. Sburlati, Heidi J. Lyneham, Carolyn A. Schniering, and Ronald M. Rapee. © 2014 John Wiley & Sons, Ltd. Published 2014 by John Wiley & Sons, Ltd.

translate EBP. Provisional evidence from Beidas and Kendall's (2010) literature review suggests that, when all levels of the systems-contextual model are addressed, therapists reach proficiency levels in competence, adherence, and skill that facilitate effective client change.

Bennett-Levy (2006) presents a cognitive model for training therapists that emphasizes changes in therapists' information processing and reflection. In Bennett-Levy's model there are three principal systems at work: declarative, procedural, and reflective (DPR). The declarative system consists of factual information typically learned through didactic teaching, observed learning, supervision, and reading assignments. The procedural system consists of applied skills; and the reflective system consists of metacognitive skills that include observations, interpretations, and evaluations of one's self in the past, present, and future. Bennett-Levy demonstrates how this model accounts for a new therapist's progressive learning until he or she becomes an expert. The new therapist begins by relying on the declarative system using didactic learning, modeling, practice, and feedback but further develops clinical expertise through the procedural system. Finally, he or she moves to the stage of clinician, as a teacher or expert, through the reflective system. The transition to becoming an expert happens when the therapist goes from reflection-on-action (retrospective review of therapeutic interventions) to reflection-in-action (reflection that occurs during therapy sessions).

Other theoretical reviews – such as Milne, Aylott, Fitzpatrick, and Ellis (2008) and Rakovshik and McManus (2010) – emphasize the relationship between trainee changes and methods of instruction. Here it is found that trainees in CBT need supervision that provides not only didactic teaching but also experiential learning methods such as role-play, cotherapy, and modeling. Further, Rakovshik and McManus (2010) provide evidence to suggest that, if supervision is removed prior to consolidation, then the learned skills can deteriorate over time.

On the basis of these learning models, many types of training have emerged. Bennett-Levy, McManus, Westling, and Fennell (2009) examine which training methods are most effective, testing the didactic versus experiential distinction described above. Although their study relies on therapists' perceptions, it does allow for predictions to be made about the effect of training methods on CBT skills and competence. In this study, 120 therapists were surveyed regarding the effectiveness of 6 popular training methods and 11 different CBT skills. Bennett-Levy and colleagues found that different methods of learning were perceived to be effective across different CBT skills. Passive training strategies such as reading manuals and books, attending lectures and workshops, and completing non-interactive online training increased declarative knowledge and some conceptual and technical skills. Active training strategies such as role-play, reflective practice, self-experiential work, graded training and supervision were found to increase the therapist–client exchange and the level of technical, interpersonal, procedural, and reflective skills.

Herschell, Kolko, Baumann, and Davis (2010) reviewed 55 different studies on training therapists in psychosocial treatments. Their review found that passive training – such as reading and workshops – develops knowledge but is not sufficient for achieving competence, as skills learnt through these methods do not reliably persist over time. The addition of skill feedback and short-term consultation or supervision after a workshop was shown to increase both knowledge and skills. In particular, clinical supervision and consultation with field experts consistently produced superior training outcomes, despite difficulties that may arise with cost and availability. Overall, Herschell and colleagues concluded that multi-component training programs are superior to other (single-component) training methods.

With the advent of online training, new hybrid training methods that incorporate both passive and active learning methods have become popular (Dimeff et al. 2009; Granpeesheh et al. 2010; Sholomskas and Carroll 2006; Sholomskas et al. 2005; Weingardt 2004; Weingardt, Cucciare, Bellotti, and Lai 2009). For example, Dimeff et al. (2009) investigated the efficacy of three different training methods for dialectical behavior therapy (DBT): (i) a 20-hour interactive online training (OLT) session; (ii) a two-day instructor-led training (ILT) session; and (iii) reading two treatment manuals. These researchers made sure the OLT was interactive and sophisticated, as they felt that variable results in other studies might be due to OLT's being presented like a book on a screen. Specifically, the OLT included audio and visual presentation as well as a fictional DBT skills group for participants to observe and learn from, expert insights, practical exercises, and knowledge quizzes. Participants were evaluated before and after training, and also in a 90-day follow-up, regarding their knowledge of DBT, satisfaction with training, referencing of materials, and clinical performance in role-play. Dimeff and colleagues found that OLT significantly out-performed both the ILT method and the method of training through manuals.

The duration of training is, potentially, a factor to be considered when investigating effective training methods. However, conclusions on duration are difficult to draw, as the majority of studies do not address this topic. Those studies that do mention training duration only give broad temporal descriptions and vary widely in approach, which makes them difficult to compare. In Rakovshik and McManus (2010), 37 different training programs are compared; but researchers point to a lack of agreement on the terminology that describes the training. For example, they argue that a comparison between a "workshop" that was didactic and interactive and contained role-play and case discussions and a "workshop" that was strictly didactic would be imprecise. Finally, specifying the nature of competence and its measurement presents its own challenges (see below). Therefore further research is needed on measuring competence and on the optimal duration of training. Nevertheless, most training studies reviewed above support multi-component programs that include active learning methods as well as didactic teaching.

Training Approaches for Treating Anxiety and Depressive Disorders

Training models in cognitive behavioral therapy (CBT) vary (see previous section), and competencies achieved by trainees are not clearly defined in all studies. Roth and Pilling (2008), however, developed a systematic model of the competencies needed by a therapist in order to treat anxiety and depression in adult populations; to do this, they used a Delphi technique that draws on sharing and refining contributions from individual field experts so as to arrive at a consensus. Roth and Pilling's model describes five increasingly specific domains of competence: general psychotherapeutic competencies; basic CBT competencies (related to the structure and content of CBT); specific CBT techniques; problem-specific competencies; and competencies that allow adaptation to individual client needs while maintaining treatment fidelity (these are termed "meta-competencies"). The authors highlight that achieving meta-competencies generally requires the highest CBT expertise and the greatest amount of experience, which makes these competencies the most challenging ones to impart to trainees.

Studies of anxious and depressed clients generally emphasize treatment methods and client outcomes (chiefly symptomatic improvement, but also client perceptions of therapy in some studies, as for instance in Hepner, Paddock, Zhou, and Watkins 2011). The therapist's competence is not consistently measured and evaluated on that basis, and, when measured, this is usually a side issue, subordinated to client outcomes rather than representing a separate goal. Training methods, in the most relevant studies, reflect the multi-component approach recommended more broadly in the training literature – an approach consisting of a blend of didactic teaching, interactive learning, and supervision. Computer-assisted training that incorporates didactic seminars with skills practice, role-play, and videos of "bad" therapy techniques, as well as training via tele-health, are becoming increasingly popular and participants show positive gains in competence and adherence (Reese and Gillam, 2001; Rose et al. 2011). Individual supervision, in particular the kind that focuses on the ongoing refinement of the trainee's skills on the basis of the supervisor's input, has shown superiority to other training methods in some studies (e.g., Mannix et al. 2006). Further to these training findings, Karlin et al. (2010), in collaboration with post-traumatic stress disorder (PTSD) therapists, found that incorporating collaborative consultation on actual cases in a training program increased therapists' competence and helped enhance the adoption of therapy into practice. It is, however, more time-consuming than other learning methods. As an alternative, group supervision models have the potential to optimize the use of a supervisor's time, but they have received limited evaluation (Manassis et al. 2009; Newton and Yardley 2007).

An approach that diverts from the multi-component recommendation is that of training through participation in cotherapy. For example, Hepner and colleagues (2011) trained addiction counselors in depression-focused CBT group by using a co-therapy model where an inexperienced therapist conducted a treatment program together with an experienced therapist prior to implementing the program independently. The authors were able to demonstrate trainees' ability to lead depression-focused CBT groups with high fidelity to treatment protocols, without training in individual CBT methods first. This cotherapy option may be a viable addition to other recommended multi-component approaches.

When direct evaluation of therapist competence has been incorporated into studies of CBT, the Cognitive Therapy Scale (Dobson, Shaw, and Vallis 1985) has been the most frequently reported measure of competence. In this measure, expert raters evaluate videotapes of CBT sessions by using an 11-item scale. Reliability of ratings increases with the number of raters and the number of videotapes rated. Other measures of therapist competence include the Cognitive Formulation Rating Scale, the Cognitive Therapy Awareness Scale, and the CBT Supervision Checklist (Sudak,

Beck, and Wright 2003). Nevertheless, there is a paucity of research into standardized measures of therapist competence.

In the depression and anxiety literature, CBT skills and the ability to structure sessions are the aspects of competence that have been regularly linked to therapeutic change (Simons et al. 2010). The literature is not entirely consistent, however, possibly due to difficulty separating the effects of therapist competence from other client- and therapist-related factors. For example, Trepka, Rees, Shapiro, Hardy, and Barkham (2004) found that the relationship between competence and depression outcome was no longer significant when controlling for therapeutic alliance, and Strunk, Brotman, DeRubeis, and Hollon (2010) found that the relationship between therapist competence and change in depressive symptoms was moderated by factors related to the client, as client anxiety, early onset of depression, and chronic course predicted lower levels of change. Kuyken and Tsivrikos (2009), however, found that therapists' high competence was associated with improved outcomes to depression regardless of clients' comorbid diagnoses. Factors related to the therapist, such as positive attitudes toward empirically supported treatments, resulted in better implementation of depression-focused CBT in community settings (Lewis and Simons, 2011), and previous cognitive therapy experience and careful case selection were linked to therapist competence in a sample of 20 postgraduate trainees working with depressed clients (James, Blackburn, Milne, and Reichfelt 2001).

Each anxiety and depressive disorder poses unique challenges to training, and this is due to the nature of the disorders themselves. Trainees need to acquire knowledge and experience related to internalizing psychopathology (see Chapter 8). Within the training context some difficulties may arise from the multiple explanations for a single behavior that may occur in anxiety and depression. For example, inconsistent attendance at appointments may occur for different reasons: depressive clients may be fatigued and feel hopeless about the possibility of improvement; anxious clients may wish to avoid the exposure to anxious situations that is integral to therapy. Helping trainees consider multiple alternatives and explanations is likely crucial for an effective training. Similarly, the psychological treatment of mood disorders is more regularly combined with medication than the psychological treatment of anxiety disorders in youth (Treatment for Adolescents with Depression Study Team, 2004). Familiarity with psychotropic medications and regular communication with the prescribing physician are therefore essential for the successful treatment of depressed clients, but not always for the treatment of anxious clients.

The nature of the skills required to treat anxiety and depression may be challenging for novice therapists. For example, encouraging client exposure to feared situations causes discomfort in many training therapists, and is thus a potential barrier to the dissemination of CBT (this is further described below, in the section on obstacles to competent practices). Harned, Dimeff, Woodcock, and Skutch (2011) investigated a solution to this potential barrier by comparing the uses of an interactive online CBT training program in two variants: with and without motivational interviewing. They found that both groups of training therapists gained knowledge, but the group receiving motivational interviewing developed more positive attitudes toward exposure. This suggested that motivational interviewing may aid dissemination through improved attitude on the part of the therapist.

Training Therapists of Children and Adolescents

Competence in CBT with anxious or depressed children and adolescents presupposes an understanding of children's social, cognitive, and emotional development and an appreciation of the impact of environmental factors on their well-being, as these are more salient in child care than in adult care (see Chapter 5). As outlined in Chapter 1, a more sophisticated understanding of competencies needed for child and adolescent CBT has been published by Sburlati, Schniering, Lyneham, and Rapee (2011). Ideally, a therapist will flexibly and skillfully integrate these various competencies to tailor CBT to the needs of each child or adolescent treated (see Chapter 10 for a detailed discussion). In addition, competence in child CBT generally entails the ability to effectively engage and collaborate with the client's parents. CBT protocols vary in the extent of parental involvement in therapy, but all are predicated on some parental engagement – at least as much of it as would be enough for parents to bring the child to sessions consistently (see Chapter 6). There is a lack of research into the effectiveness of training programs that target those who work with children and adolescents. Logically, however, successful training programs need to incorporate a broad spectrum of examples, which should not only vary in the way they present the problem but also incorporate the developmental and environmental variations that naturally occur within each age group.

Therapists training in child and adolescent CBT often find themselves in a wider variety of settings than those training to treat adults. CBT with youth is not limited to the health care sector, as schools and social service agencies provide psychotherapy as well. School- and community-based CBT training programs are among the most highly evaluated. ACTION is a gender-sensitive CBT program for depressed youth, originally developed on the basis of studies of depression in early teen girls (Stark et al. 2007). It now contains separate workbooks for each gender (20 sessions), as well as gender-specific parent workbooks (8 sessions). Weisz and colleagues (2009) trained community clinic therapists in this program in 6 hours of teaching followed by weekly supervision, and they compared its effectiveness to that of treatment as usual. Both groups of adolescents improved symptomatically, but CBT-treated youth required fewer sessions and fewer additional services than those receiving treatment as usual. The program is currently being adapted for use by school psychologists (Stark, Arora, and Funk 2011).

Manassis and colleagues (2009) also dealt with community mental health providers in their child-focused training program designed to disseminate CBT for children with anxiety disorders. Training consisted of a 20-session group supervision program that included some didactic teaching, either face to face or by videoconference. Trainees showed increased knowledge of child CBT and increased confidence in their ability to practice child CBT after training. Experienced therapists and therapists working in agencies that used a diagnostic screen at intake – which increased their chances of working with children suitable for CBT through thorough assessment – reported the greatest confidence.

The most extensive investigation into training in child CBT has been undertaken by Barrett, Farrell, Ollendick, and Dadds (2006), in their dissemination of the FRIENDS program for child anxiety. Largely a prevention program, FRIENDS is a group CBT intended for use as a universal intervention for all students in a classroom; it can be conducted by teachers or by qualified mental health staff. A single day of group training is required, and implementation occurs via manuals specific to various age groups. In several randomized trials, high-risk students (i.e., those who score above clinical cut-off for anxiety or depression on standardized measures) showed greater symptomatic improvements after intervention, and some maintenance of the gains – up to 36 months after intervention (Barrett et al. 2006). Moreover, benefits were evident regardless of whether psychologists or teachers led the CBT groups.

In summary, although studies that formally evaluate therapists' competence are lacking in the child CBT training literature, there is accumulating evidence that community- and school-based practitioners can learn and successfully implement this therapeutic modality.

Common Obstacles to Training Therapists and Potential Solutions

Knowledge translation of CBT is a multifaceted, complex process. Each level of translation (client-directed, therapist-directed, and organizational) needs to be addressed. Adding to this complexity are many barriers that exist at each level. Barriers that relate to knowledge translation of CBT can include the therapists' attitudes toward CBT and research-based therapies, the lack of access to training and supervisors, the lack of organizational support for implementation, and the therapists' level of competence.

Attitudes of therapists toward CBT and research-based therapies in general have been identified as a large obstacle to effective knowledge translation (Nelson & Steele, 2007). Training, however, appears to effectively improve these attitudes. For example, Bennett-Levy and Beedie (2007) show increased positive attitudes and self-perception of competence over a one-year cognitive therapy training course. An empirical approach to training that consisted in inviting trainees to observe and comment upon their training experience has also been linked to improved attitudes toward CBT (Sudak et al. 2003).

Due to the inherent structure of CBT, manuals are considered critical to implementation. In these manuals, instructions for the therapist are carefully outlined for each session. For example, one well-known manual for anxiety-focused child CBT is the *Coping Cat Manual* and *Coping Cat Workbook* (Kendall and Hedtke 2006a and 2006b). This program and various site-specific, adapted versions of it have been evaluated in multiple studies and have shown consistent efficacy (e.g., Compton et al. 2004; Kendall 1994; Kendall et al. 1997; Khanna and Kendall 2008; Podell, Mychailyszyn, Edmunds, Puleo, and Kendall 2010; Suveg, Sood, Comer, and Kendall 2009). Although CBT manuals have had great success in research and are clearly helpful in standardizing treatment, they have been criticized by therapists in routine clinical settings for limiting the personalization of treatment and the therapist's ability to respond to the client's needs. To address this issue, Kendall, Settipani, and Cummings (2012) explain how manuals should be implemented. They advocate employing flexibility as long as the underlying principles of CBT treatment are maintained – namely principles such as having session goals, using a CBT perspective, remaining action-oriented, and using social learning theory. Specific exercises and activities, however, can be modified and individualized to address individual client needs. These researchers believe that the mark of a competent therapist is being able to use good clinical judgment so as to work flexibly within the framework of an evidence-based treatment manual.

Another approach to increasing flexibility within treatment manuals is the modular approach to CBT. This approach breaks down CBT into basic modules such as self-calming and cognitive reframing (Chorpita, Taylor, Francis, Moffitt, and Austin 2004). While this approach to treatment can be effective, it does require a high level of expertise and clinical judgment to select, organize, and apply the most appropriate modules in a given case (Weisz et al. 2012); consequently the approach may be more appropriate for experienced clinicians and/or may require specialized training.

As mentioned above, therapists' attitudes to specific techniques such as exposure tasks can be particularly problematic in CBT. Therapists may fear that exposure would be traumatic to the child and detrimental to the therapeutic alliance, and therefore they may be hesitant to guide their clients through what could be fearful situations. These preconceived ideas about exposure are often due to misinformation. Kendall and colleagues (2009) studied the effect of exposure tasks on the therapist–client alliance. Alliance was reported by both the client and the therapist independently after every session, and it was found that exposure had no harmful effect on the therapeutic relationship. Also, Hedtke, Kendal, and Tiwari (2009) studied the effects of exposure tasks in general and the characteristics of exposure tasks used in CBT for children with anxiety and found exposure tasks to be an integral part of treating anxiety disorders effectively. Despite these findings, some therapists fear clients' unpredictable reactions to exposure, as they may not have been trained to address these challenging reactions. This problem underscores a further barrier to knowledge translation of CBT: access to effective training and supervision.

Lack of access to effective training as therapist and supervision can impede knowledge translation. CBT training methods have been discussed above; they generally support the inclusion of role-play, modeling, reflective practice, and other forms of experiential learning in addition to didactic teaching (Bennett-Levy et al. 2009). Further, programs that provide ongoing supervision with an expert have been found to result in higher levels of therapists' satisfaction and competence than those that do not (Bennett-Levy et al. 2009; Herschell et al. 2010; Rakovshik and McManus 2010; Sholomskas et al. 2005). Expert supervision is not available in all jurisdictions, however, and it is often costly and time consuming. Group supervision, including supervision via tele-health, has the potential to increase training access (Manassis et al. 2009). Although sophisticated training models that include case conceptualization and adoption of fidelity measures may further increase knowledge translation, such training models require even greater time commitments and cost.

Karlin and colleagues (2010) show how limiting the eligibility for training programs to therapists who have prior experience and high general competence skills in psychotherapy may be worthwhile, if experienced and competent trainees are available. They found increased completion and post-training success rates among trainees who met predefined competence levels before the training. Consistent with these findings, Manassis and colleagues (2009) found that more experienced therapists reported greater CBT training benefits than less experienced therapists.

Organizational barriers to knowledge translation also exist. Agencies are confronted daily with questions regarding the cost-effectiveness of implementing new treatments and of training therapists in the administration of different treatments. An organization's ability to flexibly support staff attending training, peer supervision opportunities, funding for training, private therapy space, and other requirements for evidence-based training and practice often determines the success of knowledge translation efforts there. Certain organizational mandates can also play a large role in the implementation of new treatments such as CBT. For example, the mandate to see clients on a first come–first serve basis may result in low availability of clients suitable for CBT when a CBT supervision opportunity arises. In summary, being able to reduce the cost of training and treatment without sacrificing their quality is vital if organizations are to implement CBT effectively.

In order to anticipate obstacles to implementing CBT in an organization, it is important to assess potential knowledge translation challenges. Assessment tools such as the Texas Christian University organizational readiness for change (ORC; Lehman, Greener, and Simpson 2002), the Evidence-Based Practice Attitude Scale (EBPAS), and attitudes toward treatment manuals (Bartholomew, Joe, Rowan-Szal, and Simpson 2007) have been developed to identify possible barriers to implementing new programs. These measures have shown positive results, helping leaders identify areas of need, so that they can be proactive in overcoming barriers. Further research in this area is needed, however, particularly regarding measures that are specifically for use within children's mental health organizations.

Conclusion

Effective knowledge translation must address all levels of mental health care. Training programs should educate therapists and organizations in the principles and evidence base of CBT, provide active learning styles, promote flexibility in treatment, and provide support to both the therapist and the organization. Further, knowledge translation should aid organizations in developing their own support system for the sustainability of CBT practice, whether through peer supervision, train-the-trainer models, or ongoing consultation with experts. Assessment of obstacles to implementing evidence-based care may be beneficial when one takes a proactive approach to knowledge translation.

References

Barrett, Paula M., Lara J. Farrell, Thomas H. Ollendick, and Mark M. Dadds. 2006. "Long-Term Outcomes of an Australian Universal Prevention Trial of Anxiety and Depression Symptoms in Children and Youth: An Evaluation of the Friends Program." *Journal of Clinical Child & Adolescent Psychology*, 35: 403–11. DOI: 10.1207/s15374424jccp3503_5

Bartholomew, Norma G., George W. Joe, Grace A. Rowan-Szal, and D. Dwayne Simpson. 2007. "Counselor Assessments of Training and Adoption Barriers." *Journal of Substance Abuse Treatment*, 33: 193–9. DOI: 10.1016/j.jsat.2007.01.005

Beidas, Rinad S., and Philip C. Kendall. 2010. "Training Therapists in Evidence-Based Practice: A Critical Review of Studies from a Systems-Contextual Perspective." *Clinical Psychology Review*, 17: 1–30. DOI: 10.1111/j.1468-2850.2009.01187.x

Bennett-Levy, James. 2006. "Therapist Skills: A Cognitive Model of Their Acquisition and Refinement." *Behavioural and Cognitive Psychotherapy*, 34: 57–78. DOI: 10.1017/S1352465805002420

Bennett-Levy, James, and Alexis Beedie. 2007. "The Ups and Downs of Cognitive Therapy Training: What Happens to Trainees' Perception of Their Competence During a Cognitive Therapy Training Course?" *Behavioural and Cognitive Psychotherapy*, 35: 61–75. DOI: 10.1017/S1352465806003110

Bennett-Levy, James, Freda McManus, Bengt E. Westling, and Melanie Fennell. 2009. "Acquiring and Refining CBT Skills and Competencies: Which Training Methods Are Perceived to Be Most Effective?" *Behavioural and Cognitive Psychotherapy*, 37: 571–83. DOI: 10.1017/S1352465809990270

Chorpita, Bruce F., Alissa A. Taylor, Sarah E. Francis, Catherine Moffitt, and Ayda A. Austin. 2004. "Efficacy of Modular Cognitive Behavior Therapy for Childhood Anxiety Disorders." *Behavior Therapy*, 35: 263–87.

Compton, Scott N., John S. March, David Brent, Anne M. Albano, V. Robin Weersing, John Curry. 2004. "Cognitive Behavioral Psychotherapy for Anxiety and Depressive Disorders in Children and Adolescents: An Evidence-Based Medicine Review." *Journal of American Academic Child Adolescent Psychiatry*, 43: 930–59.

Dimeff Linda A., Kelly Koerner, Eric A. Woodcock, Blair Beadnell, Milton Z. Brown, Julie M. Skutch, ... Melanie S. Harned. 2009. "Which Training Method Works Best? A Randomized Controlled Trial Comparing Three Methods of Training Clinicians in Dialectical Behavior Therapy Skills." Behaviour Research and Therapy, 47: 921–30. DOI: 10.1016/j.brat.2009.07.011

Dobson Keith S., Brian F. Shaw, and T. Michael Vallis. 1985. "Reliability of a Measure of the Quality of Cognitive Therapy." *British Journal of Clinical Psychology*, 24: 295–300. DOI: 10.1111/j.2044-8260.1985.tb00662.x

Granpeesheh, Doreen, Jonathan Tarbox, Dennis R. Dixon, Catherine A. Peters, Kathleen Thompson, and Amy Kenzer. 2010. "Evaluation of an Elearning Tool for Training Behavioral Therapists in Academic Knowledge of Applied Behavior Analysis." *Research in Autism Spectrum Disorders*, 4: 11–17. DOI: 10.1016/j.rasd.2009.07.004

Harned, Melanie S., Linda A. Dimeff, Eric A. Woodcock, and Julie M. Skutch. 2001. "Overcoming Barriers to Disseminating Exposure Therapies for Anxiety Disorders: A Pilot Randomized Controlled Trial of Training Methods." *Journal of Anxiety Disorders*, 25: 155–63. DOI: 10.1016/j.janxdis.2010.08.015

Hedtke, Kristina A., Philip C. Kendall, and Shilpee Tiwari. 2009. "Safety-Seeking and Coping Behavior during Exposure Tasks with Anxious Youth." *Journal of Clinical Child and Adolescent Psychology*, 38: 1–15. DOI: 10.1080/15374410802581055

Hepner, Kimberly A., Sarah B. Hunter, Susan M. Paddock, Annie J. Zhou, and Katharine E. Watkins. 2011. "Training Addiction Counselors to Implement CBT for Depression." *Administration Policy Mental Health*, 38: 313–23. DOI: 10.1007/s10488-011-0359-7

Herschell, Amy D., David J. Kolko, Barbara L. Baumann, and Abigail C. Davis. 2010. "The Role of Therapist Training in the Implementation of Psychosocial Treatments: A Review and Critique with Recommendations." *Clinical Psychology Review*, 30: 448–66. DOI: 10.1016/j.cpr.2010.02.005

James, Ian A., Ivy M. Blackburn, Derek L. Milne, and F. Katharina Reichfelt. 2001. "Moderators of Trainee Therapists' Competence in Cognitive Therapy." *British Journal of Clinical Psychology*, 40: 131–41. DOI: 10.1348/014466501163580

Karlin, Bradley E., Josef I. Ruzek, Kathleen M. Chard, Afsoon Eftekhari, Candice M. Monson, Elizabeth A. Hembree, Patricia A. Resick, and Edna B. Foa. 2010. "Dissemination of Evidence-Based Psychological Treatments for Posttraumatic Stress Disorder in the Veterans Health Administration." *Journal of Traumatic Stress*, 23: 663–73. DOI: 10.1002/jts.20588

Kendall, Phillip C. 1994. "Treating Anxiety Disorders in Children: Results of a Randomized Clinical Trial." *Journal of Consulting and Clinical Psychology*, 62: 100–10.

Kendall, Philip C., and Kristina Hedtke. A. 2006a. *Cognitive–Behavioral Therapy for Anxious Children: Therapist Manual* (3rd ed.). Ardmore, PA: Workbook Publishing.

Kendall, Philip C., and Kristina Hedtke. A. 2006b. *The Coping Cat Workbook* (2nd ed.). Ardmore, PA: Workbook Publishing.

Kendall, Philip C., Cara A. Settipani, and Colleen M. Cummings. 2012. "No Need to Worry: The Promising Future of Child Anxiety Research." *Journal of Clinical Child and Adolescent Psychology*, 41: 103–15. DOI: 10.1080/15374416.2012.632352.

Kendall, Philip C., Ellen Flannery-Schroeder, Susan M. Panichelli-Mindel, Michael Southam-Gerow, Aude Henin, and Melissa Warman. 1997. "Therapy for Youths with Anxiety Disorders: A Second Randomized Clinical Trial." *Journal of Consulting and Clinical Psychology*, 65: 366–80.

Kendall, Philip C., Jonathan S. Comer, Craig D. Marker, Torrey A. Creed, Anthony C. Puliafico, Alicia A. Hughes, ... Jennifer Hudson. 2009. "In-Session Exposure Tasks and Therapeutic Alliance across the Treatment of Childhood Anxiety Disorders." *Journal of Consulting and Clinical Psychology*, 77: 517–25. DOI: 0.1037/a0013686

Khanna, Muniya S., and Philip C. Kendall. 2008. "Computer-Assisted CBT for Child Anxiety: The Coping Cat CD-Rom." *Cognitive and Behavioral Practice*, 15: 159–65.

Kuyken Willem, and Dimitrios Tsivrikos. 2009. "Therapist Competence, Comorbidity and Cognitive-Behavioral Therapy for Depression." *Psychotherapy and Psychosomatics*, 78: 42–8. DOI: 10.1159/000172619

Lehman, Wayney E., Jack M. Greener, and Dwayne Simpson. 2002. "Assessing Organizational Readiness for Change." *Journal of Substance Abuse Treatment*, 22: 197–209.

Lewis, Cara C., and Anne D. Simons. 2011. "A Pilot Study Disseminating Cognitive Behavioral Therapy for Depression: Therapist Factors and Perceptions of Barriers to Implementation." *Administration and Policy in Mental Health and Mental Health Services Research*, 38: 324–34. DOI: 10.1007/s10488-011-0348-x

Manassis, Katharina, Abel Ickowicz, Erin Picard, Beverly Antle, Ted McNeill, Anu Chahauver, ... Gili Adler Nevo. 2009. "An Innovative Child CBT Training Model for Community Mental Health Practitioners in Ontario." *Academic Psychiatry*, 33: 394–9. DOI: 10.1176/appi.ap.33.5.394

Mannix, Kathryn A., Ivy M. Blackburn, Anne Garland, Jennifer Gracie, Stirling Moorey, Barbara Reid, Sally Standart, and Jan Scott. 2006. "Effectiveness of Brief Training in Cognitive Behaviour Therapy Techniques for Palliative Care Practitioners." *Palliative Medicine*, 20(6): 579–84.

Milne, Derek, Helen Aylott, Helen Fitzpatrick, and Michael V. Ellis. 2008. "How Does Clinical Supervision Work? Using a "Best Evidence Synthesis" Approach to Construct a Basic Model of Supervision." *The Clinical Supervisor*, 27: 170–90. DOI: 10.1080/07325220802487915

Nelson, Timothy D., and Ric G. Steele. 2007. "Predictors of Practitioner Self-Reported Use of Evidence-Based Practices: Practitioner Training, Clinical Setting, and Attitudes toward

Research." *Administration and Policy in Mental Health and Mental Health Services Research*, 34: 319–30. DOI: 0.1007/s10488-006-0111-x

Newton, J. Richard, and Priscilla G. Yardley. 2007. "Evaluation of CBT Training of Clinicians in Routine Clinical Practice." *Psychiatric Services*, 58: 1497. DOI: 10.1176/appi. ps.58.11.1497

Podell, Jennifer L., Matthew Mychailyszyn, Julie Edmunds, Conner M. Puleo, and Philip C. Kendall. 2010. "The Coping Cat Program for Anxious Youth: The Fear Plan Comes to Life." *Cognitive and Behavioral Practice*, 17: 132–41. DOI: 10.1016/j.cbpra.2009.11.001

Rakovshik, Sarah G., and Freda McManus. 2010. "Establishing Evidence-Based Training in Cognitive Behavioral Therapy: A Review of Current Empirical Findings and Theoretical Guidance." *Clinical Psychology Review*, 30: 496–516. DOI:10.1016/j.cpr.2010.03.004

Reese, Claire S., and D. Gillam. 2001. "A Comparison of the Cost of Cognitive–Behavioural Training for Mental Health Professionals Using Videoconferencing or Conventional, Face-to-Face Teaching." *Journal of Telemedicine and Telecare*, 7: 359–60. DOI: 10.1258/ 1357633011937010

Rose, Raphael D., Ariel J. Lang, Stacy Shaw Welch, Laura Campbell-Sills, Denise A. Chavira, Greer Sullivan, … Michelle G. Craske. 2011. "Training Primary Care Staff to Deliver a Computer-Assisted Cognitive–Behavioral Therapy Program for Anxiety Disorders." *General Hospital Psychiatry*, 33: 336–42. DOI: 10.1016/j.genhosppsych.2011.04.011

Roth, Anthony D., and Stephen Pilling. 2008. "Using an Evidence-Based Methodology to Identify the Competences Required to Deliver Effective Cognitive and Behavioural Therapy for Depression and Anxiety Disorders." *Behavioural and Cognitive Psychotherapy*, 36: 129–47. DOI: 10.1017/S1352465808004141

Sburlati, Elizabeth S., Carolyn A. Schniering, Heidi J. Lyneham, and Ronald M. Rapee. 2011. "A Model of Therapist Competencies for the Empirically Supported Cognitive Behavioral Treatment of Child and Adolescent Anxiety and Depressive Disorders." *Clinical Child and Family Psychology Review*, 14: 89–109. DOI: 10.1007/s10567-011-0083-6

Sholomskas, Diane E., and Kathleen M. Carroll. 2006. "One Small Step for Manuals: Computer-Assisted Training in Twelve-Step Facilitation." *Journal of the Studies on Alcohol*, 67: 939–45.

Sholomskas, Diane E., Gia Syracuse-Siewert, Bruce J. Rounsaville, Samuel A. Ball, Kathryn F. Nuro, and Kathleen M. Carroll. 2005. "We Don't Train in Vain: A Dissemination Trial of Three Strategies of Training Clinicians in Cognitive–Behavioral Therapy." *Journal of Consulting and Clinical Psychology*, 73: 106–15. DOI: 10.1037/0022-006X.73.1.106

Simons, Anne, Christine Padesky, Jeremy Montemarano, Cara Lewis, Jessica Murakami, Kristen Lamb, … Aaron Beck. 2010. "Training and Dissemination of Cognitive Behavior Therapy for Depression in Adults: A Preliminary Examination of Therapist Competence and Client Outcomes." *Journal of Consulting and Clinical Psychology*, 78: 751–6. DOI: 10.1037/a0020569

Stark, Kevin D., Prerna Arora, and Catherine L. Funk. 2011. "Training School Psychologists to Conduct Evidence-Based Treatments for Depression." *Psychology in the Schools*, 48: 272–82. DOI: 10.1002/pits.20551

Stark, Kevin D., Sarah Schnoebelen, Jane Simpson, Jennifer Hargrave, Johanna Molnar, and R. Glen. 2007. *Treating Depressed Youth: Therapist Manual for "Action."* Philadelphia, PA: Workbook Publishing.

Strunk, Daniel R., Melissa A. Brotman, Robert J. DeRubeis, and Steven D. Hollon. 2010. "Therapist Competence in Cognitive Therapy for Depression: Predicting Subsequent Symptom Change." *Journal of Consulting and Clinical Psychology*, 78: 429–37. DOI: 10.1037/a0019631

Sudak Donna M., Judith S. Beck, and Jessie Wright. 2003. "Cognitive Behavioral Therapy: A Blueprint for Attaining and Assessing Psychiatry Resident Competency." *Academic Psychiatry*, 27: 154–9. DOI: 10.1176/appi.ap.27.3.154

Suveg, Cynthia, Erica Sood, Jonathan S. Comer, and Philip C. Kendall. 2009. "Changes in Emotion Regulation Following Cognitive–Behavioral Therapy for Anxious Youth." *Journal of Clinical Child and Adolescent Psychology*, 38: 390–401. DOI: 10.1080/15374410902851721.

Treatment for Adolescents with Depression Study Team. 2004. "Fluoxetine, Cognitive Behavioral Therapy, and Their Combination for Adolescents with Depression: Treatment for Adolescents with Depression Study (Tads) Randomized Controlled Trial." *Journal of the American Medical Association*, 292: 807–20. DOI: 10.1001/jama.292.7.807

Trepka, Chris, Anne Rees, David Shapiro, Gillian Hardy, and Michael Barkham. 2004. "Therapist Competence and Outcome of Cognitive Therapy for Depression." *Cognitive Therapy and Research*, 28: 143–57.

Weingardt, Kenneth R. 2004. "The Role of Instructional Design and Technology in the Dissemination of Empirically Supported, Manual-Based Therapies." *Clinical Psychology: Science and Practice*, 11(3): 313–31.

Weingardt, Kenneth R., Michael A. Cucciare, Christine Bellotti, and Wen Pin Lai. 2009. "A Randomized Trial Comparing Two Models of Web-Based Training in Cognitive–Behavioral Therapy for Substance Abuse Counselors." *Journal of Substance Abuse Treatment*, 37(3): 219–27. DOI: 10.1016/j.jsat.2009.01.002

Weisz John R., Michael Southam-Gerow, Elana Gordis, Jennifer Connor-Smith, Brian Chu, David Langer, ... Bahr Weiss. 2009. "Cognitive–Behavioral Therapy versus Usual Clinical Care for Youth Depression: An Initial Test of Transportability to Community Clinics and Clinicians." *Journal of Consulting and Clinical Psychology*, 77: 383–96. DOI: 10.1037/a0013877

Weisz, John R., Bruce F. Chorpita, Laurence A. Palinkas, Sonja K. Schoenwald, Jeanne Miranda, Sarah K. Bearman, ... Robert B. Gibbons. 2012. "Testing Standard and Modular Designs for Psychotherapy Treating Depression, Anxiety, and Conduct Problems in Youth: A Randomized Effectiveness Trial." *Archives of General Psychiatry*, 69: 274–82. DOI: 10.1001/archgenpsychiatry.2011.147

Further Reading

Frueh, B. Christopher, Anouk L. Grubaugh, Karen J. Cusack, Matthew O. Kimble, Jon D. Elhai, and Rebecca G. Knapp. 2007. "Therapist Adherence and Competence with Manualized Cognitive–Behavioral Therapy for PTSD Delivered via Videoconferencing Technology." *Behavior Modification*, 31: 856–66. DOI: 10.1016/j.janxdis.2009.02.005

Jungbluth, Nathaniel J., and Stephen R. Shirk. 2009. "Therapist Strategies for Building Involvement in Cognitive–Behavioral Therapy for Adolescent Depression." *Journal of Consulting and Clinical Psychology*, 77: 1179–84. DOI:10.1037/a0017325

Khanna, Muniya S., and Philip C. Kendall. 2009. "Exploring the Role of Parent Training in the Treatment of Childhood Anxiety." *Journal of Consulting and Clinical Psychology*, 77: 981–6. DOI: 10.1037/a0016920

Manassis, Katharina. 2009. *Cognitive Behavioral Therapy with Children: A Guide for the Community Practitioner*. New York: Routledge.

Part I

Generic Therapeutic Competencies

3

Self-Assessment of Our Competence as Therapists

Elizabeth S. Sburlati and James Bennett-Levy

Introduction

The gold standard for ensuring therapists have an acceptable and sustainable level of competence is generally achieved through objective measurement of a therapist's competency by an experienced assessor, clinical supervision, continued targeted professional development, and positive outcomes with clients. However, in routine clinical practice, the most usual and most readily available method of quality control on a daily basis is self-assessment.

Research has shown that therapists are often inaccurate in their estimations of their level of competence. Less competent therapists have been reported to overrate their level of competence when their own ratings were compared to ratings made by objective observers (Brosan, Reynolds, and Moore 2008). One of the reasons, it is suggested, is that less competent therapists often "don't know what they don't know" (Bennett-Levy and Beedie 2007; McManus, Rakovshik, Kennerley, Fennell, and Westbrook 2012, p. 301). On rare occasions it has been found that more competent therapists underestimate their abilities by comparison with supervisor ratings (McManus et al. 2012). Generally, however, therapists tend to have an overly positive view of their own abilities (Walfish, McAlister, O'Donnell, and Lambert 2012), which may compromise the standard of practice among the therapist workforce (Brosan et al. 2008).

Since research shows problems with therapists' self-assessment, the purpose of this chapter is to assist with improving self-assessment, both in general and in the specific area of the treatment of child and adolescent anxiety and depressive disorders. In order to do this, the chapter includes four sections, which cover (i) suggested methods for competent self-assessment of therapeutic knowledge and skills; (ii) self-assessment in relation to working with anxiety and depressive disorders; (iii) self-assessment in

Evidence-Based CBT for Anxiety and Depression in Children and Adolescents: A Competencies-Based Approach,
First Edition. Edited by Elizabeth S. Sburlati, Heidi J. Lyneham, Carolyn A. Schniering, and Ronald M. Rapee.
© 2014 John Wiley & Sons, Ltd. Published 2014 by John Wiley & Sons, Ltd.

relation to working with children and adolescents; and (iv) common obstacles to self-assessment and methods to overcome them.

We should make it clear from the outset that, although self-assessment may be commonly used, it is a far from perfect method of assessing therapist competence. While in this chapter we suggest some ways to assist therapists in assessing themselves, it is important to note that far more research is required in this area. Self-assessment is probably best used in combination with other methods of therapist competence assessment, such as objective competence assessment, client process and outcome data, 360-degree evaluations, pen-and-paper tests, and oral examinations (Kaslow et al. 2009).

Key Features of Self-Assessment and Professional Development Competencies

Definition of self-assessment

Self-assessment of competence is the practice of validly assessing one's professional competencies in an area of practice, with the purpose of determining competency strengths and weaknesses (Kaslow et al. 2007; Kaslow et al. 2009). Following self-assessment, therapists should identify their competency limitations, make plans to improve these competencies by engaging in appropriate professional development study, supervision/consultation, and deliberate practice (Ericsson, 2009), and monitor progress toward their competency goals (Belar et al. 2001; Caverzagie, Shea, and Kogan 2008; Kaslow et al. 2007; Kaslow et al. 2009).

Methods of self-assessment

We recommend the following methods of self-assessment: measurement of client outcomes and process; use of a guiding model of therapist competencies; use of valid and reliable assessment tools; active review and reflection on audio or video recording of therapy sessions; engagement in reflective practice; and active participation in clinical supervision and professional development, so as to increase one's knowledge and refine self-assessment skills. These six methods are described below.

Measurement of client outcomes and process
A useful metric of therapist performance is whether clients are improving in line with expectations, or whether they are failing to improve. Research shows that therapists tend to be poor judges of client progress and outcomes and have an overly optimistic perspective and a biased appraisal of their own skill level (Newnham and Page 2010; Walfish et al. 2012). These biases suggest the need for accurate feedback on client progress.

The adult psychotherapy literature indicates that the best way to judge client progress accurately is to measure outcomes on a routine basis (e.g., every session) and compare the results against population benchmarks and expected outcomes (Lambert 2010). An additional refinement is to get direct feedback from clients about the process of therapy: Are the client's needs (therapeutic bond, tasks, and goals) being adequately met? Routine monitoring of the client's experience of therapy, with a particular emphasis on elements with which the client is dissatisfied, has been shown to enhance therapy outcomes (Lambert 2010).

The conclusion from the adult psychotherapy literature is that the assessment of client outcomes and therapeutic process provides an important foundation for making both positive adjustments to the therapeutic intervention (where these are necessary) and accurate self-assessment. In order to assess the therapeutic process and its outcomes, clinicians working with children and adolescents can use a range of available measures. Chapter 7 provides information on a number of evidence-based measures for assessing anxiety and depression that allow for an evaluation of client outcomes in terms of return to nonclinical range. Chapter 6 provides information on process-oriented measures that can be used to identify whether changes may be needed in the therapeutic process in order to enhance the likelihood of positive gains.

Unlike the adult literature, however, the child and adolescent literature does not yet have client outcome benchmarks against which a therapist can compare his or her client's progress *during* therapy. In consequence, a therapist can only determine whether all his or her clients' outcome scores are improving or not, but cannot determine whether the degree of improvement of an individual client is at the expected level during therapy. In the absence of appropriate benchmarks, data concerning the outcomes of a number of clients treated by a therapist could be compared with the expected outcomes that are based on meta-analyses. In anxiety disorders, for all clients who begin treatment, the response rate expected immediately after treatment would be about 59 percent – assuming that, if there are drop-outs, these did not improve (James, James, Cowdrey, Soler, and Choke 2013). Comparisons for depression are only available on the basis of effect sizes; however, response rates for the larger treatment trials would indicate an expected response of between 43 and 65 percent at the 12–18 week mark (March et al. 2007). Although this is a crude comparison, it will provide useful evidence for a therapist's self-reflection, until such time as research yields appropriate benchmarks for children and adolescents.

Having a model of therapist competencies as a guide
Without clear competency guidelines, therapists are unlikely to have a good understanding of the competencies required to implement a particular therapy with a given population. Further, the evidence suggests that, when left to their own devices, therapists prefer to focus on self-assessing and improving conceptual knowledge and technical skills rather than interpersonal skills (Niemi and Tiuraniemi 2010).

One way of ensuring that therapists are aware of the depth and breadth of the required competencies is to develop therapist competencies guidelines that list and describe in detail the competencies required when one is using a particular therapeutic orientation with a specific population. For example, there are guidelines in the form of therapist competencies models for treating anxiety and depression using CBT in adults (Roth and Pilling 2008) and in children and adolescents (Sburlati, Schniering, Lyneham, and Rapee 2011). Such models should be made readily available for those therapists who are attempting to learn the competencies required for a given therapy and population.

Use of reliable, valid, objectively rated assessment tools

Self-assessment practices tend to be non-standardized. One way to make self-assessment more standardized would be to use reliable and valid therapist competence assessment tools. This has been done in a number of research trials (e.g., Bennett-Levy and Beedie 2007; McManus et al. 2012). These assessment tools include a number of items that correspond to necessary competencies in a given area of practice, and also a Likert scale of competency-related anchor points (e.g., incompetent, novice, advanced beginner, competent, proficient, expert) for each item (see Blackburn, James, Milne, and Reichelt 2001). An overall label is given for each competency item and more detailed descriptions are provided for how that competency might look at each level of competence.

While the vast majority of these tools are observer-rated – that is, a supervisor or some other observer rates the competence of a therapist, either *in vivo* or from a recording – the self-assessing therapist can record selected therapy sessions and simply change any reference to "the therapist" in the assessment measure to "I." The validity of therapist self-assessment ratings might be increased when these ratings are made in conjunction with observer ratings on the same therapy sessions (Bennett-Levy and Beedie 2007).

Two examples of observer-rated CBT competency measures that have been psychometrically validated are the following:

1. the Cognitive Therapy Scale (Vallis, Shaw, and Dobson 1986; Young and Beck 1980);
2. the Cognitive Therapy Scale – Revised (Blackburn, James, Milne, Baker, et al. 2001; Blackburn, James, Milne, and Reichelt 2001).

A problem is that the above competency tools are measures of CBT in treating adults. Measures of competencies in treating children and adolescents with anxiety and depressive disorders are required. A measure based on the Sburlati and colleagues (2011) model is currently under development.

Audio or video recording of therapy sessions

Neither self-assessment nor objective assessment of competencies can take place in a systematic manner without sessions being audio- or video-recorded. Competency measures typically have a number of dimensions (e.g., conceptual, technical, interpersonal), and assess specific skills (e.g., identification of negative automatic thoughts, case formulation). Recording one's sessions enables therapists to review their microskills at a level of detail that is simply impossible when conducting a session *in vivo* (Brown, Moller, and Ramsey-Wade 2013).

Reviewing a recorded session enables a therapist to assess him- or herself carefully at specific times in the therapy (e.g., when developing a shared conceptualization of the problem) and to determine how well this was enacted and whether it could have been carried out better (Brown et al. 2013). It is frequently the experience of therapists that, as they listen to a session recording, they pick up on details and nuances of the session of which they were quite unaware at the time. After a therapy session, therapists are sometimes left with a vague feeling that they "missed the point," or that there was discomfort or a mini-rupture at some juncture in the session (Bennett-Levy and Thwaites, 2007, pp. 264–5). As we will describe in the next section, such experiences represent perfect opportunities to enhance our skills by engaging in reflective practice.

Engaging in reflective practice
Bennett-Levy and Thwaites (2007) and Bennett-Levy, Thwaites, Chaddock, and Davis (2009) propose that reflective practice is an integral part of self-assessment. Listening to a session recording and using a competency scale is one aspect of reflective practice that requires an objective assessment of performance against defined criteria. This kind of objective, detached reflection, which these authors termed "general reflection" (Bennett-Levy and Thwaites 2007), is important in the assessment of one's own skills, particularly conceptual and technical ones.

However, equally important for therapists is another type of reflection: "self-reflection." As defined by Bennett-Levy and colleagues (2009), the content of self-reflection is self-referenced to one's thoughts, feelings, behaviors, or personal history. Self-reflection is particularly important where there is discomfort or a therapeutic rupture in the relationship. At such times we need to "go inside" and both feel our own feelings and reflect on the feelings and experiences of the client, in order to gauge them accurately and to determine whether any of our own preconceptions, emotions, or experiences from past events have been unwittingly triggered by the client. Self-reflection is more emotionally demanding and more personal than "general reflection" – but just as necessary for therapists who wish to assess themselves accurately, and particularly important for enhancing their interpersonal skills (Bennett-Levy and Thwaites, 2007).

An "on the run" useful way to engage in reflective practice is spending 5–10 minutes to reflect on a session immediately after it has finished and answering the following questions: "What did I do well?" "What could I have improved? How?" This is particularly useful once the therapist has internalized the required competencies and can mentally cross-check them against the actual performance.

Actively participating in supervision and accessing professional development
Supervision, or consultation, is now considered to be an integral part of training and professional development (e.g., Beidas, Edmunds, Marcus, and Kendall 2012; Rakovshik and McManus 2010). Engagement in supervision may be enhanced by recording one's therapy sessions and giving the supervisor these recordings for review and feedback; by agreeing on a competence assessment method with the supervisor; by comparing observer-rated and self-rated competence results; and by analyzing the discrepancies between these assessments – as well as various strengths and weaknesses. Once areas of weakness are identified, a learning plan can be developed, along with a method of tracking improvement over time; and the plan should highlight the learning needs and the professional development training methods to achieve them (Belar et al. 2001; Caverzagie, Shea, and Kogan 2008; Kaslow et al. 2007; Kaslow et al. 2009).

Competence in Self-Assessment when Treating Anxiety Disorders and Depression

While the *process* of therapist self-assessment appears to be broadly similar for anxiety disorders and for depression, the therapist should be mindful that evidence-based treatment in anxiety disorders and in depression includes some different *techniques*. This means that the competencies or techniques on which therapists are assessing themselves when they treat anxiety will be slightly different from the ones they are assessing themselves on when they treat depression. For instance, in the CBT treatment of both anxiety disorders and depressive disorders, cognitive restructuring would likely be indicated for both. However, while exposure therapy would be indicated for anxiety, it would not usually be indicated for depression. On the other hand, pleasant events scheduling or behavioral activation might be suggested for depression, but not usually for anxiety.

Given the high degree of comorbidity between anxiety disorders and depression (Angold, Costello and Erkanli, 1999), therapists must be aware of the need to combine, in their treatment planning, evidence-based techniques for treating anxiety with evidence-based techniques for treating depression. It follows from the example above that, on seeing a child with both anxiety and depression, the therapist ought to make use of cognitive restructuring applied to both anxiolytic and depressogenic thoughts and may utilize aspects of exposure to enable that client to engage in pleasant events scheduling or behavioral activation. This skill, which is related to treatment planning, is an additional competency for the therapist to assess him- or herself in (see Chapter 9 for more details about treatment planning for anxiety and depression).

Competence in Self-Assessment of Skills when Treating Children and Adolescents

While the *process* of self-assessment is likely the same for therapists treating children and for therapists treating adolescents, the *strategies, techniques,* and *interpersonal skills* that the therapist assesses him- or herself on when treating these different age groups can differ. As is highlighted throughout this book, there are important differences in the therapeutic competencies required for treating anxiety and/or depression in different age groups. When working with children and adolescents, therapists need to understand how a child's age and other characteristics of children impact on therapy (see Chapter 5), and be capable of making age-appropriate accommodations for therapy procedures (e.g., structure, pace, use of age-appropriate activities) and techniques (e.g., limiting cognitive requirements in cognitive restructuring) (Kingery et al. 2006; Ollendick and Hovey 2010; Sauter, Heyne, and Westenberg 2009; Sburlati et al. 2011).

Unlike those engaged in the treatment of adults, therapists treating children and adolescents are required to develop and maintain a therapeutic alliance with both the client (the child or the adolescent) and the parent(s) (see Chapter 6 for a more detailed discussion). In addition, the therapist needs to be capable of judging the appropriate level of parental involvement in therapy on the basis of the child's or the adolescent's developmental level (Kingery et al. 2006; Sauter, Heyne, and Westenberg 2009). Therefore therapists of children and adolescents need the ability to develop and maintain multiple alliances – which can be difficult when the aims of the client and those of their parents differ.

As part of their self-reflection process, therapists may reflect on how their experiences as parents impact on their therapeutic alliances with parent and child and on how their own parenting beliefs, practices, and relationship with children may be impacting the therapeutic relationship. In addition, whether a therapist is a parent or not may influence the parent's perception of that therapist's competence. Hence the therapist's handling of the question "Do you have children?" is worth reflecting on: it may have significant implications for building and maintaining the desired alliance.

Common Obstacles to Self-Assessment and Professional Development Practice and Methods to Overcome Them

There are many obstacles to a therapist assessing his or her competence in an effective way. Below we describe some common obstacles and methods to overcome them.

Monitoring client progress and gaining client feedback

Although weekly monitoring of progress and getting feedback from the client are associated with better outcomes (Lambert 2010; Newnham and Page 2010) – and, quite probably, with enhanced self-assessment – many therapists are reluctant to use these procedures. Therapists would do well to study the empirical literature on process and outcome monitoring and, if they are still reluctant, to ask themselves self-reflectively: What concerns (e.g., ideas about therapy or about myself as a therapist) are getting in the way of a regular monitoring of process and outcome with my clients? Having addressed these concerns, therapists who make a decision to change their practice should determine what measures would work best for their clients' age group and population and how best to seek accurate feedback about process from clients who may be reluctant to articulate negative opinions.

Recording therapy sessions

As indicated earlier, one of the key methods for assessing one's own competence is the use of recorded therapy sessions. However, both therapists and clients may show reluctance to being recorded – and for similar reasons: fear of negative evaluation. Therapists may be reluctant to expose their "mistakes" to supervisors. Self-reflective practice may be helpful to determine what thoughts and ideas are getting in the way. Clients may be apprehensive about how the recording may be used in the future, or they may fear negative evaluation from observers (this might be particularly true for self-conscious adolescents). In order to overcome client apprehension, the therapist could:

1. develop a system that will ensure the confidentiality of recordings (e.g., by keeping physical copies in a locked filing cabinet and digital copies in a password-protected environment, and by ensuring that only authorized individuals can obtain access to them);
2. generate an official information and consent form outlining the specific purpose and uses of the recording, as well as the procedure in place for maintaining confidentiality;
3. assure the client that the aim of the recording is to assess the therapist, not the client;
4. direct the recording device away from the client onto him- or herself, to diminish fear of negative evaluation from viewers;
5. offer the client a choice between audio only and video recording, as the former may be seen as less threatening.

In addition to these modifications, the therapist may also offer to give the child or adolescent – and maybe the parent(s) if they are actively involved in therapy – a copy of the recorded session, so that they may listen to it again, if they wish. Adult clients are reported to find this beneficial, particularly as they do not recall everything said in a session (Shepherd, Salkovskis, and Morris 2009).

Accessing supervision

It can be difficult for therapists to obtain supervision from a clinical expert in their area of practice; this may be due to a lack of experts, geographical distance from them, and costs associated with obtaining expert consultation. Therefore therapists may not always be able to make use of supervision to assist with their self-assessment and professional development choices. One method of overcoming the geographical obstacle is the use of web conferencing (Abbass et al. 2011). This tool is advantageous given the increased availability of easy to use and affordable internet applications that allow face-to-face communication across the globe. Group supervision methods are also sometimes used (e.g., Abbass et al. 2011; Riva and Erickson Cornish 2008): these could reduce the cost associated with expert supervision.

Accessing training

Once the therapist has assessed his or her own level of competence and has identified the nature of the training required, a possible obstacle to obtaining this training is its inaccessibility due to geographical distance from face-to-face workshops (Weingardt, Villafranca, and Levin 2006). This is particularly true in countries with widely dispersed populations (e.g., Australia, USA). Recently some training programs have been made accessible online, with research to date demonstrating promising results (e.g., Bennett-Levy, Hawkins, Perry, Cromarty, and Mills 2012; Kobak, Craske, Rose, and Wolitsky-Taylor 2013). By having training programs online, therapists may be more likely to obtain the training that will help them to meet their self-assessed learning needs. However, research also suggests that, in order for training to be more effective, follow-up reflective practice (Bennett-Levy and Padesky 2014) and consultation (Beidas, Edmonds, Marcus and Kendall 2012) are prime requirements.

Conclusion

This chapter has discussed the importance of therapists' self-assessment of their competence and professional development; methods for improving self-assessment; ways of assessing one's own skills when one is treating child and adolescent anxiety and depressive disorders; and common obstacles to self-assessment and professional development. It is hoped that, by improving self-assessment and ensuring therapists receive effective training and supervision, individuals seeking assistance for psychological problems will receive a better standard of care.

References

Abbass, Allan, Stephen Arthey, Jason Elliott, Tim Fedak, Dion Nowoweiski, Jasmina Markovski, and Sarah Nowoweiski. 2011. "Web-Conference Supervision for Advanced Psychotherapy Training: A Practical Guide." *Psychotherapy*, 48: 109–18. DOI: 10.1037/a0022427

Angold, Adrian, E. Jane Costello, and Alaattin Erkanli. 1999. "Comorbidity." *Journal of Child Psychology and Psychiatry*, 40: 57–87. DOI: 10.1111/1469-7610.00424

Beidas, Rinad S., Julie M. Edmunds, Steven C. Marcus, and Philip C. Kendall. 2012. "Training and Consultation to Promote Implementation of an Empirically Supported Treatment: A Randomized Trial." *Psychiatric Services*, 63: 660–5. DOI: 10.1176/appi.ps.201100401

Belar, Cynthia D., Robert A. Brown, Lee E. Hersch, Lynne M. Hornyak, Ronald H. Rozensky, Edward P. Sheridan, … and Geoffrey W. Reed. 2001. "Self-Assessment in Clinical Health Psychology: A Model for Ethical Expansion of Practice." *Professional Psychology: Research and Practice*, 32: 135–41. DOI: 10.1037/0735-7028.32.2.135

Bennett-Levy, James, and Alexis Beedie. 2007. "The Ups and Downs of Cognitive Therapy Training: What Happens to Trainees' Perception of Their Competence during a Cognitive Therapy Training Course?" *Behavioural and Cognitive Psychotherapy*, 35: 61–75. DOI: 10.1017/S1352465806003110

Bennett-Levy, James, Russell Hawkins, Helen Perry, Paul Cromarty, and Jeremy Mills. 2012. "Online Cognitive Behavioural Therapy Training for Therapists: Outcomes, Acceptability, and Impact of Support." *Australian Psychologist*, 47: 174–82. DOI: 10.1111/j.1742-9544.2012.00089.x

Bennett-Levy, James, and Christine Padesky. 2014. "Use It or Lose It: Post-workshop Reflection Enhances Learning and Utilization of CBT Skills." *Cognitive and Behavioral Practice*, 21, 12–19. DOI: 10.1016/j.cbpra.2013.05.001.

Bennett-Levy, James, and Richard Thwaites. 2007. "Self and Self-Reflection in the Therapeutic Relationship: A Conceptual Map and Practical Strategies for the Training, Supervision and Self-Supervision of Interpersonal Skills." In Paul Gilbert and Robert L. Leahy (Eds.), *The therapeutic relationship in the cognitive behavioral psychotherapies* (pp. 255–82). New York: Routledge.

Bennett-Levy, James, Richard Thwaites, Anna Chaddock, and Melanie Davis. 2009. "Reflective Practice in Cognitive Behavioural Therapy: The Engine of Lifelong Learning." In Jacqui Stedmon and Rudi Dallos (Eds.), *Reflective practice in psychotherapy and counselling* (pp. 115–35). Maidenhead, England: Open University Press.

Blackburn, Ivy-Marie, Ian A. James, Derek L. Milne, and F. Katharina Reichelt. 2001. Cognitive Therapy Scale – Revised (CTS-R). Unpublished manuscript. Newcastle upon Tyne, England.

Blackburn, Ivy-Marie, Ian A. James, Derek L. Milne, Chris Baker, Sally Standart, Anne Garland, and F. Katharina Reichelt. 2001. "The Revised Cognitive Therapy Scale (CTS-R): Psychometric Properties." *Behavioural and Cognitive Psychotherapy*, 29: 431–46. DOI: 10.1017/S1352465801004040

Brosan, Lee, Shirley Reynolds, and Richard G Moore. 2008. "Self-Evaluation of Cognitive Therapy Performance: Do Therapists Know How Competent They Are?" *Behavioural and Cognitive Psychotherapy*, 36: 581–7. DOI: 10.1017/S1352465808004438

Brown, Ellie, Naomi Moller, and Christine Ramsey-Wade. 2013. "Recording Therapy Sessions: What Do Clients and Therapists Really Think?" *Counselling and Psychotherapy Research: Linking Research with Practice*, 13: 254–62. DOI: 10.1080/14733145.2013.768286

Caverzagie, Kelly J., Judy A. Shea, and Jennifer R. Kogan. 2008. "Resident Identification of Learning Objectives after Performing Self-Assessment Based upon the ACGME Core Competencies." *Journal of General Internal Medicine*, 23: 1024–7. DOI: 10.1007/s11606-008-0571-7

Ericsson, K. Anders (Ed.). 2009. *Development of Professional Expertise: Toward Measurement of Expert Performance and Design of Optimal Learning Environments*. Cambridge: Cambridge University Press.

James, Anthony C., Georgina James, Felicity A. Cowdrey, Angela Soler, and Aislinn Choke. 2013. "Cognitive Behavioural Therapy for Anxiety Disorders in Children and Adolescents." *Cochrane Database of Systematic Reviews*, 6: 1–104. DOI: 10.1002/14651858. CD004690.pub3

Kaslow, Nadine J., Catherine L. Grus, Linda F. Campbell, Nadya A. Fouad, Robert L. Hatcher, and Emil R. Rodolfa. 2009. "Competency Assessment Toolkit for Professional Psychology." *Training and Education in Professional Psychology*, 3: S27–S45. DOI: 10.1037/a0015833

Kaslow, Nadine J., Nancy J. Rubin, Linda Forrest, Nancy S. Elman, Barbara A. Van Horne, Sue C. Jacobs, ... Beverly E. Thorn. 2007. "Recognizing, Assessing, and Intervening with Problems of Professional Competence." *Professional Psychology: Research and Practice*, 38: 479–92. DOI: 10.1037/0735-7028.38.5.479

Kingery, Julie N., Tami L. Roblek, Cynthia Suveg, Rachel L. Grover, Joel T. Sherrill, and R. Lindsay Bergman. 2006. "They're Not Just "Little Adults": Developmental Considerations for Implementing Cognitive–Behavioral Therapy with Anxious Youth." *Journal of Cognitive Psychotherapy: An International Quarterly*, 20: 263–73. DOI: 10.1891/jcop.20.3.263

Kobak, Kenneth A., Michelle G. Craske, Raphael D. Rose, and Kate Wolitsky-Taylor. 2013. "Web-Based Therapist Training on Cognitive Behavior Therapy for Anxiety Disorders: A Pilot Study." *Psychotherapy*, 50: 235–47. DOI: 10.1037/a0030568

Lambert, Michael J. 2010. *Prevention of Treatment Failure: The Use of Measuring, Monitoring, and Feedback in Clinical Practice*. Washington, DC: American Psychological Association. DOI: 10.1037/12141-000

March, John S., Susan Silva, Stephen Petrycki, John Curry, Karen Wells, John Fairbank, ... Joanne Severe. 2007. "The Treatment for Adolescents with Depression Study (TADS): Long-Term Effectiveness and Safety Outcomes." *Archives of General Psychiatry*, 64: 1132–43. DOI: 10.1001/archpsyc.64.10.1132

McManus, Freda, Sarah Rakovshik, Helen Kennerley, Melanie Fennell, and David Westbrook. 2012. "An Investigation of the Accuracy of Therapists' Self-Assessment of Cognitive-Behaviour Therapy Skills." *British Journal of Clinical Psychology*, 51: 292–306. DOI: 10.1111/j.2044-8260.2011.02028.x

Newnham, Elizabeth A., and Andrew C. Page. 2010. "Bridging the Gap between Best Evidence and Best Practice in Mental Health." *Clinical Psychology Review*, 30: 127–42. DOI: 10.1016/j.cpr.2009.10.004

Niemi, Päivi M., and Juhani Tiuraniemi. 2010. "Cognitive Therapy Trainees' Self-Reflections on Their Professional Learning." *Behavioural and Cognitive Psychotherapy*, 38: 255–74. DOI: 10.1017/S1352465809990609

Ollendick, Thomas H., and Laura D. Hovey. 2010. "Anxiety Disorders." In Jay C. Thomas and Michel Hersen (Eds.), *Handbook of Clinical Psychology Competencies* (pp. 1219–44). New York: Springer.

Rakovshik, Sarah G., and Freda McManus. 2010. "Establishing Evidence-Based Training in Cognitive Behavioral Therapy: A Review of Current Empirical Findings and Theoretical Guidance." *Clinical Psychology Review*, 30: 496–516. DOI: 10.1016/j.cpr.2010.03.004

Riva, Maria T., and Jennifer A. Erickson Cornish. 2008. "Group Supervision Practices at Psychology Predoctoral Internship Programs: 15 Years Later." *Training and Education in Professional Psychology*, 2: 18–25. DOI: 10.1037/1931-3918.2.1.18.

Roth, Anthony D., and Stephen Pilling. 2008. "Using an Evidence-Based Methodology to Identify the Competences Required to Deliver Effective Cognitive and Behavioural Therapy for Depression and Anxiety Disorders." *Behavioural and Cognitive Psychotherapy*, 36: 129–47. DOI: 10.1017/S1352465808004141

Sauter, Floor M., David Heyne, and P. Michiel Westenberg. 2009. "Cognitive Behavior Therapy for Anxious Adolescents: Developmental Influences on Treatment Design and Delivery." *Clinical Child and Family Psychology Review*, 12: 310–35. DOI: 10.1007/s10567-009-0058-z

Sburlati, Elizabeth S., Carolyn A. Schniering, Heidi J. Lyneham, and Ronald M. Rapee. 2011. "A Model of Therapist Competencies for the Empirically Supported Cognitive Behavioral Treatment of Child and Adolescent Anxiety and Depressive Disorders." *Clinical Child and Family Psychology Review*, 14: 89–109. DOI: 10.1007/s10567-011-0083-6

Shepherd, Laura, Paul M. Salkovskis, and Martin Morris. 2009. "Recording Therapy Sessions: An Evaluation of Patient and Therapist Reported Behaviours, Attitudes and Preferences." *Behavioural and Cognitive Psychotherapy*, 37: 141–50. DOI: 10.1017/S1352465809005190

Vallis, T. Michael, Brian F. Shaw, and Keith S. Dobson. 1986. "The Cognitive Therapy Scale: Psychometric Properties." *Journal of Consulting and Clinical Psychology*, 54: 381–5. DOI: 10.1037/0022-006X.54.3.381

Walfish, Steven, Brian McAlister, Paul O'Donnell, and Michael J. Lambert. 2012. "An Investigation of Self-Assessment Bias in Mental Health Providers." *Psychological Reports*, 110: 639–44. DOI: 10.2466/02.07.17.PR0.110.2.639-644

Weingardt, Kenneth R., Steven W. Villafranca, and Cindy Levin. 2006. "Technology-Based Training in Cognitive Behavioral Therapy for Substance Abuse Counselors." *Substance Abuse*, 27: 19–25. DOI: 10.1300/J465v27n03_04

Young, Jeffrey, and Aaron T. Beck. 1980. *Cognitive Therapy Scale: Rating Manual*. Unpublished Manuscript. University of Pennsylvania, Philadelphia, PA.

4

Professional Evidence-Based Practice with Children and Adolescents

Rinad S. Beidas, Matthew Ditty, Margaret Mary Downey, and Julie Edmunds

Introduction

Sburlati, Schniering, Lyneham, and Rapee (2011) have outlined a model of therapist competencies for the cognitive behavioral treatment (CBT) of pediatric anxiety and depressive disorders. CBT for these disorders is considered an evidence-based practice (EBP) given the significant empirical evidence it has garnered from randomized controlled trials. The authors have delineated three main categories of competencies: (i) generic therapeutic competencies (e.g., practicing professionally); (ii) CBT competencies (e.g., collaboratively conducting CBT sessions); and (iii) specific CBT techniques (e.g., changing maladaptive behaviors). These categories contribute to a deeper understanding of what competencies and techniques are necessary for appropriate delivery of CBT for pediatric anxiety and depressive disorders, which assists in closing the chasm between research and practice. This chapter describes generic therapeutic competencies related to professional practice that are relevant to CBT for pediatric anxiety and depressive disorders. The specific sub-competencies that fall under practicing professionally are outlined in Box 4.1.

Key Features of Competencies

Attitudes and ability to utilize research

The first aspect to professional practice as delineated by Sburlati and colleagues (2011) includes open and positive attitudes toward EBPs and the ability to access, evaluate, and apply research to inform practice.

Evidence-Based CBT for Anxiety and Depression in Children and Adolescents: A Competencies-Based Approach, First Edition. Edited by Elizabeth S. Sburlati, Heidi J. Lyneham, Carolyn A. Schniering, and Ronald M. Rapee. © 2014 John Wiley & Sons, Ltd. Published 2014 by John Wiley & Sons, Ltd.

> ## Box 4.1   Practicing professionally
>
> - Possession of an open attitude toward psychotherapy research, and the ability to access, critically evaluate, and utilize this research to inform practice.
> - Knowledge of and ability to operate within professional, ethical, and legal codes of conduct relevant to working with children and adolescents and their families (e.g., providing a duty of care).
> - Ability to actively participate in supervision.
>
> Source: Sburlati, Schniering, Lyneham, and Rapee (2011, p. 94).

Attitudes

The importance of therapists' attitudes has long been recognized in the professional practice of evidence-based treatments. Early research identified the role of individual therapists' attitudes in the dissemination and implementation of EBPs (Aarons 2004), and subsequently a number of studies surveyed therapist attitudes toward EBPs. One study found that therapists held favorable attitudes toward EBPs (Najavits, Weiss, Shaw, and Dierberger 2000) whereas another found that therapists held largely unfavorable attitudes toward EBPs (Addis and Krasnow 2000). One potential explanation for these conflicting results refers to therapist theoretical orientation. In the first study participants identified themselves as cognitive behavioral, the modality that has arguably received the greatest support in the EBP movement. In the second study a number of theoretical orientations were surveyed. Another potential explanation may be clinical experience. Therapists at an earlier stage in their careers may hold more favorable attitudes toward EBPs than therapists who are at a later stage (Aarons 2004). This may be due to increasing emphasis on training in EBP in graduate programs, or to more openness to varying viewpoints before identifying with a particular theoretical orientation.

An early interest in therapist attitudes led to the development of the now widely used Evidence-Based Practice Attitude Scale (EBPAS), a 15-item psychometrically validated questionnaire that assesses participants' attitudes toward the adoption and implementation of EBP via four subscales: appeal, requirements, openness, and divergence (Aarons 2004). Appeal refers to the extent to which a therapist will adopt a new practice if it is intuitively appealing. Requirements refer to the extent to which a therapist will adopt a new practice if it is required by his or her organization. Openness is the extent to which a therapist is generally receptive to using new interventions. Divergence is the extent to which a therapist perceives research-based treatments as lacking clinical utility.

Given that positive attitudes toward EBPs predict the use of such practices (Nelson and Steele 2007), we recommend two ways supervisors can work to increase the likelihood that trainees will have more positive attitudes toward EBPs. First, we recommend that supervisors assess these attitudes regularly, in order to facilitate an open overall attitude toward psychotherapy research. In addition, the evidence suggests that training in EBPs may be associated with a greater appreciation of the value of evidence-based interventions (Beidas and Kendall 2010). It is likely that regularly monitoring openness and other attitudes toward EBPs, while providing feedback to trainees, will increase openness and diminish negative attitudes. Second, the delivery mode impacts the way EBP information is perceived by therapists. For example, providing a research summary of the most appropriate EBP alongside a case study increases the likelihood that a therapist will use an EBP rather than relying soley upon clinical experience (Stewart and Chambless 2007), so this could be a potential strategy used in supervision to modify attitudes and improve utilization of EBPs.

Evidence consumers

Having an open attitude toward EBPs is likely necessary, but not sufficient for the successful implementation of EBPs. Another critical competency for therapists to master and for supervisors to foster is that of being "evidence consumers" (Spring 2007), which refers to the ability to identify, evaluate, and utilize research evidence to engage in evidence-based decision-making regarding treatment for individual clients. The process of being an evidence consumer is comprised of five steps, each of which is a separate skill necessary for evidence-based decision-making (Spring 2007). These steps are: ask the clinical question, acquire the evidence, appraise the evidence, apply the results, and assess the outcomes (Strauss, Richardson, Glasziou, and Haynes 2005).

To develop as an evidence consumer, therapists must have the ability to identify, evaluate, and utilize resources so as to stay current with innovations and EBPs. Given the rapid proliferation of interest in EBPs, new resources are continuously being added that can guide therapists in the use of CBT for youth anxiety and depressive disorders. To keep abreast of the latest innovations for patient care, therapists can access websites such as http://www.nrepp.samhsa.gov/, http://www.effectivechild-therapy.com/, and http://www.iapt.nhs.uk/. Further, a number of online free training opportunities on how to provide EBPs are available (e.g., http://tfcbt.musc.edu/). These are just a few of many resources available on the internet. Therapists should learn how to find such resources, as new websites and resources constantly emerge and older material becomes outdated.

To give an example of engaging in decision-making as an evidence consumer, imagine a therapist who meets with a new patient. She is a 12-year-old African American female with symptoms of anxiety in relation to an experienced trauma, as well as with some unrelated obsessions and compulsions. The first step, following evidence-based assessment, is to ask the clinical question, which in this case might be: "What interventions have empirical evidence supporting efficacy or effectiveness with African American youth with post-traumatic stress disorder (PTSD) and obsessive–compulsive disorder (OCD)?" The next step would be to acquire the evidence. One could visit a website such as http://www.effectivechildtherapy.com/ or PubMed, PsycInfo, or Google Scholar to search for treatment outcome trials. If a therapist searched for the terms "youth," "PTSD," and/or "OCD" together with the phrase "treatment outcome," a number of studies documenting EBPs for these presenting difficulties would emerge (e.g., trauma focused-CBT; TF-CBT, exposure with response prevention). The therapist might also include the phrase "ethnic minority," to check whether any studies have examined differential treatment outcome response based on ethnicity and/or race. After conducting this review, the therapist would need to appraise the evidence on the basis of the quality of the studies that were found. Typically, randomized controlled trials are considered the gold standard with regard to determining efficacy of interventions. In step 4, the therapist applies the results to the youth s/he is working with. In this case, the therapist would determine the primary disorder and begin there. For example, if the PTSD symptoms were primary, the therapist would start with TF-CBT and then move on to the OCD symptoms with exposure and response prevention. In the final step, the therapist would assess outcomes. In this case, administering self-report rating scales and tracking symptoms before, during, and after treatment would be important steps in the EBP process.

Operating within professional, ethical, and legal codes

Professional practice
In addition to having an open attitude and acting as an evidence consumer, professional competence involves awareness of other aspects of one's own behavior, appearance, and communication style. Many of these attributes are not specified in CBT treatment manuals, yet they potentially impact the provision of effective care. Inappropriate self-disclosures, offensive language, messy office space, chronic lateness, inappropriate physical contact, or disrespectful attitudes toward colleagues could have similarly negative impact. Avoiding such behaviors requires introspection and judgment based on each client and context. For example, professional dress may differ greatly between agencies and according to the function of the worker. Appropriate boundaries can vary across cultural contexts. Not all behaviors pertinent to professionalism can be outlined here, yet consideration of them must not be ignored, given their potential impact on clinician effectiveness.

Luckily, several attempts to outline succinct yet exhaustive lists of core generic professional competencies have been undertaken by organizations such as the American Psychological Association (APA), the Council on Social Work Education (CSWE), and the British Psychological Society (BPS). The "Competency Benchmarks Document" provides a particularly extensive resource for the APA (Fouad et al. 2009). The "Educational Policy 2.1" (Council on Social Work Education 2008) and the "Required Competencies Mapping Document for Doctoral Programmes in Clinical Psychology" (British Psychology Association, n.d.) similarly outline each organization's behavioral expectations of professionals. While designed for academic use, such documents can be used as checklists for clinicians to consider the broad array of competencies necessary for professional practice, and each reference can easily be located with the help of an internet search. Further, supervisors can use these checklists to provide feedback to trainees about their professional practice.

Ethical practice
All three documents described above discuss ethics as a vital aspect of professional competence. Professional organizations such as the APA, the BPS, the Australian Psychological Society, the European Federation of Psychologists' Associations, and the International Federation of Social Workers (IFSW) have formal ethical codes. Most include professionalism and evidence utilization in their definitions of ethical

competence, while urging clinicians to respect and uphold human rights. Given the differences between nations and professions, all clinicians must be familiar with and abide by their respective professional organization's ethics code.

Legal practice

Professional competence also encompasses the ability to operate within legal parameters. Particularly relevant concerns for clinicians working with children are informed consent, privacy, and mandatory reporting. The specifics of these, such as the age at which a child can legally consent to treatment, what information a parent is entitled to, and the legal definition of abuse vary between countries and states. Clinicians must be aware of the laws to the best of their ability. However, knowing every local statute can be challenging, as laws are often difficult to locate and interpret, especially for clinicians lacking legal training. Therefore an important aspect of legal competence is connecting with helpful resources. Most of the professional organizations previously mentioned offer online guidelines and telephone assistance in legal matters for their members. Some clinical settings have their own attorney or knowledgeable individuals available for consultation. Supervisors can help guide clinicians to locate such resources as part of their training.

Supervision/consultation

A number of literature reviews (Beidas and Kendall 2010; Herschell, Kolko, Baumann, and Davis 2010; Rakovshik and McManus 2010) have suggested the importance of ongoing support in the form of supervision and/or consultation as a critical component in training therapists. We will use "consultation" as an umbrella term, to encompass the numerous others used for ongoing support – for instance supervision, coaching, and audit with feedback (Edmunds, Beidas, and Kendall 2013). Emerging empirical literature has demonstrated that the number of hours spent in consultation after training predicts therapist fidelity, above and beyond the type of training method (Beidas, Edmunds, Marcus, and Kendall 2012). Therapist fidelity involves adherence to an EBP – in other words, use of specified procedures – and competence in delivery – that is, skill (Perepletchikova, Treat, and Kazdin 2007). Thus a critical competency for therapists at all levels is to seek out and participate in regular consultation. This is required from trainees prior to licensure, but it is also a competency therapists of all levels must display, particularly when faced with a difficult case or a difficulty that presents itself outside of their competence area and where referrals are not possible (American Psychological Association 2002). Consultation's mechanism of change is unknown, but it likely provides therapists with a venue for clarification and experiential practice with concepts, massed practice, case consultation, and problem solving of implementation barriers.

One model of mental health consultation is a useful framework for categorizing the varying types of consultation (Caplan and Caplan 1993). Four types of consultation can be provided, although a consultant–consultee relationship may encompass all four types. In type 1 consultation the client is the target. This type (client-centered case consultation) involves the consultant's expert assessment of the client's problem, treatment recommendations, and other support included in the provision of client care. Type 2 (consultee-centered case consultation) targets the consultee's professional functioning and involves identifying and remedying consultee difficulties, such as a therapist's development of a skill. Type 3 consultation (program-centered administrative consultation) provides support and an effective course of action for program implementation; a treatment developer working with an agency to implement an EBP would fall in this category. Type 4 consultation (consultee-centered administrative consultation) targets difficulties or barriers encountered by consultees when implementing a new program.

When one is specifically applying CBT on youth anxiety and depressive disorders, ongoing support and consultation from peers and experts is critical. This is especially true for novices – that is, trainees who are new to the implementation of CBT. For example, when one is learning exposure procedures, a core ingredient of CBT for child anxiety, consultation is critical due to the heightened anxiety produced in both child and therapist and to the considerable skill required to perform the procedure (exposure is discussed in detail in Chapter 14). For example, during one of my first cases, I – Rinad Beidas – selected an exposure that was too difficult for my client, who was just starting to tackle the challenges listed on his fear hierarchy. He was to take an elevator by himself to another floor, to find a prize, and then come back to me. He forgot how to get back to the clinic's floor, and I could hear him crying in the elevator. I tried to model for him that I coped with the anxiety of not knowing where he was, when he eventually found the correct floor; but the episode certainly elicited a large amount of anxiety in us both. Without debriefing and support from my supervisor, I may have never attempted another exposure! Consultation is also beneficial for those more advanced in their career who seek to refine their skills, work with difficult cases, and expand areas of expertise. For example, if an anxiety expert began working with a severely depressed patient, consultation on CBT for depression would be the recommended and most ethical course of action.

Competence in Treating the Anxiety Disorders and Depression

The competencies discussed in this chapter are nonspecific and apply equally to both anxiety and depressive disorders.

Competence in treating both children and adolescents

The generic competencies outlined so far must also be developmentally appropriate. For example, the process of becoming an evidence consumer requires careful consideration of a client's age and maturity when one is searching for evidence, as a treatment of teenagers that has a strong empirical base may be ineffective for 6-year-olds. When a treatment lacks age-relevant evidence, therapists must determine whether and how to adopt or adapt treatment protocol so as to ensure developmentally appropriate care. Unfortunately, little is known about how to modify treatments for effective use across developmental stages (Holmbeck, Devine, and Bruno 2010). Therefore therapists must stay current with developmental literature in order to adapt EBPs for particular age groups.

Developmental considerations should also be made when engaging in alliance building, assessment, and other professional competencies. Clinicians must be able to set the stage for effective care by engaging minors in developmentally appropriate ways (Kingery et al. 2006). Offices filled with toys may foster a therapeutic alliance with young children while deterring teens. Employment of complex language may communicate respect for teens while confusing small children. All clinicians working with children and adolescents must possess a basic understanding of how to best communicate with them.

Because age and development also determine a client's decision-making ability, maturity, and legal status, such considerations directly impact professional competence when one is obtaining informed consent and determining the optimal degree of caregiver involvement. For example, the adult caregivers of many minors may best be conceptualized as co-clients, whose involvement is required beyond the consenting process (Koocher and Daniel 2012). Older adolescents are also known to take risks with substance use, bullying, sexual activity, and criminal behavior. In addition to the need to understand laws of mandatory reporting, determining who is entitled to what information presents the challenge that one has to balance confidentiality with an ethical responsibility to clients who lack maturity (Koocher and Daniel 2012). Given the complexities and responsibilities involved in child and adolescent treatment, as well as the current gaps in the evidence available for every nuanced scenario, therapy with minors particularly requires regular and intensive consultation with individuals who have expertise in dealing with relevant age groups. Chapter 5 offers a broader discussion of developmental considerations in child and adolescent therapy, and Chapter 6 gives more details about engaging in and developing a therapeutic alliance within this kind of therapy.

Common Obstacles to Competent Practice and Methods to Overcome Them

Obstacles to favorable attitudes toward EBPs

Experience is more valuable than evidence
For over fifty years, psychologists have wrestled with the debate over which method is more effective at predicting patient outcomes, clinical judgment, or statistical algorithms and research-based evidence. Dr. Paul Meehl's (1954) *Clinical Versus Statistical Prediction* sparked controversy by declaring that statistical algorithms were more accurate about predicting behavior than clinical judgment. Psychologists are still wrestling with this assertion, and particularly with the last decade's EBP movement, which promotes the use of manualized treatments that are based upon research evidence (Kendall and Beidas 2007). Even as the catalogue of EBPs expands, it can still take up to 17 years for a treatment to move from research to practice (Balas and Boren 2000). Clinicians' belief that experience is more valuable than evidence remains an obstacle, as many are skeptical of research-based models that seek to summarize the deeply personal, experiential nature of a disorder and its treatment (e.g., anxiety) into a manualized treatment (Addis, Wade, and Hatgis 1999; Stiles 2006). Recent qualitative data demonstrate this perspective, as some clinicians report difficulties in trusting research-based evidence and perceive the manipulated conditions and the exclusion criteria of clinical

trials – for example, the exclusion of children with comorbid externalizing disorders when one tests a treatment for internalizing disorders – as lacking in generalizability: the settings of these trials cannot be generalized (Nelson, Steele, and Mize 2006).

The belief that experience overrides evidence can be illustrated through the example of CBT for child anxiety. CBT is now widely identified as an EBP for youth anxiety (Silverman, Pina, and Viswesvaran 2008), yet some community therapists have expressed concerns that CBT may not be appropriate for anxious youth in community settings. The literature indicates that there may be some differences between anxious youth who come for treatment to a research clinic and anxious youth who come for treatment to a community clinic. Although youth in community settings are similar to youth in research settings with regard to symptoms and diagnoses, they are more likely to belong to ethnic minorities and to have lower family incomes (Ehrenreich-May et al. 2011; Southam-Gerow, Silverman, and Kendall 2006). However, a recent meta-analysis found that EBPs such as CBT for child anxiety can, without significant modifications, remain efficacious in addressing the needs of ethnic minority youth (Huey and Polo 2008). Thus, despite differences between anxious youth in research and in community settings, evidence suggests that CBT remains the optimal EBP of choice for both.

Attitudes toward manualized treatment

Although guidelines in the use of EBPs carefully highlight the importance of taking into account the best evidence, clinical judgment, and patient preferences, many therapists conflate the use of EBPs with strict adherence to a manualized treatment (American Psychological Association 2006). Attitudes toward manualized EBPs include a number of concerns regarding a perceived inflexibility, a lack of attention to the therapeutic alliance, and a perceived "coldness" of approach, where technique is emphasized over care (Addis and Krasnow 2000; Borntrager, Chorpita, Higa-McMillan, and Weisz 2009; Castonguay, Goldfried, Wiser, Raue, and Hayes 1996). Given data demonstrating that strict adherence can negatively impact therapeutic alliance (Castonguay et al. 1996), we suggest flexibility within fidelity (Kendall and Beidas 2007), which gives clinicians freedom from rigidly following manuals at the expense of responding creatively.

Adaptation or "flexibility within fidelity" is an important means to overcome obstacles related to clinician attitudes toward EBPs. Flexibility within fidelity refers to maintaining high treatment integrity while also individualizing the treatment to the particular client and his or her context. For example, a clinician working with an anxious youth with secondary depressive symptoms would integrate components of CBT for depression (e.g., cognitive restructuring for anxious and depressive thoughts, behavioral activation; Beidas, Benjamin, Puleo, Edmunds, and Kendall 2010). CBT for pediatric anxiety and depressive disorders is designed to allow for treatment individualization for each patient while maintaining fidelity to core components.

Relationship between organizational characteristics and provider attitudes

A provider's work setting can influence his or her attitudes toward EBPs (Aarons 2004; Aarons et al. 2012; Nelson et al. 2006). Expectations of behavior, levels of stress, and managerial support are all examples of factors that may make EBP adoption easier or harder. For example, a high-stress work environment could overwhelm providers who attempt to learn a new intervention, and this may result in negative attitudes toward EBPs and reluctance to use them. Alternatively, a provider may work in a low-resource setting (say, with poor technology or lack of adequate work space) that makes obtaining manuals or completing exposures essential to EPBs – like CBT for youth anxiety – seem unrealistic. Proficient organizational cultures are those that actively promote client well-being and up-to-date knowledge, and they have the highest levels of EBP adoption (Aarons et al. 2012). Resistant organizational cultures are critical, suppressive, and do not expect clinicians to change or to adopt new ways of providing service. Rigid cultures contain clinicians with little decision-making authority, flexibility, or discretion. Interestingly, such contexts were not significantly related to clinician attitudes toward EBPs, which indicates that clinician-level commitment to EBPs and to problem solving may surmount difficult organizational characteristics (Aarons et al. 2012).

Obstacles to professional practice

Legal considerations
Occasionally, legal considerations represent challenges to professional competence. For example, when the client is a child with PTSD and a car-accident survivor, that client may benefit from exposure to riding in an actual car; yet many clinicians are reluctant to drive with a child, due to associated legal risks. To overcome such obstacles, therapists may consider creative ways to optimize therapeutic duties while minimizing legal risk, such as imaginal exposures or recruiting a caregiver to drive with the client.

Compliance with mandatory reporting can also raise legal barriers to the exercise of professional competence, as real-life scenarios are often complex and difficult to navigate. For example, when a client is intensely afraid of reporting abuse, how long (if at all) should a therapist delay filing, in order to ease client concerns and preserve the therapeutic alliance? At what point, if any, does bullying from a peer meet the legal definition of abuse? To deflate potential conflicts as much as possible, mandatory reporting procedures should be clearly articulated at the outset of treatment and, when "gray area" situations are encountered, consultation with legal and therapeutic experts in order to explore creative ways to balance therapeutic and legal duties is imperative.

Consent to treatment and privacy issues
Obtaining consent and sharing information with caregivers also represent barriers to professional competence when one is working with minors. For example, a set of divorced parents with a divisive relationship may contain a parent reluctant to consent to treatment. To avoid being entangled in parental feuds, clinicians must employ assertiveness skills and obtain legal consent from both parents, while maintaining clear rules and boundaries throughout treatment. Therapists must also mindfully consider the flow of information between all parties and how it will be used.

Obstacles to consultation

Despite the importance of engaging in consultation in order to improve fidelity (Beidas et al. 2012), clinicians encounter obstacles when accessing and utilizing consultation, particularly after they obtain licensure, at which time ongoing support is no longer to be required. Examples of such obstacles are the clinician's own failure to recognize the need for consultation, the limited time available for it, its high cost, and limited access to consultants.

Recognizing the need

Clinicians often seek to develop clinical expertise over time. Whereas some clinicians aim to develop expertise in a specific treatment modality or disorder, other clinicians consider themselves generalists and desire competence across a variety of disorders, populations, and modalities. Regardless of the route, all clinicians will encounter clients for whom an optimal treatment is difficult to identify, let alone implement. It is important for clinicians to recognize when consultation is needed and to be willing to ask for it. Lack of openness to feedback may prevent clinicians from seeking such help. Thus it is recommended that clinicians regularly reflect on their ability to implement particular treatments with particular clients and to seek consultation when they encounter an impasse. It is also recommended that clinicians routinely gather standardized data on client progress and that they seek consultation when clients fail to progress or achieve therapy goals; doing so will assist clinicians in reflecting on the ability described above.

Time and cost

When one is a trainee or a pre-licensed clinician, supervision is a required activity often built into the work week. Once licensure is obtained, consultation can be viewed as valuable, yet it is not something that a clinician can currently bill for. Additional fees can be incurred depending on the financial arrangement with consultants. Nonetheless, it is ethically appropriate for clinicians to carve out time for consultation in order to enhance optimal care. For example, one EBP, dialectical behavior therapy, includes consultation as a required component of competent practice in reducing therapist burnout. Regularly scheduled consultation times are recommended, whether they are weekly, fortnightly, or monthly. Consultation can be scheduled at times that do not interfere with clinical work (e.g., during school hours). In order to overcome costs that may be associated with the payment of consultants, therapists can organize peer consultation partnerships or groups. Another solution is for therapists to lobby for policy change, so that insurance companies may reimburse the consultation time so as to foster improved care.

Consultant availability

It is possible that a clinician is willing to commit time and money toward consultation but does not have a readily available consultant. One option for addressing this problem is to develop a peer support network, which can take the form of meetings, scheduled either regularly or as needed. Meetings can involve pairs or groups and can occur face to face, via teleconferencing, or in web-conferencing formats (e.g., Beidas et al. 2012; Weingardt, Cucciare, Bellotti, and Lai 2009). Additional options include seeking consultation via peer-mediated online discussion boards (Moore and Marra 2005) and via LISTSERV mailing lists of professional organizations (e.g., the Association of Behavioral and Cognitive Therapies). These platforms allow clinicians to post general and specific questions related to de-identified cases and to benefit from the collective wealth of knowledge and expertise of members. Other online learning collaboratives (such as www.practiceground.org) provide opportunities to access materials and set up peer consultation in order to improve competence in delivering EBPs.

Conclusion

In this chapter we have discussed three sub-competencies gathered under the umbrella of practicing professionally. We have provided behavioral markers, examples of professional practice, strategies to improve upon competency from the supervisor's and the therapist's perspective, developmental considerations, and obstacles to achieving each sub-competency. Specifically, we have reviewed the importance of: (i) open attitudes toward psychotherapy research that allow therapists to develop the ability to seek out resources and to become a thoughtful "evidence consumer"; (ii) operation within professional, ethical, and legal codes; and (iii) active participation in ongoing consultation. Although these competencies are likely nonspecific to EBPs, they are absolutely critical for the professional practice of EBPs, particularly in the case of therapists practicing CBT on anxiety and depression in youth.

References

Aarons, Gregory A. 2004. "Mental Health Provider Attitudes toward Adoption of Evidence-Based Practice: The Evidence-Based Practice Attitude Scale (EBPAS)." *Mental Health Services Research*, 6: 61–74.

Aarons, Gregory A., Charles Glisson, Phillip D. Green, Kimberly Hoagwood, Kelly J. Kelleher, and John A. Landsverk. 2012. "The Organizational Social Context of Mental Health Services and Clinician Attitudes toward Evidence-Based Practice: A United States National Study." *Implementation Science*, 7 (1): 56. DOI: 10.1186/1748-5908-7-56

Addis, Michael E., and Aaron D. Krasnow. 2000. "A National Survey of Practicing Psychologists' Attitudes toward Psychotherapy Treatment Manuals." *Journal of Consulting and Clinical Psychology*, 68: 331–9.

Addis, Michale E., Wendy A. Wade, and Christina Hatgis. 1999. "Barriers to Evidence Based Practices: Addressing Practitioners' Concerns about Manual Based Psychotherapies." *Clinical Psychology: Science and Practice*, 6: 430–41.

American Psychological Association. 2002. APA Ethical principles of Psychologists and Code of Conduct, http://www.apa.org/ethics/code2002.html (accessed February 20, 2013).

American Psychological Association. 2006. "Evidence-Based Practice in Psychology: APA Presidential Task Force on Evidence-Based Practice." *American Psychologist*, 61: 271–85. DOI: 10.1037/0003-066X.61.4.271

Balas, E. Andrew, and Suzanne A. Boren. 2000. *Managing Clinical Knowledge for Health Care Improvement*. Stuttgart, Germany: Schattauer.

Beidas, Rinad S., and Philip C. Kendall. 2010. "Training Therapists in Evidence-Based Practice: A Critical Review of Studies From a Systems-Contextual Perspective." *Clinical Psychology: Science and Practice*, 17: 1–30. DOI: 10.1111/j.1468-2850.2009.01187.x

Beidas, Rinad S., Julie E Edmunds, Steven C. Marcus, and Philip C. Kendall. 2012. "Training and Consultation to Promote Implementation of an Empirically Supported Treatment: A Randomized Trial." *Psychiatric Services*, 63: 660–5. DOI: 10.1176/appi.ps.201100401

Beidas, Rinad S., Courtney L. Benjamin, Connor M. Puleo, Julie M. Edmunds, and Philip C. Kendall. 2010. "Flexible Applications of the Coping Cat Program for Anxious Youth." *Cognitve and Behavioral Practice*, 17: 142–53. DOI: 10.1016/j.cbpra.2009.11.002

Borntrager, Cameo F., Bruce F. Chorpita, Charmaine Higa-McMillan, and John R. Weisz. 2009. "Provider Attitudes toward Evidence-Based Practices: Are the Concerns with the Evidence or with the Manuals?" *Psychiatric Services*, 60: 677–81. DOI: 10.1176/appi.ps.60.5.677

British Psychology Association. (n.d.). Required Competencies Mapping Document for Doctoral Programmes in Clinical Psychology, http://www.bps.org.uk/sites/default/files/documents/required_competencies_-_counselling_psychology.doc (accessed November 25, 2013).

Caplan, Gerald, and Ruth B. Caplan. 1993. *Mental Health Consultation and Collaboration.* San Francisco, CA: Jossey-Bass Publishers.

Castonguay, Louis G., Marvin R. Goldfried, Susan Wiser, Patrick J. Raue, and Adele M. Hayes. 1996. "Predicting the Effect of Cognitive Therapy for Depression: A Study of Unique and Common Factors." *Journal of Consulting and Clinical Psychology*, 64: 497–504.

Council on Social Work Education. 2008. Educational Policy and Accreditation Standards. *Educational Policy*, 2 (1): 3–7, http://www.cswe.org/File.aspx?id=13780 (accessed February 20, 2013).

Edmunds, Julie E., Rinad S. Beidas, and Philip C. Kendall. 2013. "Dissemination and Implementation of Evidence-Based Practices: Training and Consultation as Implementation Strategies," http://onlinelibrary.wiley.com/doi/10.1111/cpsp.12031/abstract (accessed December 10, 2013).

Ehrenreich-May, Jill, Michael A. Southam-Gerow, Shannon E. Hourigan, Lauren R. Wright, Donna B. Pincus, and John R. Weisz. 2011. "Characteristics of Anxious and Depressed Youth Seen in Two Different Clinical Contexts." *Administration and Policy in Mental Health and Mental Health Services*, 38: 398–411. DOI: 10.1007/s10488-010-0328-6

Fouad, Nadya A., Catherine L. Gus, Robert L. Hatcher, Nadine J. Kaslow, Philinda S. Hutchings, Michael B. Madson, Frank L. Collins, and Raymond E. Crossman. 2009. "Compentency Benchmarks: A Developmental Model for Understanding and Measuring Competence in Professional Psychology." *Training and Education in Professional Psychology*, 3: S5–S26.

Herschell, Amy D., David J. Kolko, Barbara L. Baumann, and Abigail C. Davis. 2010. "The Role of Therapist Training in the Implementation of Psychosocial Treatments: A Review and Critique with Recommendations." *Clinical Psychology Review*, 30: 448–66. DOI: 10.1016/j.cpr.2010.02.005

Holmbeck, Grayson, Katie A. Devine, and Elizabeth F. Bruno. 2010. "Developmental Issues and Considerations in Research and Practice." In John R. Weisz and Alan E. Kazdin (Eds.), *Evidence-Based Psychotherapies for Children and Adolescents* (2nd ed., pp. 28–39). New York: Guilford Press.

Huey, Stanley J., and Antonio J. Polo. 2008. "Evidence-Based Psychosocial Treatments for Ethnic Minority Youth." *Journal of Clinical Child and Adolescent Psychology*, 37: 262–301. DOI: 10.1080/15374410701820174

Kendall, Philip C., and Rinad S. Beidas. 2007. "Smoothing the Trail for Dissemination of Evidence-Based Practices for Youth: Flexibility within Fidelity." *Professional Psychology: Research and Practice*, 38: 13–20. DOI: 10.1037/0735-7028.38.1.13

Kingery, Julie N., Tami L. Roblek, Cynthia Suveg, Rachel L. Grover, Joel T. Sherrill, and R. Lindsey Bergman. 2006. "They're Not Just 'Little Adults': Developmental Considerations for Implementing Cognitive–Behavioral Therapy with Anxious Youth." *Journal of Cognitive Psychotherapy: An Internation Quarterly*, 20: 263–73.

Koocher, Gerald P., and Jessica H. Daniel. 2012. "Treating Children and Adolescents." In Samuel J. Knapp (Ed.), *APA Handbook of Ethics in Psychology*. Volume 2: *Practice, Teaching, and Research* (pp. 3–14). Washington, DC: American Psychological Association.

Moore, Joi L., and Rose M. Marra (2005). "A Comparative Analysis of Online Discussion Participation Protocols." *Journal of Research on Technology in Education*, 38: 191–212.

Meehl, Paul E. 1954. *Clinical versus Statistical Prediction: A Theoretical Analysis and a Review of the Evidence*. Minneapolis: University of Minnesota Press.

Najavits, Lisa, Roger D. Weiss, Sarah R. Shaw, and Amy Dierberger. 2000. "Psychotherapists' Views of Manuals." *Professional Psychology: Research and Practice*, 31: 404–8.

Nelson, Timothy D., and Ric G. Steele. 2007. "Predictors of Practitioner Self-Reported Use of Evidence-Based Practices: Practitioner Training, Clinical Setting, and Attitudes Toward Research." *Administration and Policy in Mental Health and Mental Health Services*, 34: 319–30. DOI: 10.1007/s10488-006-0111-x

Nelson, Timothy D., Ric G. Steele, and Jennifer A. Mize. 2006. "Practitioner Attitudes toward Evidence-Based Practice: Themes and Challenges." *Administration and Policy in Mental Health and Mental Health Services*, 33: 398–409. DOI: 10.1007/s10488-006-0044-4

Perepletchikova, F., Teresa A. Treat, and Alan E. Kazdin. 2007. "Treatment Integrity in Psychotherapy Research: Analysis of the Studies and Examination of the Associated Factors." *Journal of Consulting and Clinical Psychology*, 75, 829–41. DOI: 10.1037/0022-006X.75.6.829

Rakovshik, Sarah G., and Freda McManus. 2010. "Establishing Evidence-Based Training in Cognitive Behavioral Therapy: A Review of Current Empirical Findings and Theoretical Guidance." *Clinical Psychology Review*, 30: 496–516. DOI: 10.1016/j.cpr.2010.03.004

Sburlati, Elizabeth S., Carolyn A. Schniering, Heidi J. Lyneham, and Ronald M. Rapee. 2011. "A Model of Therapist Competencies for the Empirically Supported Cognitive Behavioral Treatment of Child and Adolescent Anxiety and Depressive Disorders." *Clinical Child and Family Psychology Review*, 14: 89–109. DOI: 10.1007/s10567-011-0083-6

Silverman, Wendy, Armando A. Pina, and Chockalingam Viswesvaran. 2008. "Evidence-Based Psychosocial Treatments for Phobic and Anxiety Disorders in Children and Adolescents." *Journal of Clinical Child and Adolescent Psychology*, 37: 105–30. DOI: 10.1080/15374410701817907

Southam-Gerow, Michael A., Wendy K. Silverman, and Philip C. Kendall. 2006. "Client Similarities and Differences in Two Childhood Anxiety Disorders Research Clinics." *Journal of Clinical Child and Adolescent Psychology*, 35: 528–38. DOI: 10.1207/s15374424jccp3504_4

Spring, Bonnie. 2007. "Evidence-Based Practice in Clinical Psychology: What It Is, Why it Matters; What You Need To Know." *Journal of Clinical Psychology*, 63: 611–31. DOI: 10.1002/jclp.20373

Stewart, Rebecca E., and Dianne L. Chambless. 2007. "Does Psychotherapy Research Inform Treatment Decisions in Private Practice?" *Journal of Clinical Psychology*, 63: 267–81. DOI: 10.1002/jclp.20347

Stiles, William B. 2006. "Case Studies." In John C. Norcross, Larry E. Beutler, and Ronald F. Levant (Eds.), *Evidence-Based Practices in Mental Health: Debate and Dialogue on the Fundamental Questions* (pp. 57–73). Washington, DC: American Psychological Association.

Strauss, Sharon E., W. Scott Richardson, Paul Glasziou, and R. Brian Haynes. 2005. *Evidence-Based Medicine: How to Practice and Teach EBM* (3rd ed.). New York: Elsevier.

Weingardt, Kenneth R., Michael A. Cucciare, Christine Bellotti, and Wen Pin Lai. 2009. "A Randomized Trial Comparing Two Models of Web-Based Training in Cognitive–Behavioral Therapy for Substance Abuse Counsellors." *Journal of Substance Abuse Treatment*, 37 (3): 219–27. DOI: 10.1016/j.jsat.2009.01.002

5

Child and Adolescent Characteristics that Impact on Therapy

Caroline L. Donovan and Sonja March

Introduction

This chapter describes background knowledge that a therapist should possess when working with youth who experience internalizing disorders. The chapter has four major foci. First it will discuss knowledge about the internalization of psychopathology, its presentation in youth, and the impact of comorbidity on treatment. The influence of cognitive, social, and emotional developmental issues on therapy will be presented next. Then the discussion will center around the impact of individual differences among young people on therapy, with a particular focus on demographic variables, health conditions, and learning disorders. Finally, the chapter will examine the impact on therapy of environmental factors (parental psychopathology, parenting style, and conflict) and life events (stressful life events, trauma, and bullying).

Internalizing Psychopathology in Young People

Presentation in youth

Young people, like adults, may be afflicted with any of the anxiety and mood disorders outlined in the fourth edition of the *Diagnostic and Statistical Manual of Mental Disorders* (DSM-IV; APA 1994) as well as with separation anxiety disorder and selective mutism, which are placed in the section "Disorders Usually First Diagnosed in Infancy, Childhood, or Adolescence." Males and females are equally likely to have mood disorders in pre-adolescence, but by adolescence females are twice as likely to experience depression (Avenevoli, Knight, Kessler, and Merikangas 2008). With respect to anxiety disorders, girls are more likely to have an anxiety disorder than boys, although the differences are not large (Costello, Egger, and Angold 2005).

Evidence-Based CBT for Anxiety and Depression in Children and Adolescents: A Competencies-Based Approach,
First Edition. Edited by Elizabeth S. Sburlati, Heidi J. Lyneham, Carolyn A. Schniering, and Ronald M. Rapee.
© 2014 John Wiley & Sons, Ltd. Published 2014 by John Wiley & Sons, Ltd.

The presentation of mood and anxiety disorders may be somewhat different in youth from what it is in adults. For instance, for youth with mood disorders, DSM-IV adjusts time and symptom requirements. For dysthymia, symptoms need only be present for one year rather than two, while for depression youth may show irritability rather than depressed mood and failure to make expected weight gain rather than weight loss during depressive episodes. It has also been found that depressed children are more likely to present with somatic complaints than adolescents and adults, that girls tend to display more hypersomnia and reduced appetite during adolescence, and that suicide risk peaks during middle adolescence for girls and during late adolescence for boys (Avenevoli et al. 2008). Finally, for preschool children, anhedonia may manifest itself as a difficulty to enjoy play activities, and preoccupation with negative thoughts may manifest themselves as preoccupation with play themes (Luby 2010).

DSM-IV also suggests differences in the presentation of anxiety disorders in youth by comparison with adults. In specific phobia (SP) crying, tantrums, freezing, or clinging may be evident; the child may not realize that his or her fear is excessive or unreasonable; and the duration of symptoms must be at least six months. The "other" category of phobias may include avoidance of loud sounds or of costumed characters. For social phobia (SoP) crying, tantrums, freezing, or shrinking away from social situations with unfamiliar people may occur; there must be evidence that the child can develop and maintain social relationships with familiar others; the anxiety must be triggered by same-age peers as well as by adults; the child may not realize that his or her anxiety is unreasonable or excessive; and the symptoms must be present for at least 6 months. In obsessive compulsive disorder (OCD) the child may not recognize that the obsessions and compulsions are excessive or unreasonable, while in generalized anxiety disorder (GAD) only one of the six core symptoms must be present for diagnosis. For post-traumatic stress disorder (PTSD) the response may be expressed through disorganized or agitated behavior, and the re-experiencing of the event may be evidenced by repetitive play involving the trauma theme, frightening dreams where the child fails to recall or recognize the content, or episodes of re-enactment of the trauma. Thus it is evident that there are differences between the presentation of mood and anxiety disorders in youth and the presentation of the same disorders in adults.

Comorbidity

When youth show symptoms of anxiety or depression, they frequently show symptoms of other disorders as well. For anxiety disorders, comorbidity with other anxiety disorders is most common (Ollendick, Jarrett, Grills-Taquechel, Hovey, and Wolff 2008), and our own research suggests that 89 percent of the youth involved in treatment for anxiety disorders hold more than one clinical-level anxiety diagnosis. Comorbid mood disorders are also common: 10 to 15 percent of anxious youth display comorbid depression (Garber and Weersing 2010). When comorbid depression is present in anxious youth, the young person tends to be somewhat older, the anxiety is more severe, and family dysfunction is higher (O'Neil, Podell, Benjamin, and Kendall 2010). Finally, externalizing disorders such as attention deficit hyperactivity disorder (ADHD), oppositional defiant disorder (ODD) and conduct disorder (CD) are commonly comorbid with youth anxiety (Ollendick et al. 2008). Angold, Costello, and Erkanli (1999) suggest that around 10 percent of youth with an anxiety disorder have comorbid CD or ODD and that anxiety and ADHD co-occur at a rate three times higher than what would be predicted by chance.

Comorbidity is also very common in youth with mood disorders. Comorbidity with anxiety disorders is most commonplace, with 25–75 percent of depressed youth also being diagnosed with an anxiety disorder (Angold et al. 1999, Garber and Weersing 2010). Rates of comorbid externalizing disorders seem to vary considerably across studies: ranges between 0 and 79 percent are found for CD and ODD, and rates of 0 and 5 percent are found for ADHD (Angold et al. 1999). Of particular concern is the high rate of suicidal ideation and attempts evidenced in depressed teenagers (Kovacs, Goldston, and Gatsonis 1993). Indeed, when youth with depression have comorbid disorders, the onset of depression tends to be earlier and suicidal behavior tends to be more common (Lewinsohn, Rohde, and Seeley 1998). Furthermore, when depressed youth also demonstrate suicidality, both depression severity and impairment are greater (Barbe, Bridge, Birmaher, Kolko, and Brent 2004).

From the above discussion it would seem that comorbidity is associated with greater severity and impairment, or at least with more complex diagnostic profiles. But how does this impact on treatment? For anxiety disorders, the news is relatively good. The results of two large reviews suggest that, for the vast majority of studies, comorbidity is not predictive of poorer treatment outcome for youth with anxiety disorders (Nilsen, Eisemann, and Kvernmo 2012; Ollendick et al. 2008). Furthermore, it has been found that focusing treatment on the primary anxiety disorder also results in the reduction of comorbid anxiety disorders and of other comorbid disorders such as depression, ADHD, and ODD (see, e.g., Kendall, Brady, and Verduin 2001). It may therefore not be necessary (or efficient) for clinicians to attempt to incorporate treatment components for comorbid conditions; they should rather focus on treating the primary anxiety disorder and determine later whether additional treatment is required.

For youth suffering from mood disorders, the presence of comorbidity seems less clear in terms of its effect on treatment outcome. Some reviews and large-scale studies have concluded that comorbidity, and particularly comorbidity with anxiety, is associated with poorer outcome (e.g., Emslie, Kennard, and Mayes 2011; Ollendick et al. 2008), while others have found little effect (Nilsen et al. 2012). What is clear is that suicidality predicts poorer treatment outcome and is associated with dropout, and that treating depression does not necessarily lead to a reduction in suicidality or vice-versa (Barbe et al. 2004). Furthermore, it has been found that focusing on adolescent depression has the effect of also reducing anxiety symptoms, but not externalizing problems (e.g., Weisz, McCarty, and Valeri 2006). Thus it may not be necessary for clinicians to target comorbid anxiety in depression treatment (at least not initially), but treatment should include strategies aimed at reducing comorbid externalizing problems and should allow for specific considerations related to the importance of suicidality.

Developmental Issues

Children demonstrate numerous developmental changes as they mature. With respect to youth and development and its impact on therapy, questions that are often asked include: "At what age can you use CBT with children?" and "Do older children benefit more from CBT than younger children?" Overall, for youth with anxiety and depression, age does not seem to have a large effect on treatment outcome or dropout (Berman, Weems, Silverman, and Kurtines 2000; Emslie et al. 2011; Gonzalez, Weersing, Warnick, Scahill, and Woolston 2011; Nilsen et al. 2012), perhaps because it is a proxy for developmental level (Bolton and Graham 2005).

There is some consensus that children as young as 7 years – an age that roughly corresponds with Piaget's concrete operational stage – can benefit from CBT (Stallard 2004). During this stage children learn to classify objects and put them in series, their mathematical abilities develop, they can play games that have rules, and they can use logic to solve problems. Children at this level begin to understand reversibility and generalizability and their previous egocentrism is reduced, so that they are able to view things from the perspective of another. Also around the age of 7–10 years, the child begins to regulate his or her emotions autonomously, is able to employ distancing strategies to manage them, has a better ability to use emotional expression to regulate his or her relationships, and becomes aware of being able to feel multiple emotions about the same person. Furthermore, the child becomes able to use information he or she has acquired about his or her own emotions and those of others across contexts, for the purpose of developing and maintaining friendships (Carr 2006). Hence many important cognitive and emotional changes occur around 7 years of age.

The various changes that occur around the age of 7 may allow for a more successful implementation of particular CBT strategies. For instance, the ability to self-regulate or regulate his/her emotion autonomously may allow the child to engage in relaxation strategies when required. The emerging ability to move from the specific to the more general means that examples used during session might be more easily generalized to life outside the session. The child's ability to take the perspective of others and to use the information learned about his/her own and others' emotions may assist him/her in the successful learning and implementation of interpersonal skills, problem-solving strategies, and cognitive restructuring procedures.

Although 7 years is most commonly agreed upon as the age around which CBT may become useful, Stallard (2004) has argued that children as young as 5 years may also benefit. He suggests that, although CBT can be quite complex, it often is not when applied to children. Children of 5–6 years can articulate their thoughts and are able to talk to themselves. Furthermore, around the age of 5–7 children are beginning to regulate their emotions themselves and to use social skills to deal with their own emotions and those of others (Carr 2006). Thus Stallard (2004) suggests that children of 5 years can be taught less sophisticated, specific, and concrete cognitive techniques such as positive self-talk. Furthermore, given that children of this age have not yet mastered the ability to generalize, Stallard suggests providing them with information that helps them reach conclusions about specific problems they are experiencing outside the session. Thus clinicians should not necessarily reject out of hand the idea of simple cognitive techniques when working with 5–6-year-old children.

Rather than speak of age, or even of developmental level, it is perhaps more important for therapists to develop a sound conceptualization of the individual child case, as there is enormous variation in ability and developmental level among children. Indeed, it has been suggested by Bolton and Graham (2005: 17) that asking "What cognitive developmental level is needed for CBT?" is less useful than asking "What cognition is involved in the production and maintenance of the problem in the particular case?" For instance, if a child is not yet of a developmental level where he or she can engage in metacognition, then metacognitive processes will not be maintaining his or her anxiety or depression, and hence strategies targeting metacognitve processes will be unnecessary. In other words, "don't fix it if it ain't broke." This points to the importance of both good assessment and strong case conceptualization. A thorough assessment of symptoms and of causal and maintaining factors is imperative, so that a sound case conceptualization can be made. For good CBT therapists, treatment is always based on conceptualization, and thus only cognitive and behavioral factors that are found to be contributing to the child's issues should be targeted. Chapter 9 gives more details concerning case formulation and treatment planning.

Individual Differences

Regardless of developmental level, children display a myriad of individual differences that the therapist must take into account. In particular, the literature highlights the importance of familial culture and learning disabilities as potential determinants of treatment outcome.

Ethnicity

It is important for therapists to be aware of the ways in which a child's ethnicity may impact upon the treatment of his or her internalizing disorder. There is some evidence to suggest that particular ethnic groups have higher rates of internalizing disorders (e.g., Twenge and Nolen-Hoeksema 2002) and are more likely to drop out of treatment (Gonzalez et al. 2011). Furthermore, although research is limited, it would seem that ethnicity is not highly associated with poorer treatment outcome for anxiety, but may be so for depression (Nilsen et al. 2012).

There are no exact guidelines as to how clinicians should work with clients who are from a culture that is different from their own. However, Harmon and colleagues (2006) discuss a number of issues that therapists should be aware of. Symptom expression may vary acoss cultures, and the family's belief about the origins of a disorder may affect both treatment compliance and treatment outcome. In addition, the anxiety or the depressive disorder may be the result of prejudice or discrimination, and a history of prejudice or discrimination may lead to suspicion and lack of trust in the therapist. Therapists should also be aware of the family's cultural practices in terms of organization and decision-making and should have knowledge of the child's religion and acculturation. Indeed particular opinions, emotions, and behaviors may be prohibited or encouraged in various cultures, and attempts on the part of the therapist to increase or minimize these factors may result in a poor therapeutic alliance and in problems with treatment compliance and outcome. Thus therapists should educate themselves in the culture from which their clients come and should be aware of the various ways in which cultural beliefs and practices may impact on clients and on their progression through treatment.

Learning disorders

Youth may suffer from a variety of learning disorders (LDs), dyslexia being the most common and the most researched one. It has been suggested that around 20–25 percent of all dyslexic young people across the span from grade 1 to university have internalizing problems (Mugnaini, Lassi, La Malfa, and Albertini 2009); and the results of meta-analyses support the notion that, compared to youth without learning disorders, youth with dyslexia demonstrate higher rates of anxious and depressive symptoms (Maag and Reid 2006; Nelson and Harwood 2011). It should be noted, however, that some researchers have failed to find an association between LDs and internalizing problems in children (see, e.g., Miller, Hynd, and Miller 2005) and that there is more evidence for internalizing *symptoms* than for clinical-level internalizing *disorders* (Maag and Reid 2006; Nelson and Harwood 2011).

Mugnaini and colleagues (2009) suggest that children with dyslexia have poor self-efficacy, are not motivated to do homework, demonstrate poor social integration, and have a sense of learned helplessness. They also note that youth with dyslexia are more likely to have insecure attachment styles, a lower sense of coherence, greater loneliness, to experience more bullying, and to be dissatisfied with the level of support they receive from parents, teachers and peers. The authors also discuss risk factors for the development of internalizing issues in the LD child, suggesting that greater LD severity, the presence of more than one LD, comorbid ADHD, borderline intellectual capacity, non-inclusion in mainstream classes, female gender, and inappropriate management of the learning disorder all place a LD child at greater risk of internalizing problems.

In addition to the psychosocial reasons for the link described above between LDs and internalizing problems, the clinician should also be aware of evidence that common brain etiology may account for at least some of the comorbidity between LDs and internalizing problems. Furthermore, the presence of internalizing issues in LD children can serve to worsen their academic achievement, as these youth are already more likely to have problems with particular cognitive functions, such as working memory and metacognition (Nelson and Harwood 2011). For example, when a young person becomes anxious, his or her attention is diverted and anxious cognitions can take up important space in working memory, which will in turn lead to even less efficient information processing (Eysenck, Derakshan, Santos, and Calvo 2007). Thus anxiety in a child with a LD may have a "double whammy" effect on his or her abilities. Clinicians should therefore look for both psychosocial and cognitive processes that might contribute to, or exacerbate, internalizing disorders in the LD child, or indeed they should check whether the internalizing symptoms are the result of unidentified learning difficulties.

Environmental Factors and Life Events

In addition to the many and varied diagnostic and individual characteristics that may impact on therapy, specific environmental factors and life events have been associated with anxiety and depression in children and adolescents.

Environmental factors

Socioeconomic status

There are many stressors inherent to lower socioeconomic status (SES): lack of material and social resources, frequent chronic and uncontrollable stressful life events, health problems, dangerous neighborhoods, crowded and noisier homes, family conflict and instability, crime and exposure to violence, and frequent moves and transitions (Evans 2004; Lorant et al. 2003; Santiago, Wadsworth, and Stump 2011). The relationship between SES and youth anxiety or depression is not quite as straightforward as that demonstrated in the adult literature, and it has received significantly less empirical attention. Some studies have reported no association between SES and the internalizing disorders (e.g., Twenge and Nolen-Hoeksema 2002); some have shown that lower SES is negatively associated with internalizing disorders (e.g., Cronk, Slutske, Madden, Bucholz, and Heath 2004); some have shown mixed results within one and the same study, depending on the measure of SES (e.g., Ozer, Fernald, and Roberts 2008); and some have shown that higher SES is associated with greater anxiety (e.g., Merikangas et al. 2010).

The reasons for differences in findings pertaining to the association of SES with internalizing disorders are likely to be complex. For example, Vine et al. (2012) found different results depending on type of anxiety symptom, distinction between family and neighborhood incomes, and gender. Furthermore, although research is scant, there is some evidence to suggest that SES may impact in various ways upon the treatment of child anxiety and depressive disorders. For example, it has been found that higher SES may be related to better treatment outcome, at least for adolescent depression (Emslie et al. 2011); that disadvantage may be significantly related to dropout (Kazdin, Mazurick, and Bass 1993); and that lower income and lower social class may be more strongly related to dropout for younger than for older children (Pekarik and Stephenson 1988). Thus the relationship between SES and internalizing disorders in youth is complex, and clinicians should not only be aware of the child's SES, but also assess and take into account the broader implications and bidirectional impact associated with it.

Family structure and conflict

Living in a single-parent household has been inconsistently associated with higher dropout from treatment (e.g., Gonzalez et al. 2011) but has not been found relevant to treatment outcome. There is evidence to suggest, however, that family conflict, whether between parent and child, mother and father, or child and sibling, is associated with anxiety and depression (Drake and Ginsburg 2012; Kane and Garber 2004; Sheeber, Davis, Leve, Hops, and Tildesley 2007). Interparental conflict in particular has received considerable empirical attention, being consistently associated with youth anxiety and depression (Drake and Ginsburg 2012; Restifo and Bögels 2009). Indeed, it has been suggested that interparental conflict, rather than marital discord, marital status or divorce per se, affects child internalizing disorders (Drake and Ginsburg 2012; Rapee 2012). Furthermore, the effects of parental conflict have been found to be worse when there is aggression or the threat of aggression, when a parent is angry and withdrawn, and when the parent uses avoidant conflict tactics (Restifo and Bögels 2009).

The scant evidence conducted to date suggests that family conflict and dysfunction are associated with poorer treatment outcome for depression (Emslie et al. 2011) and anxiety (Crawford and Manassis 2001) in youth. Various mechanisms through which interparental conflict has its effect on internalizing disorders have been suggested: impairment of parenting practices; disruption of the youth–parent bond; parental modeling of anxiety, withdrawal, poor coping, and maladaptive conflict resolution; child appraisals of self-blame; and threat associated with the conflict (Drake and Ginsburg 2012). It is thus important for clinicians to look for family conflict (child–parent, interparent, and child–sibling conflict) and to incorporate it into the conceptualization and treatment plans for youth with internalizing issues.

Life events

Stressful life events have been found to be associated with internalizing and externalizing symptoms in the vast majority of studies (Grant, Compas, Thurm, McMahon, and Gipson 2004), even those investigating preschool-age children (Luby 2010). This section discusses particular types of life events, trauma, chronic health issues, and bullying, with respect to their relationship with youth anxiety and depression.

Trauma

Unfortunately, young people may be exposed to numerous types of trauma, and consequently go on to develop anxiety and depression in response to them. One of the most studied forms of trauma is childhood sexual abuse (CSA). With respect to the effect of CSA on childhood internalizing disorders, it would seem that mood rather than anxiety disorders are a more common result. In his review, Rapee (2012) concluded that CSA increases the risk of anxiety disorders in children, but that the link is not as strong as it is with other disorders. The effects of CSA on the development of depression appear somewhat stronger: there are higher rates of depression in abused compared to non-abused children and the severity of the resulting depression is higher when there has been sexual abuse with contact, when the child knows the perpetrator, and when the child is male (Putnam 2003).

With respect to trauma more generally, the clinician should be aware that, when adolescents experience it, trauma tends to result in specific mood and anxiety disorders, whereas in younger children the effects on mood and anxiety are more diffuse and can take on a variety of internalizing difficulties (De Young, Kenardy, Cobham, and Kimble 2012; Yule 2001). Furthermore, it has been suggested that adverse effects following trauma are more likely to develop in children when the events are ongoing, when the events lead to longer term disruptions in the child's life, when the child has had a high level of exposure, when the child is female, and when the child has less social support, or when the child's social support networks are disrupted due to the trauma (Pine and Cohen 2002). Clinicians should therefore look for trauma and the risk factors associated with it, so that a thorough case conceptualization and treatment plan can be made.

Chronic health issues

Unfortunately many children have to contend with a chronic illness, and chronic illness has been associated with internalizing disorders. Youth with chronic illnesses such as epilepsy, asthma, diabetes, or migraine demonstrate higher levels of depression (Pinquart and Shen 2011). It would seem that this link is evident even in very young children, as chronic illness is also associated with the early onset of depression in preschool children (Curtis and Luby 2008).

When one considers the difficulties faced by youth beset by chronic illness, it is not surprising that they frequently develop internalizing disorders. Although a full review of health conditions is beyond the scope of this small section, it may be illustrative to take the example of the child suffering from type 1 diabetes. Diabetes can have numerous serious and potentially lethal medical complications if one does not adhere to the regime very closely, and the burden of treatment is heavy on youth afflicted by this disease. A number of areas that young people with diabetes tend to find stressful have been identified (Rubin and Peyrot 2001). First, dietary restrictions can be worrisome and upsetting for youth. Birthday parties and other social events frequently revolve around foods such as sweets, which diabetic children are unable to consume. As a result, these children may feel different from others, deprived, and anxious that they may appear to be "weird" in the eyes of their peers. Second, there can be stress associated with monitoring blood glucose levels, the unpredictability of blood sugar levels being a strong cause of stress and frustration. The finger prick itself, required to monitor blood glucose levels, can be painful and become associated with behavioral problems and anxiety. Third, insulin delivery can be very stressful, both in terms of needle phobia on behalf of the child and in terms of concern around inducing hyperglycemia by administering too much insulin. Finally, there can be much conflict around diabetic management, as the developing need for autonomy in the adolescent, the fear of injections, the deprivation of particular foods, and the concern about being "different" from peers leads to resistance to the diabetic regime and distress around it.

This example highlights a number of areas that the clinician should be aware of when working with a child with chronic health concerns and comorbid anxiety or depression. First, the clinician should be aware that depression and anxiety are *common* in chronic illness and should be assessed for. Second, given that chronic health conditions are often associated with physical pain, the clinician should ascertain whether the anxiety or the depression is associated (even in part) with pain in some way. Third, the clinician should assess for, and be aware of, any links (uni- or bidirectional) between the required medical regime and the child's experience of anxiety or depression.

Bullying

Unfortunately bullying among children is highly prevalent and is associated with a number of deleterious consequences, including anxiety and depression (O'Brennan,

Bradshaw, and Sawyer 2009). It has been suggested that childhood is an important time for the development of cognitive vulnerabilities for depression and that bullying might be one pathway in which these depressive cognitions develop (Gibb, Stone, and Crossett 2012; Sinclaire 2011).

Within the bullying area there are distinctions made between bullies, victims, and those who are referred to as bully-victims (those who have been both a bully and victim). Unsurprisingly perhaps, victims of bullying are at high risk of developing internalizing problems, while bullies are not (Juvonen, Graham, and Schuster 2003; Nansel, Craig, Overpeck, Saluja, and Ruan 2004). Interestingly, however, it has also been found that bully-victims are the most likely to display internalizing symptoms and disorders (O'Brennan et al. 2009). Clinicians should be aware that internalizing problems associated with bullying seem to increase as youth get older, that the association is stronger for boys, and that social support has been found to be an important buffer between bullying and the development of internalizing disorders (Sinclaire 2011).

A distinction between direct and indirect bullying is also made in the literature. Direct bullying involves physical contact or threat thereof, while indirect (or relational) bullying involves covert social manipulation, such as exclusion of the victim and rumor spreading. Interestingly, youth seem to be more at risk of developing internalizing issues if they are the victim of indirect rather than direct bullying (Marini, Dane, Bosacki, and Cura 2006), indirect bullying being more directly related to changes in depressive cognitions than direct bullying (Sinclaire 2011). Thus clinicians should ensure that they assess for bullying, both indirect and direct, when working with youth with internalizing disorders, so that appropriate strategies can be included within treatment.

Conclusion

It is hoped that this chapter has provided the clinician with some important background knowledge regarding particular child characteristics that may impact on therapy. The take-home message we want to impart is that a thorough assessment of psychopathology, developmental issues, individual child characteristics, and environmental factors is essential. Through knowledge and subsequent assessment of the factors that may impact on youth internalizing disorders and treatment, the clinician can develop a more accurate case conceptualization, which will ultimately lead to greater therapeutic success.

References

Angold, Adrian, E. Jane Costello, and Alattin Erkanli. 1999. "Comorbidity." *Journal of Child Psychology and Psychiatry*, 40: 57–87. DOI: 10.1111/1469-7610.00424

APA. 1994. Diagnostic and Statistical Manual of Mental Disorders. Washington, DC: American Psychiatric Association.

Avenevoli, Shelley, Erin Knight, Ronald C. Kessler, and Kathleen R. Merikangas. 2008. "Epidemiology of Depression in Children and Adolescents." In John R. Z. Abela and Benjamin L. Hankin (Eds.), *Handbook of depression in children and adolescents* (pp. 6–32). New York: Guilford Press.

Barbe, Remy P., Jeffery Bridge, Boris Birmaher, David Kolko, and David A Brent. 2004. "Suicidality and Its Relationship to Treatment Outcome in Depressed Adolescents." *Suicide and Life-Threatening Behavior*, 34: 44–55. DOI: 10.1521/suli.34.1.44.27768

Berman, Stephen L., Carl F. Weems, Wendy K. Silverman, and William M. Kurtines. 2000. "Predictors of Outcome in Exposure-Based Cognitive and Behavioral Treatments for Phobic and Anxiety Disorders in Children." *Behavior Therapy*, 31: 713–31. DOI: org/10.1016/S0005-7894(00)80040-4

Bolton, Derek, and Philip Graham. 2005. "Cognitive Behaviour Therapy for Children and Adolescents: Some Theoretical and Developmental Issues." In Philip Graham (Ed.), *Cognitive behaviour therapy for children and families* (pp. 9–24). Cambridge: Cambridge University Press.

Carr, A. 2006. *The Handbook of Child and Adolescent Clinical Psychology: A Contextual Approach* (2nd ed.). New York: Routledge.

Costello, E. Jane, Helen L. Egger, and Adrian Angold. 2005. "The Developmental Epidemiology of Anxiety Disorders: Phenomenology, Prevalence, and Comorbidity." *Child and Adolescent Psychiatric Clinics of North America*, 14 (4): 631–48. DOI: 10.1016/j.chc.2005.06.003

Crawford, A. Melissa, and Katharina Manassis. 2001. "Familial Predictors of Treatment Outcome in Childhood Anxiety Disorders." *Journal of the American Academy of Child & Adolescent Psychiatry*, 40: 1182–9. DOI: 10.1097/00004583-200110000-00012

Cronk, Nikole J., Wendy S. Slutske, Pamela A. F. Madden, Kathleen K. Bucholz, and Andrew C. Heath. 2004. "Risk for Separation Anxiety Disorder among Girls: Paternal Absence, Socioeconomic Disadvantage, and Genetic Vulnerability." *Journal of Abnormal Psychology*, 113: 237–47. DOI: 10.1037/0021-843x.113.2.237

Curtis, Carmen E., and Joan L. Luby. 2008. "Depression and Social Functioning in Preschool Children with Chronic Medical Conditions." *The Journal of Pediatrics*, 153: 408–13. DOI: 10.1016/j.jpeds.2008.03.035

De Young, Alexandra C., Justin A. Kenardy, Vanessa E. Cobham, and Roy Kimble. 2012. "Prevalence, Comorbidity and Course of Trauma Reactions in Young Burn-Injured Children." *Journal of Child Psychology and Psychiatry*, 53: 56–63. DOI: 10.1111/j.1469-7610.2011.02431.x

Drake, Kelly L., and Golda S. Ginsburg. 2012. "Family Factors in the Development, Treatment, and Prevention of Childhood Anxiety Disorders." *Clinical Child and Family Psychology Review*, 15 (2): 1–19. DOI: 10.1007/s10567-011-0109-0

Emslie, Graham J., Betsy D. Kennard, and Taryn L. Mayes. 2011. "Predictors of Treatment Response in Adolescent Depression." *Pediatric Annals*, 40: 300–6. DOI: 10.3928/00904481-20110512-05

Evans, Gary W. 2004. "The Environment of Childhood Poverty." *American Psychologist*, 59 (2): 77–92. DOI: 10.1037/0003-066X.59.2.77

Eysenck, Michael W., Nazanin Derakshan, Rita Santos, and Manuel G. Calvo. 2007. "Anxiety and Cognitive Performance: Attentional Control Theory." *Emotion*, 7: 336–53. DOI: 10.1037/1528-3542.7.2.336

Garber, Judy, and V. Robin Weersing. 2010. "Comorbidity of Anxiety and Depression in Youth: Implications for Treatment and Prevention." *Clinical Psychology: Science and Practice*, 17: 293–306. DOI: 10.1111/j.1468-2850.2010.01221.x

Gibb, Brandon E., Lindsay B. Stone, and Sarah E. Crossett. 2012. "Peer Victimization and Prospective Changes in Children's Inferential Styles." *Journal of Clinical Child & Adolescent Psychology*, 41: 561–9. DOI: 10.1080/15374416.2012.703124

Gonzalez, Araceli, V. Robin Weersing, Erin M. Warnick, Lawrence D. Scahill, and Jospeh L. Woolston. 2011. "Predictors of Treatment Attrition among an Outpatient Clinic Sample of Youths with Clinically Significant Anxiety." *Administration and Policy in Mental Health and Mental Health Services Research*, 38: 356–67. DOI: 10.1007/s10488-010-0323-y

Grant, Kathryn E., Bruce E. Compas, Audrey E. Thurm, Susan D. McMahon, and Polly Y. Gipson. 2004. "Stressors and Child and Adolescent Psychopathology: Measurement Issues and Prospective Effects." *Journal of Clinical Child and Adolescent Psychology*, 33: 412–25. DOI: 10.1207/s15374424jccp3302_23

Harmon, Holly, Audrey Langley, and Golda S. Ginsburg. 2006. "The Role of Gender and Culture in Treating Youth with Anxiety Disorders." *Journal of Cognitive Psychotherapy*, 20: 301–10. DOI: http://dx.doi.org/ 10.1891/088983906780644000

Juvonen, Jaana, Sandra Graham, and Mark A. Schuster. 2003. "Bullying among Young Adolescents: The Strong, the Weak, and the Troubled." *Pediatrics*, 112: 1231–7. DOI: 10.1542/peds.112.6.1231

Kane, Peter, and Judy Garber. 2004. "The Relations among Depression in Fathers, Children's Psychopathology, and Father–Child Conflict: A Meta-Analysis." *Clinical Psychology Review*, 24: 339–60.

Kazdin, Alan E., Jennifer L. Mazurick, and Debra Bass. 1993. "Risk for Attrition in Treatment of Antisocial Children and Families." *Journal of Clinical Child Psychology*, 22: 2–16. DOI: 10.1207/s15374424jccp2201_1

Kendall, Philip C., Erika U. Brady, and Timothy L. Verduin. 2001. "Comorbidity in Childhood Anxiety Disorders and Treatment Outcome." *Journal of the American Academy of Child & Adolescent Psychiatry*, 40: 787–94. DOI: 10.1097/00004583-200107000-00013

Kovacs, Maria, David Goldston, and Constantine Gatsonis. 1993. "Suicidal Behaviors and Childhood-Onset Depressive Disorders: A Longitudinal Investigation." *Journal of the American Academy of Child & Adolescent Psychiatry*, 32: 8–20. DOI: 10.1097/00004583-199301000-00003

Lewinsohn, Peter M., Paul Rohde, and John R. Seeley. 1998. "Major Depressive Disorder in Older Adolescents: Prevalence, Risk Factors, and Clinical Implications." *Clinical Psychology Review*, 18: 765–94. DOI: http://dx.doi.org/10.1016/S0272-7358(98)00010-5

Lorant, Vincent, Denise Deliege, William Eaton, Annie Robert, Pierre Philippot, and Marc Ansseau. 2003. "Socioeconomic Inequalities in Depression: A Meta-Analysis." *American Journal of Epidemiology*, 157: 98–112. DOI: 10.1093/aje/kwf182

Luby, Joan L. 2010. "Preschool Depression: The Importance of Identification of Depression Early in Development." *Current Directions in Psychological Science*, 19: 91–5. DOI: 10.1177/0963721410364493

Maag, John W., and Robert Reid. 2006. "Depression among Students with Learning Disabilities: Assessing the Risk." *Journal of Learning Disabilities*, 39: 3–10. DOI: 10.1177/00222194060390010201

Marini, Zopito A.., Andrew V. Dane, Sandra L. Bosacki, and Y. Cura. 2006. "Direct and Indirect Bully-Victims: Differential Psychosocial Risk Factors Associated with Adolescents Involved in Bullying and Victimization." *Aggressive Behavior*, 32: 551–69. DOI: 10.1002/ab.20155

Merikangas, Kathleen R., Jian P. He, Debra Brody, Prudence W. Fisher, Karen Bourdon, and Doreen S. Koretz. 2010. "Prevalence and Treatment of Mental Disorders among US Children in the 2001–2004 NHANES." *Pediatrics*, 125: 75–81. DOI: 10.1542/peds.2008-2598

Miller, Carlin J., George W. Hynd, and Scott R. Miller. 2005. "Children with Dyslexia: Not Necessarily at Risk for Elevated Internalizing Symptoms." *Reading and Writing*, 18: 425–36. DOI: 10.1007/s11145-005-4314-4

Mugnaini, Daniel, Stefano Lassi, Giampaolo La Malfa, and Giorgio Albertini. 2009. "Internalizing Correlates of Dyslexia." *World Journal of Pediatrics*, 5: 255–64. DOI: 10.1007/s12519-009-0049-7

Nansel, Tonja R., Wendy Craig, Mary D. Overpeck, Gitanjali Saluja, and W. June Ruan. 2004. "Cross-National Consistency in the Relationship between Bullying Behaviors and Psychosocial Adjustment." *Archives of Pediatrics & Adolescent Medicine*, 158: 730. DOI: 10.1001/archpedi.158.8.730

Nelson, Jason M., and Hannah R. Harwood. 2011. "A Meta-Analysis of Parent and Teacher Reports of Depression among Students with Learning Disabilities: Evidence for the Importance of Multi-Informant Assessment." *Psychology in the Schools*, 48: 371–84. DOI: 10.1002/pits.20560

Nilsen, Toril S., Martin Eisemann, and Siv Kvernmo. 2012. "Predictors and Moderators of Outcome in Child and Adolescent Anxiety and Depression: A Systematic Review of Psychological Treatment Studies." *European Child & Adolescent Psychiatry*, 22 (2): 1–19. DOI: 10.1007/s00787-012-0316-3

O'Brennan, Lindsay M., Catherine P. Bradshaw, and Anne L. Sawyer. 2009. "Examining Developmental Differences in the Social–Emotional Problems among Frequent Bullies, Victims, and Bully/victims." *Psychology in the Schools*, 46: 100–15. DOI: 10.1002/pits.20357

O'Neil, Kelly A., Jennifer L. Podell, Courtney L. Benjamin, and Philip C. Kendall. 2010. "Comorbid Depressive Disorders in Anxiety-Disordered Youth: Demographic, Clinical, and Family Characteristics." *Child Psychiatry & Human Development*, 41: 330–41. DOI: 10.1007/s10578-009-0170-9

Ollendick, Thomas H., Matthew A. Jarrett, Amy E. Grills-Taquechel, Laura D. Hovey, and Jennifer C. Wolff. 2008. "Comorbidity as a Predictor and Moderator of Treatment Outcome in Youth with Anxiety, Affective, Attention Deficit/Hyperactivity Disorder, and Oppositional/Conduct Disorders." *Clinical Psychology Review*, 28: 1447–71. DOI: 10.1016/j.cpr.2008.09.003

Ozer, Emily J., Lia C. H. Fernald, and Sarah C. Roberts. 2008. "Anxiety Symptoms in Rural Mexican Adolescents." *Social Psychiatry and Psychiatric Epidemiology*, 43: 1014–23. DOI: 10.1007/s00127-008-0473-3

Pekarik, Gene, and Laura A. Stephenson. 1988. "Adult and Child Client Differences in Therapy Dropout Research." *Journal of Clinical Child Psychology*, 17: 316–21. DOI: 10.1207/s15374424jccp1704_3

Pine, Daniel S., and Judith A. Cohen. 2002. "Trauma in Children and Adolescents: Risk and Treatment of Psychiatric Sequelae." *Biological Psychiatry*, 51: 519–31. DOI: http://dx.doi.org/10.1016/S0006-3223(01)01352-X

Pinquart, Martin, and Yuhui Shen. 2011. "Depressive Symptoms in Children and Adolescents with Chronic Physical Illness: An Updated Meta-Analysis." *Journal of Pediatric Psychology*, 36: 375–84. DOI: 10.1093/jpepsy/jsq104

Putnam, Frank W. 2003. "Ten-Year Research Update Review: Child Sexual Abuse." *Journal of the American Academy of Child & Adolescent Psychiatry*, 42: 269–78. DOI: 10.1097/00004583-200303000-00006

Rapee, Ronald M. 2012. "Family Factors in the Development and Management of Anxiety Disorders." *Clinical Child and Family Psychology Review*, 15 (1): 69–80. DOI: 10.1007/s10567-011-0106-3

Restifo, Kathleen, and Susan Bögels. 2009. "Family Processes in the Development of Youth Depression: Translating the Evidence to Treatment." *Clinical Psychology Review*, 29 (4): 294–316. DOI: 10.1016/j.cpr.2009.02.005

Rubin, Richard R., and Mark Peyrot. 2001. "Psychological Issues and Treatments for People with Diabetes." *Journal of Clinical Psychology*, 57: 457–78. DOI: 10.1002/jclp.1041

Santiago, Catherine D. C., Martha E. Wadsworth, and Jessica Stump. 2011. "Socioeconomic Status, Neighborhood Disadvantage, and Poverty-Related Stress: Prospective Effects on Psychological Syndromes among Diverse Low-Income Families." *Journal of Economic Psychology*, 32: 218–30. DOI: 10.1016/j.joep.2009.10.008

Sheeber, Lisa B., Betsy Davis, Craig Leve, Hyman Hops, and Elizabeth Tildesley. 2007. "Adolescents' Relationships with Their Mothers and Fathers: Associations with Depressive Disorder and Subdiagnostic Symptomatology." *Journal of Abnormal Psychology*, 116: 144. DOI: 10.1037/0021-843x.116.1.144

Sinclaire, Jane. 2011. *Hidden Side to the Story*. Victoria, Australia: Palmer Higgs Pty.

Stallard, Paul. 2004. Cognitive Behaviour Therapy with Prepubertal Children. In Philip J. Graham (Ed.), *Cognitive Behaviour Therapy for Children and Families* (pp. 121–35). Cambridge: Cambridge University Press.

Twenge, Jean M., and Susan Nolen-Hoeksema. 2002. "Age, Gender, Race, Socioeconomic Status, and Birth Cohort Difference on the Children's Depression Inventory: A Meta-Analysis." *Journal of Abnormal Psychology*, 111: 578. DOI: 10.1037/0021-843X.111.4.578

Vine, Michaela, Anne V. Stoep, Janice Bell, Isaac C. Rhew, Gretchen Gudmundsen, and Elizabeth McCauley. 2012. "Associations between Household and Neighborhood Income and Anxiety Symptoms in Young Adolescents." *Depression and Anxiety*, 29: 824–32. DOI: 10.1002/Da.21948

Weisz, John R., Carolyn A. McCarty, and Silvia M. Valeri. 2006. "Effects of Psychotherapy for Depression in Children and Adolescents: A Meta-Analysis." *Psychological Bulletin*, 132: 132–49. DOI: 10.1037/0033-2909.132.1.132

Yule, William. 2001. "Post-traumatic Stress Disorder in Children and Adolescents." *International Review of Psychiatry*, 13: 194–200. DOI: 10.1080/09540260120074064

6

Building a Positive Therapeutic Relationship with the Child or Adolescent and Parent

Ruth C. Brown, Kimberly M. Parker, Bryce D. McLeod, and Michael A. Southam-Gerow

Introduction

Although there is debate about the relative importance and influence of the therapeutic relationship in psychological treatments for children and adolescents, few assert that the relationship is not important. Evidence-based treatments assume that a strong therapeutic relationship with the child and parent is critical. Further, workgroups and task forces have underscored that the therapeutic relationship is a key component of evidence-based practice (e.g., Castonguay and Beutler 2005; Norcross 2011).

The therapeutic relationship is also believed to play an instrumental role in cognitive behavioral therapy (CBT) for children with anxiety and depressive disorders. For one, a strong therapeutic relationship is believed to promote positive outcomes by increasing child engagement in the skill-building tasks that are a hallmark of CBT. A strong therapeutic relationship is also believed to facilitate child engagement in the emotionally challenging tasks of CBT, such as exposure tasks. Considered a key component of CBT for child anxiety, exposure tasks are challenging and emotionally demanding. Children who feel a strong connection to their therapist may be more willing to engage in exposure tasks and thus experience greater symptom improvement (Chu and Kendall 2004).

The ability to form a strong therapeutic relationship with a child and parent depends in part on a therapist's ability to tailor treatment to the unique needs of the client. This requires a thorough understanding of the core CBT interventions and of how to adapt the delivery of these interventions to fit the personal, developmental, and cultural needs of particular clients. It also requires an understanding of how to help children and parents agree on the tasks and goals of treatment. Ultimately, treatment success depends on the therapist's ability to convince the child and parent

Evidence-Based CBT for Anxiety and Depression in Children and Adolescents: A Competencies-Based Approach,
First Edition. Edited by Elizabeth S. Sburlati, Heidi J. Lyneham, Carolyn A. Schniering, and Ronald M. Rapee.
© 2014 John Wiley & Sons, Ltd. Published 2014 by John Wiley & Sons, Ltd.

that the different elements of a CBT program are important and that participating in treatment will lead to symptom reduction.

In this chapter we describe competencies that are relevant for building and maintaining a positive therapeutic relationship with child or adolescent clients and their parent(s). Specifically, we will focus on four aspects of the therapeutic relationship by (i) describing key competencies that contribute to therapists fostering positive therapeutic relationships; (ii) discussing how those competencies are specifically applied in treating anxiety and depression in children/adolescents; (iii) outlining how those competencies are adjusted for clients of different developmental levels (e.g., younger children vs. adolescents) and different cultural background; and (iv) delineating obstacles to building a positive therapeutic relationship and outlining methods for overcoming those obstacles.

Key Features of Competencies

Sburlati, Schiering, Lyneham, and Rapee (2011) identified four broad competencies associated with building a positive therapeutic relationship: (i) building alliance with children; (ii) building alliance with parents; (iii) instillation of hope and optimism for change; and (iv) engaging children in developmentally appropriate activities. In this chapter we discuss each of these competencies, beginning with alliance-building behaviors. Before we dive into these issues, it is important to note that cultural and diversity issues must be carefully considered when building a therapeutic relationship. A number of factors relevant to the therapeutic relationship can be influenced by a client's cultural background. Such factors may be the degree of formality of the therapeutic relationship, expectations for treatment, and treatment goals (e.g., expression of distress). Thus a key part of building a therapeutic relationship with a parent and a child is understanding how their cultural values may impact the process and the outcome of therapy. This information should be used in turn to inform efforts to build and maintain the alliance.

Alliance building

It is important to build a positive alliance early in treatment and to maintain a strong alliance throughout treatment. The alliance is often conceptualized as being comprised of three related but distinct dimensions: bond, tasks, and goals. *Bond* refers to the affective aspects of the client–therapist relationship. *Tasks* constitute agreement and participation in the activities of therapy. *Goals* represent the agreement between the client and the therapist on the desired outcome of treatment. A challenge for child therapists is building and maintaining a strong alliance with both the child and the parent. And, of course, the therapist should carefully consider the client's cultural background, as this can influence a number of factors relevant to forming the alliance (the therapist's stance, the target of treatment, and so on).

Alliance building with children

Children rarely refer themselves for therapy, so their motivation to participate in therapeutic activities can vary. A key task of a therapist is to engage children in treatment and to keep them motivated throughout treatment. With children the alliance-building process often starts with forming a strong affective bond and working to achieve agreement on the goals and tasks of therapy.

The affective bond is one of the most important components of the alliance with children who derive motivation to participate in therapeutic tasks from a positive relationship with the therapist. It is therefore important to establish with a child a relationship marked by warmth and openness, and to do so early in treatment. Interventions traditionally associated with client-centered psychotherapy can facilitate alliance building. Rapport-building behaviors that elicit information, provide emotional understanding and support, and explore the child's subjective feelings help foster an affective bond (Karver, Handelsman, Fields, and Bickman 2008). Therapists' use of collaborative language (e.g., *we, us, let's*) can also help build the bond by helping to establish therapy as a collaborative effort (Creed and Kendall 2005). Attending to and tracking client affect (e.g., fear, disappointment) and the use of validating statements help clients feel understood and supported. In all, client-centered interventions such as these help form an affective bond and ensure that the child will present him-/herself to treatment ready to engage in the hard work ahead.

As children get older, agreement on the tasks and goals of treatment becomes increasingly important. Young children do not have the cognitive capacity to understand long-term goals, so the affective aspect of the alliance is more important for young children (Shirk and Saiz 1992). However, adolescents have an increased need for autonomy, so it is essential that they have a say in establishing the goals and tasks of treatment. Of course, treatment goals and tasks should be presented in developmentally appropriate terms. Young children may find the simplest explanation suitable (e.g., "Today we are going to learn how to talk back to your anxiety"), whereas adolescents may benefit from a more detailed rationale of the treatment strategies to be used (e.g., "Today we are going to talk about two kinds of thoughts: anxious thoughts and coping thoughts because it is important to understand how our thoughts can influence our feelings"). Collaborative approaches that allow the child to have input into the selection of goals and tasks help to strengthen the alliance. Indeed, children who feel like they have some say in establishing treatment goals and tasks are more motivated and willing to engage in treatment (Meyer et al. 2002). Therapists must be aware that parents and children may have different goals for treatment. Parents often initiate treatment and have treatment goals that the child client may not share. The therapist must therefore work to resolve discrepancies or to identify common goals by following ethical and professional standards.

Alliance building with the parents

The therapist must build and maintain a strong alliance with the parents. Parents play a critical role in child psychotherapy. While it is important to establish a strong affective bond with them, it may be more important that both parties – therapist

> **Box 6.1   Summary for alliance building with children and parents**
>
> - Consider how cultural and diversity factors may influence alliance formation and maintenance with the child and parent.
> - Prioritize establishing an emotional bond with children at the beginning of treatment.
> - To establish the bond, therapists can
>   - (a)   make use of reflective and validating statements;
>   - (b)   use collaborative language (e.g., *we*, *us*, and *let's*); and
>   - (c)   track and validate feelings.
> - Work with children and parents to achieve mutually agreed-upon treatment goals and tasks.
> - Provide a treatment rationale that links the purpose of the treatment tasks to the larger treatment goal; provide such a rationale when each new treatment task is introduced.
> - Ensure that treatment tasks and goals are put into developmentally appropriate terms.
> - Regularly check in with the parents regarding the treatment's tasks and goals.

and parents – agree on the tasks and goals ahead. As many parents give consent and provide transportation for their children, failure to agree on the goals and tasks of treatment can result in premature termination. Taking the time to understand the parent's treatment goals, drawing a clear connection between tasks and goals, and setting realistic treatment expectations can help form a strong alliance with a parent. It is also important to check in with the parents throughout treatment, to ensure that no problems related to tasks and goals arise.

Parents play various roles in treatment. In some cases they may be asked to take responsibility for homework activities that give a child the opportunity to practice skills. In other cases parents may be asked to alter behaviors that contribute to the development and/or maintenance of a child's symptoms. Parents may not expect to participate in treatment without understanding why their participation will help achieve treatment goals. It is therefore important to clearly explain why a parent is being asked to participate in treatment, and also to detail how his or her participation will help achieve treatment goals.

Instilling hope and optimism for change

Parents and children who come to treatment with low expectations about its potential advantages can benefit from a sense of hope. Thus, early in treatment therapists must ascertain what expectations parents and children have for treatment. This work can occur when they discuss the treatment's tasks and goals. Any sign of unrealistic treatment expectancies indicates the need to instill a sense of hope for change. Providing psycho-education about the therapy process, the typical timeline for treatment, and

> **Box 6.2**   Summary for instilling hope and optimism
>
> - Assess for unrealistic treatment expectancies.
> - Provide psycho-education about the typical length and outcome of treatment.
> - Provide an explanation or rationale of the treatment.
> - Provide statements and set up therapeutic tasks that help the client build a sense of self-efficacy.

the expected outcomes can instill hope and generate a set of realistic expectancies. To help maintain hope, therapists should foster the development of client self-efficacy regarding his/her ability to successfully accomplish the tasks and goals of treatment. And, to foster this development, therapists can highlight accomplishments and normalize "set-backs" by reminding clients that change is not a linear process.

Competence in Treating Anxiety Disorders and Depression

Although the competencies described up to this point apply to working with children who suffer from anxiety or depressive disorders (or both), there are some disorder-specific suggestions to consider.

Anxiety

Some children with anxiety are inhibited. A few issues arise from this state of affairs. First, these children may be slow to form an alliance; in fact interacting with the therapist may be an exposure task for inhibited children. Second, with inhibited children, therapists may struggle to gauge the quality and progress of the alliance, which makes it important to regularly assess that alliance from the child's and the parent's perspectives.

Exposure tasks are a key ingredient of CBT for anxiety. These tasks are challenging and emotionally demanding for children. A strong alliance may facilitate client involvement in exposure tasks. Existing evidence suggests that exposure tasks do not have a negative impact on the alliance, particularly in the context of an established positive alliance (Kendall et al. 2009). It is therefore important to establish a strong alliance with a child before starting on the exposure tasks, so as to maximize child involvement. Providing encouragement and praise during exposure tasks can help maintain the alliance and build client self-efficacy.

Children with anxiety disorders are likely to have parents who suffer from anxiety too. Anxious parents may inadvertently interfere with treatment by negatively reinforcing escape behaviors or by "rescuing" their children from challenging tasks. Therefore the therapist must help parents understand how their behavior impacts treatment progress. In the context of a supportive parent–therapist alliance, parents may feel more comfortable to express concerns or difficulty in watching their children face distressing situations. Therapists may also find the need to provide the parents with strategies for coping with their own anxiety, or they may recommend that the parents seek their own treatment.

> **Box 6.3   Summary for alliance building with anxious children**
>
> - Therapists may need to spend extra time helping shy or inhibited children feel comfortable with the therapist.
> - Therapists should establish the alliance before engaging in exposure tasks for anxiety.
> - Therapists should use encouragement and praise, often during exposure tasks, to build self-efficacy.
> - Therapists may need to look out for and address parental behaviors that interfere with treatment progress.

Depression

Children with depression tend to be irritable. An irritable client can punish help-giving behaviors and can be a tough challenge for a therapist aiming to form an alliance. Indeed, clients with depression provide lower levels of reinforcement in response to alliance-building behaviors. Therapists thus need to be vigilant and maintain their alliance-building efforts despite the lack of reinforcement from the child.

Children's irritability can make reinforcement difficult for their parents as well (Dietz et al. 2008). Parents of depressed children may therefore need increased support to appropriately reinforce the tasks and skills the child is acquiring in treatment. Feedback to parents will be easier to give and better received in the context of a supportive parent–therapist alliance.

The therapist should also be aware that parents of depressed children may suffer from depression and other psychiatric disorders themselves. Depressed parents may be difficult to engage in treatment. If parental psychopathology interferes with treatment progress, it may be necessary to refer a parent to treatment. Indeed recent studies have shown that the treatment of parental depression can lead to improvements in the child's depression (Wickramaratne et al. 2011).

> **Box 6.4   Summary for alliance building with depressed children**
>
> - Therapists should make frequent use of reinforcement with depressed children.
> - Therapists should maintain a supportive stance, despite irritability or lack of reciprocal reinforcement from depressed children.
> - Therapists may need to look out for parental psychopathology and refer parents for therapy.
> - Parents of depressed children may need extra support from the therapist to follow through with the therapeutic tasks at home.

Competence in Treating both Children and Adolescents

CBT with children and adolescents can be conceptualized as a skill-building therapeutic approach. As such, it relies on children and on their parents to engage in in-session, homework, and out-of-session activities (Chorpita and Daleiden 2009). The alliance is a key mechanism in engaging children in treatment and facilitating their active involvement in skill-building tasks. However, different skills and activities are needed to establish and maintain the alliance with children of different developmental levels.

It is essential that clinicians consider the developmental level of children in the delivery of CBT, in order to foster and maintain a positive alliance. Development can refer to a variety of characteristics, including chronological age, cognitive developmental level, and emotional developmental level. Here we present guidelines to consider when building an alliance with children and adolescents; but therapists should always be aware of the particular developmental needs and preferences of their clients. Flexibility and creativity are valued qualities in designing and delivering developmentally appropriate strategies to strengthen the child–therapist alliance.

Children

With children, encouraging collaboration and engagement can be accomplished through the use of activities. Children often find direct questions uncomfortable, so therapists should consider delivering interventions via play-based activities. For example, the therapist and the child can make up stories about a superhero who uses CBT skills to face and conquer his/her fears. Therapists can use a variety of activities to deliver interventions; such activities may involve children's books, artwork, puppets, or dolls. It is also important to provide age-appropriate rewards – for example, comics, books, or stickers – for participating in therapeutic tasks. To maintain motivation, therapists can provide rewards for in-session efforts as well as for accomplishing treatment goals (e.g., for achieving a certain mark on the fear ladder).

Adolescents

The focus and delivery of therapy must shift when one works with adolescents. Individuation and autonomy are important for most adolescents, so confidentiality takes on greater importance. Adolescents may prefer that their parents not be privy to any information disclosed to the therapist. Therapists should therefore have an open and frank discussion with parents and adolescents at the outset of therapy about the limits of confidentiality. Alliance formation may be difficult for adolescents if they believe that the therapist will talk to the parents about what transpires in treatment.

It is also important to discuss treatment goals and tasks with adolescents. Adolescents may not believe that they need treatment, or they may have different treatment goals from those of their parents. It may be difficult to motivate them if they do not agree on treatment goals and tasks. Compared to children, adolescents may need the therapist to spend more time discussing treatment goals and explaining

---

Box 6.5   Summary of competences in treating children and adolescents

- Be aware of the developmental level of the client.
- Adapt language and activities to meet the appropriate developmental level. Therapists may need to engage children through the use of play, art, fantasy, or games.
- Be clear about the limits of confidentiality between therapist, parent, and child, particularly when working with adolescents.
- Use developmentally appropriate reinforcers such as candy, stickers, small toys for children; movie tickets, music downloads, or magazines for adolescents.

---

the treatment rationale. Collaboration between therapist and adolescent can be enhanced by encouraging the latter to identify treatment goals and to suggest his/her own solutions to therapeutic problems (Diamond, Liddle, Hogue, and Dakof 1999). Sufficient time should be spent working with the parent and the adolescent to set mutually agreed-upon goals.

Just as with younger children, therapists should choose age-appropriate activities and rewards for engaging adolescents. When choosing fun therapeutic tasks, therapists can have adolescents make collages with cutouts from teen-relevant magazines, use workbooks, and provide personal examples from their own life. Therapists should determine if an adolescent is comfortable with talk-based therapy or prefers to participate in other activities (e.g., collages, workbooks). Age-relevant rewards for adolescents may include items such as gift certificates for magazines, music, or clothing stores or social rewards such as spending additional time with friends.

Common Obstacles to Competent Practice and Methods to Overcome Them

Building an alliance with children and their parents is not always a simple task. Several factors can present hurdles to developing and maintaining a positive alliance. Here we describe some common obstacles to forming an alliance and methods for overcoming them: (i) discrepancies between children and parents; (ii) low motivation; (iii) poor treatment expectations; (iv) lack of treatment credibility or acceptability; and (v) alliance ruptures.

Discrepancies between children and parents

Children and parents can have different perspectives on the problems that brought them to treatment, and thus on the goals and methods of treatment (Yeh and Weisz 2001). Parents may conceptualize the cause of the presenting problem as lying solely within the child, and they may anticipate limited involvement in treatment. In contrast, youth may view their parents (or teachers, peers, etc.) as the problem and may resent being the focus of treatment. When discrepancies exist, the therapist must work with the child and the parent to identify them and to work toward consensus.

Difficulties may also arise when there is a discrepancy between the problem the parent and/or the child has identified and the therapist's conceptualization of the problem. For example, a parent may bring a child into treatment on account of disruptive behavior problems, but the therapist may identify anxiety as the treatment target. When such a discrepancy exists, the therapist must attempt to build consensus about the treatment goals and tasks. This collaborative work can be made easier by establishing from the outset a strong affective bond with both child and parent, along with developing an understanding of the client's cultural values. Sometimes this requires working with the child and the parent separately before bringing them together to discuss the treatment's tasks and goals.

Low motivation

Signs of low motivation may include poor engagement in session, frequent cancellations, or resistant behavior. Low motivation to participate in treatment can contribute to premature dropout. Anxious or depressed children may also fear or expect failure, or rejection from the therapist, and this would reduce their motivation to engage in treatment tasks. Alliance ruptures may occur if the therapist charges ahead in treatment rather than addressing the cause of the low motivation. Therapists should assess motivational levels early in treatment and quickly address any motivational issues as they arise, even if this means a delay in getting to the core content of treatment. As discussed above, establishing agreed-upon goals and building the child's sense of self-efficacy and positive expectations both play a vital role in enhancing motivation and engagement. Youth may have low motivation for treatment when they believe that others are the source of the problem. This is a common issue in therapy, as youth rarely refer themselves for treatment. For youth ambivalent about change, motivational interviewing and enhancement strategies have been shown to increase the motivation to engage in behaviors that bring about change, for instance by attending treatment sessions, engaging in in-session tasks, and completing therapeutic homework (Miller and Rollnick 2002).

Parents, too, may exhibit low motivation for treatment. Since parents may be involved in the maintenance of the target problem or may be responsible for ensuring that children attend sessions, addressing low motivation in parents may be necessary. If a parent is not motivated for treatment, then it is important to identify the reason. For example, when a youth has been referred by the school or child welfare system, the parent may not perceive a problem and may thus have low motivation for treatment. Or again, if parents have limited resources or experience a number of barriers to participating in treatment (Nock and Photos 2006), they may have less motivation to attend treatment. Finally, parents who believe that treatment should be child-focused may not be motivated to participate personally in it. Alliance ruptures may occur if a therapist does not recognize and address the source of low motivation for treatment. If a parent feels that a therapist is not aware of or concerned about practical or financial barriers, then an alliance rupture may occur. To the extent that such barriers are contributing to low motivation, therapists may need to engage in problem solving with the parent (McKay and Bannon 2004). Helping parents overcome these barriers may enhance both the motivation and the alliance, by demonstrating that the therapist is a concerned and capable ally. To the extent that low motivation is due to ambivalence, therapists may need to engage in motivational enhancement strategies to get parents to participate in their child's treatment. Fortunately, motivational interventions have been demonstrated to enhance treatment retention and outcomes in treatments with parents with low motivation as well (Chaffin et al. 2009; Erickson, Gerstle, and Feldstein 2005).

Treatment expectations

Clients come to therapy with expectations about what will happen during sessions, how long treatment will take, and what benefits they will gain. In some cases, clients have expectations that are unrealistic. For example, a parent might expect complete recovery of his or her child within just a few weeks. These clients are at risk of becoming frustrated with any lack progress in treatment, and also at increased risk of dropping out of it. On the other hand, some clients might have very low expectations concerning the benefit of treatment, and hence they may be difficult to engage in it. As discussed earlier, collaborative discussions with clients, conducted at an early stage, about what they do expect and what they should expect from treatment can establish positive expectations and facilitate a positive alliance.

Addressing treatment expectations at the beginning of treatment is important; but it is also essential to monitor these expectations throughout treatment. As treatment unfolds, expectations may change. New complexities may emerge (e.g., identification of comorbid disorders) or crises may occur (e.g., job loss, illness, marital discord, child abuse) that alter the treatment's trajectory or focus. When changes occur, the therapist should discuss how the events may influence that trajectory, together with the expected outcomes and duration of treatment. Aside from such changes, therapists should check in periodically with the clients by discussing their expectations – positive and negative. Finally, as the end of treatment draws near, it is important to talk about the client's expectations and address any concerns that (s)he may have about his/her ability to maintain treatment gains on his/her own.

Treatment credibility/acceptability

Treatment acceptability is another factor that can influence the alliance. A mismatch between the types of treatment a client expects and the treatment being offered can weaken the alliance. For example, some clients may expect the therapist to simply listen empathetically, and they become frustrated when the therapist challenges their maladaptive beliefs or pushes them to face their fears. Or some clients may expect that a therapist will be directive and not open to a collaborative approach. As discussed before, socializing clients into therapy is an important part of the treatment process – one that helps establish a collaborative therapeutic relationship. This socializing process includes providing clients with a clear, developmentally appropriate treatment rationale.

Children and adolescents who are familiar with coaches in schools and with recreational sports may easily understand the metaphor of the therapist as a coach. This metaphor triggers other relevant concepts and images applicable to treatment, such as the concepts of active involvement and frequent practice, both of which are much needed, or the metaphor of "cheerleading" from the therapist and parents, which brings many benefits.

Although offering a treatment rationale at the beginning of treatment is valuable, it is also important to discuss that rationale when a new task is introduced, or when the client exhibits resistance. The therapist might be met with resistance if the child does not understand the purpose of an in-session activity. Very young children do not require a complex treatment rationale, they simply need to understand that a given task will help them feel better or fight back against anxiety. Adolescents do, however, benefit from a credible treatment rationale. Of course, when they provide a treatment rationale, therapists need to adjust their language and activities to the developmental level of their clients.

Some clients may not find CBT acceptable or feasible, even after a clear treatment rationale has been provided. For example, certain parenting skills featured in CBT programs may not be consistent with the cultural values of certain parents. Therapists who forge ahead with therapeutic interventions that are not acceptable to clients may be faced with resistance or dropout. Therapists may therefore need to shift to methods that are acceptable to clients in order to maintain the alliance or to enhance their motivation to participate in treatment. Therapists may also have to address more practical barriers to treatment, such as issues of costs, transportation, or time (McKay and Bannon 2004).

Alliance ruptures

An alliance rupture is defined as tension on, or dissolution of, the collaborative aspects of the therapeutic relationship (Safran, Muran, and Eubanks-Carter 2011). An alliance rupture can occur at any point in therapy and therapists can take a number of steps to guard against ruptures. Failure to track affect, being pushy, appearing overly formal, and failing to recall relevant information may hinder alliance formation or lead to an alliance rupture (Creed and Kendall 2005; Karver et al. 2008). Accurate, well-timed therapeutic interpretations can enhance the therapeutic relationship by helping a child feel understood. However, excessive questioning or inaccurate interpretations can cause problems with the alliance (Karver et al. 2006). If a rupture occurs, encouraging clients to talk openly about the negative feelings they have about treatment or the therapist may help repair alliance ruptures (Safran, Muran, and Samstag 1994; Safran, Muran, Samstag, and Stevens 2001). In therapy, it is therefore important to strike the right balance between asking questions and reflecting emotions, so that the client may share relevant information without being pushed past his/her comfort zone.

Failed exposures run the risk of creating an alliance rupture, especially in the early phases of exposure treatment. Starting with exposures that guarantee success can help build a client's confidence and trust in the therapist. Should an exposure fail, the therapist must assess for an alliance rupture and re-evaluate the fear hierarchy. Using a sports metaphor may be helpful: even the best teams do not win every game, or the best players do not make every shot. Effort should be praised and reinforced even if the desired outcome was not achieved.

Monitoring for signs of resistance is important. Resistance can emerge due to a number of factors, for instance an alliance rupture, skill deficits, goal discrepancies, or avoidance patterns (Turkat and Meyer 1982). Identifying the factors that contribute to the resistance is critical. For example, to deal with resistance that results from a skill deficit (e.g., poor conversation skills), skill-building interventions would be introduced. On the other hand, resistance arising from goal discrepancies would require a return to treatment planning (Turkat and Meyer 1982). Therefore it is important to identify the underlying cause of the resistance. Regular assessment of the alliance can be a powerful tool for monitoring progress, eliciting feedback, and opening dialogue on the therapeutic process.

Issues Related to Training and Supervision

In teaching therapists how to deliver CBT for child anxiety and depression, attention must focus on the technical and relational elements of treatment. Training materials focus the appropriate amount of attention on the technical aspects of CBT. However, it is important to place equal emphasis on the skills needed to develop and maintain a strong therapeutic relationship with children and parents over the course of a treatment. Therapists should have exposure to graduate courses in developmental psychopathology, developmental processes, minority mental health, and CBT theory. The knowledge gleaned from these courses will help them understand how to adapt the technical elements of CBT to fit the unique developmental and cultural needs of each client. It is also important that therapists learn early on in their training how to deliver client-centered interventions, engage in collaborative goal setting, and explain therapeutic tasks. Supervision can then help therapists understand how best to modify the delivery of therapeutic interventions to meet the developmental and cultural needs of children and parents.

A Final Note on the Use of Assessment Tools to Inform Training and Treatment

A number of assessment tools focused upon the therapeutic relationship can be used to inform training and treatment. A growing body of evidence indicates that providing feedback to therapists about the therapeutic relationship can improve client outcomes (Lambert and Shimokawa 2011). We believe that the systematic collection of data on the therapeutic relationship can also play a role in therapist training. During treatment, therapists can collect data that can be used to inform both treatment and training. For example, collecting data on the child alliance in each session can help identify potential ruptures in the alliance. Supervisors can use observational measures to generate data from taped sessions about the therapeutic relationship that can be used to inform the training. For example, an observational alliance measure can be used to characterize the quality of the child–therapist alliance during supervision. Below we present some measures that can be used at pre-treatment and during treatment to quantify processes related to the therapeutic relationship.

Processes assessed at pre-treatment

Collecting data at the intake about treatment expectations, motivation for treatment, and about barriers to treatment can be used to inform treatment planning and training. It is important to address problems with motivation and expectations directly and early on, as well as to identify potential barriers to subsequent treatment participation. Collecting data on these processes early on in treatment can help therapists determine whether they need to spend more time engaging the family during the intake in order to retain its members in treatment. Therapists can also review the data with their supervisor. Of course, these measures can be administered during treatment as well. The following measures have demonstrated reliability and validity:

- the Parent Motivation Inventory (Nock and Photos 2006);
- the Parent Expectations for Treatment Scale (Nock and Kazdin 2001);
- the Credibility/Expectancies Questionnaire – Parent version (Nock, Ferriter, and Holmberg 2007);
- the Barriers to Treatment Participation Scale (Kazdin, Holland, and Crowley 1997).

Processes assessed during treatment

Two processes related to the therapeutic relationship can be assessed during treatment: alliance and client involvement. As noted before, feedback systems are increasingly including therapeutic relationship measures designed to help therapists identify ruptures in the alliance. These measures can therefore be administered on a weekly or monthly basis. A number of child-, parent-, therapist-, and observer-rated alliance measures exist for child psychotherapy. Observer-rated alliance measures can be used by supervisors to rate the quality of the child–therapist and/or parent–therapist alliance during supervision. A good option for this purpose is the Therapy Process Observational Scale for Child Psychotherapy – Alliance scale (McLeod and Weisz 2005). Self-report alliance measures can be used to identify potential problems in the alliance. The Therapeutic Alliance Scale for Children (Shirk and Saiz 1992) is a good option for collecting self-report alliance data, as it has child, parent, and therapist versions. Supervisors can also use the Child Involvement Rating Scale (Chu and Kendall 2004) to rate child behavioral involvement in therapeutic tasks. These measures can be used as part of a feedback system designed to identify potential problems with the therapeutic relationship that can be used to inform treatment and to guide training.

Conclusion

The therapeutic relationship plays an important role in CBT for child anxiety and depressive disorders. A strong therapeutic relationship is an important ingredient in successful treatment because it helps to maximize client involvement in treatment activities. To form a strong therapeutic relationship, therapists must understand how developmental and cultural factors influence the different facets of the therapeutic relationship and tailor CBT interventions to fit each unique client. It is important that training and supervision focus upon the skills needed to form a strong therapeutic relationship. Therapists need to be exposed to the right combination of coursework, training, and supervision in order to learn how to flexibly deliver the core components of CBT in a way that maximizes client motivation and engagement.

References

Castonguay, Louis G., and Larry E. Beutler. 2005. *Principles of Therapeutic Change that Work.* New York: Oxford University Press.

Chaffin, Mark, Linda A. Valle, Beverly Funderburk, Robin Gurwitch, Jane Silovsky, David Bard, Carol McCoy, and Michelle Kees. 2009. "A Motivational Intervention can Improve Retention in PCIT for Low-Motivation Child Welfare Clients." *Child Maltreatment,* 14: 356–68. DOI: 10.1177/1077559509332263

Chorpita, Bruce F., and Eric L. Daleiden. 2009. "Mapping Evidence-Based Treatments for Children and Adolescents: Application of the Distillation and Matching Model to 615 Treatments from 322 Randomized Trials." *Journal of Consulting and Clinical Psychology,* 77 (3): 566–79. DOI: 10.1037/a0014565

Chu, Brian C., and Philip C. Kendall. 2004. "Positive Association of Child Involvement and Treatment Outcome within a Manual-Based Cognitive-Behavioral Treatment for Children with Anxiety." *Journal of Consulting and Clinical Psychology,* 72: 821–9. DOI: 10.1037/0022-006X.72.5.821

Creed, Torrey A., and Philip C. Kendall. 2005. "Therapist Alliance-Building Behavior within a Cognitive-Behavioral Treatment for Anxiety in Youth." *Journal of Consulting and Clinical Psychology,* 73: 498–505. DOI: 10.1037/0022-006X.73.3.498

Diamond, Gary M., Howard A. Liddle, Aaron Hogue, and Gayle A. Dakof. 1999. "Alliance-Building Interventions with Adolescents in Family Therapy: A Process Study." *Psychotherapy: Theory, Research, Practice, Training,* 36: 355.

Dietz, Larua J., Boris Birmaher, Douglas E. Williamson, Jennifer S. Silk, Ronald E. Dahl, David A. Axelson, Mary Ehmann, and Neal D. Ryan. 2008. "Mother–Child Interactions in Depressed Children and Children at High Risk and Low Risk for Future Depression." *Journal of the American Academy of Child and Adolescent Psychiatry,* 47: 574–82. DOI: 10.1097/CHI.0b013e3181676595

Erickson, Sarah J., Melissa Gerstle, and Sarah W. Feldstein. 2005. "Brief Interventions and Motivational Interviewing with Children, Adolescents, and Their Parents in Pediatric Health Care Settings: A Review." *Archives of Pediatrics and Adolescent Medicine,* 159: 1173. DOI: 10.1001/archpedi.159.12.1173

Karver, Marc S., Jessica B. Handelsman, Sherecce Fields, and Len Bickman. 2006. "Meta-analysis of Therapeutic Relationship Variables in Youth and Family Therapy: The Evidence for Different Relationship Variables in the Child and Adolescent Treatment Outcome Literature." *Clinical Psychology Review,* 26: 50–65. DOI: 10.1016/j.cpr.2005.09.001

Karver, Marc, Stephen Shirk, Jessica B. Handelsman, Sherecce Fields, Heather Crisp, Gretchen Gudmundsen, and Dana McMakin. 2008. "Relationship Processes in Youth Psychotherapy Measuring Alliance, Alliance-Building Behaviors, and Client Involvement." *Journal of Emotional and Behavioral Disorders,* 16: 15–28. DOI: 10.1177/1063426607312536

Kazdin, Alan E., and Lisa Holland. 1991. *Parent Expectancies for Therapy Scale*. New Haven, CT: Yale University, Child Conduct Clinic. Unpublished manuscript.

Kazdin, Alan E., Lisa Holland, and Michael Crowley. 1997. "Family Experience of Barriers to Treatment and Premature Termination from Child Therapy." *Journal of Consulting and Clinical Psychology*, 65: 453–63. DOI: 10.1037/0022-006X.65.3.453

Kendall, Philip C., Jonathan S. Comer, Craig D. Marker, Torrey A. Creed, Anthony C. Puliafico, Alicia A. Hughes, … Jennifer Hudson. 2009. "In-session Exposure Tasks and Therapeutic Alliance across the Treatment of Childhood Anxiety Disorders." *Journal of Consulting and Clinical Psychology*, 77: 517–25. DOI: 10.1037/a0013686

Lambert, Michael J., and Kinichi Shimokawa. 2011. "Collecting Client Feedback." *Psychotherapy*, 48: 72–9. DOI: 10.1037/a0022238

McKay, Mary M., and William M. Bannon. 2004. "Engaging Families in Child Mental Health Services." *Child and Adolescent Psychiatric Clinics of North America*, 13: 905–21. DOI: 10.1016/j.chc.2004.04.001

McLeod, Bryce D., and John R. Weisz. 2005. "The Therapy Process Observational Coding System – Alliance Scale: Measure Characteristics and Prediction of Outcome in Usual Clinical Practice." *Journal of Consulting and Clinical Psychology*, 73: 323–33. DOI: 10.1037/0022-006X.73.2.323

Meyer, Bjorn, Paul A. Pilkonis, Janice L. Krupnick, Matthew K. Egan, Samuel J. Simmens, and Stuart M. Sotsky. 2002. "Treatment Expectancies, Patient Alliance and Outcome: Further Analyses from the National Institute of Mental Health Treatment of Depression Collaborative Research Program." *Journal of Consulting and Clinical Psychology*, 70: 1051–5. DOI: 10.1037/0022-006X.70.4.1051

Miller, William R., and Stephen P. Rollnick. 2002. *Motivational Interviewing: Preparing People for Change*. New York: Guilford Press.

Nock, Matthew K., and Allan E. Kazdin. 2001. "Parent Expectancies for Child Therapy: Assessment and Relation to Participation in Treatment." *Journal of Child and Family Studies*, 10 (2): 155–80.

Nock, Matthew K., and Valerie Photos. 2006. "Parent Motivation to Participate in Treatment: Assessment and Prediction of Subsequent Participation." *Journal of Child and Family Studies*, 15: 333–46. DOI: 10.1007/s10826-006-9022-4

Nock, Matthew K., Caitlin Ferriter, and Elizabeth Holmberg. 2007. "Parent Beliefs about Treatment Credibility and Effectiveness: Assessment and Relation to Subsequent Treatment Participation." *Journal of Child and Family Studies*, 16: 27–38. DOI: 10.1007/s10826-006-9064-7

Norcross, John C. 2011. *Psychotherapy Relationships that Work: Evidence-Based Responsiveness*. New York: Oxford University Press.

Safran, Jeremy D., J. Christopher Muran, and Catherine Eubanks-Carter. 2011. "Repairing Alliance Ruptures." *Psychotherapy*, 48: 80. DOI: 10.1037/a0022140

Safran, Jeremy D., J. Christopher Muran, and Lisa W. Samstag. 1994. "Resolving Therapeutic Alliance Ruptures: A Task Analytic Investigation." In A. O. Horvath and L. S. Greenberg (Eds.), *The Working Alliance: Theory, Research, and Practice* (pp. 225–55). New York: Wiley.

Safran, Jeremy D., J. Christopher Muran, Lisa W. Samstag, and Christopher Stevens. 2001. "Repairing Alliance Ruptures." *Psychotherapy: Theory, Research, Practice, Training*, 38: 406.

Sburlati, Elizabeth S., Carolyn A. Schniering, Heidi J. Lyneham, and Ronald Rapee. 2011. "A Model of Therapist Competencies for the Empirically Supported Cognitive Behavioral Treatment of Child and Adolescent Anxiety and Depressive Disorders." *Clinical Child and Family Psychology Review*, 14: 89–109. DOI: 10.1007/s10567-011-0083-6

Shirk, Stephen R., and Christopher C. Saiz. 1992. "Clinical, Empirical, and Developmental Perspectives on the Therapeutic Relationship in Child Psychotherapy." *Development and Psychopathology*, 4: 713–28. DOI: 10.1017/S0954579400004946

Turkat, Ira D., and Victor Meyer. 1982. "The Behavior-Analytic Approach." In P. L. Wachtel (Ed.), *Resistance: Psychodynamic and Behavioral Approaches* (157–84). New York: Plenum.

Wickramaratne, Priya, Marc J. Gameroff, Daniel J. Pilowsky, Carroll W. Hughes, Judy Garber, Erin Malloy, … Jonathan E. Alpert. 2011. "Children of Depressed Mothers 1 Year after Remission of Maternal Depression: Findings from the STAR*D-Child Study." *The American Journal of Psychiatry*, 168: 593–602. DOI: 10.1176/appi.ajp.2010.10010032

Yeh, May, and John R. Weisz. 2001. "Why are We Here at the Clinic? Parent–Child (Dis)agreement on Referral Problems at Outpatient Treatment Entry." *Journal of Consulting and Clinical Psychology*, 69: 1018–25. DOI: 10.1037/0022-006X.69.6.1018

7

Assessing Child and Adolescent Internalizing Disorders

Jennifer L. Hudson, Carol Newall, Sophie C. Schneider, and Talia Morris

Introduction

Internalizing disorders, including anxiety and depression, typically begin early in life and are one of the most common forms of psychopathology found in children and adolescents (Rapee, Schniering, and Hudson 2009). It can be difficult to assess for these disorders in children, as the symptoms are often unseen and can be dismissed as simply a "phase" or part of the child's personality. In contrast to other childhood disorders, such as oppositional defiant disorder, internalizing disorders can sometimes be missed by parents and teachers as the symptoms are not always observable and children may underreport their experience, to avoid causing trouble. It is vital that clinicians are able to competently detect and assess internalizing disorders, given the considerable interference caused by them within the family and across the lifespan (Merikangas et al. 2010). Undertaking a competent assessment is a fundamental step when determining the child's diagnostic profile. Moreover, it is during assessment that the therapist will develop a better understanding of the disorder-related maintaining factors, thereby becoming able to select the most appropriate intervention for the child.

Our aim in this chapter is to describe therapist competencies required for conducting a competent and thorough assessment of children and adolescents with anxiety and depressive disorders. First we will outline each of the individual competencies and discuss them in detail. Next we will outline issues that arise when conducting a competent assessment of anxiety and depression. Finally we will discuss some common obstacles to conducting a competent assessment and strategies for overcoming them.

Evidence-Based CBT for Anxiety and Depression in Children and Adolescents: A Competencies-Based Approach, First Edition. Edited by Elizabeth S. Sburlati, Heidi J. Lyneham, Carolyn A. Schniering, and Ronald M. Rapee. © 2014 John Wiley & Sons, Ltd. Published 2014 by John Wiley & Sons, Ltd.

Key Features of Competencies in Assessing Children and Adolescents

Over the last 15 years, clinical psychology has witnessed a paradigm shift toward the use of empirically supported treatments (Chambless and Hollon 1998). Not too far behind this movement is the shift toward adopting evidence-based assessments (EBAs). An evidence-based assessment framework (Hunsley and Mash 2007) demands that the therapist rely on both theory and empirical research in his or her choice of assessment procedures. As a result of this movement, a few key papers have emerged that have documented guidelines for the evidence-based assessment of anxiety and depressive disorders in children and adolescents (Klein, Dougherty, and Olino 2005; Silverman and Ollendick 2005). These guidelines are based on the rich body of research devoted to developing and evaluating assessment procedures for children and adolescents diagnosed with internalizing disorders.

Recently, Sburlati, Schniering, Lyneham, and Rapee (2011, p. 94) have added to these guidelines by outlining five key therapist competencies for conducting a thorough assessment of child and adolescent anxiety and depressive disorder. These competencies are:

1. the ability to undertake an evidence-based multi-method (e.g., self-report, observational), multi-informant (e.g., child; parent; teacher or allied health professional) psychological assessment of the disorder presentation;
2. the ability to integrate assessment reports from both the child (or adolescent) and the parent (or other parties);
3. the ability to determine a clinical diagnosis, with consideration of differential diagnosis;
4. the ability to undertake a generic assessment of the child's or adolescent's current functioning, family functioning, peer relationships, developmental history and stage, and suitability for the intervention;
5. the ability to assess and manage risk of self-harm and suicide.

Each of these competencies will be discussed in detail.

An evidence-based multi-method, multi-informant psychological assessment of the disorder presentation

Evidence-based assessment

Applying the EBA framework to psychological assessment is a crucial therapist competency, without which the success of treatment cannot be properly established. As mentioned above, there is an abundance of publications detailing different assessment methods for anxiety and depression in children and adolescents (Beidel and Alfano 2011; Brown-Jacobsen, Wallace, and Whiteside 2011; Schniering, Hudson, and Rapee 2000). The large number of assessment tools and the variation in tested populations, however, make it difficult for therapists to judge which assessment methods they should use in clinical practice for any given client. Fortunately, there has been a growing focus in recent years on providing criteria to evaluate the utility of psychological assessment measures by using the EBA framework (Hunsley and Mash 2007). EBA requires that a psychologist's choice of assessment methods should be guided by a broad set of considerations. First, for a psychological assessment method to accurately capture an internalizing disorder, it must be *highly reliable*. The reliability of a measure refers to the consistency of a client's score across differing clinicians (inter-rater reliability), across time points (test–retest reliability), and within the measure itself (internal consistency). For example, if an assessment measure does not have high test–retest reliability, a clinician is unable to conclude whether treatment changes over time reflect real changes for their client or are due to an unreliable measure.

Second, it is important that the assessment measure selected by the therapist has *established normative data* or criterion-related cut-off scores to aid a clinician in correctly interpreting his or her client's score against a larger relevant population. Norms may be used to compare a client to the general population or to specific subgroups. It is important, too, that these norms have been created from both clinical and nonclinical samples and are sensitive to age and gender. A clinician also needs to consider the child's cultural background, as norms can differ across cultures, some behaviors being considered desirable in one culture and atypical in another. Furthermore, without these norms, it is difficult for a clinician to competently conclude if his or her client's symptoms or functioning differ from those of the general population.

Third, the EBA framework requires that an assessment method have *high validity*. Specifically, is it measuring what it purports to measure? For instance, a scale that purports to measure anxiety might merely be capturing state arousal. A competent clinician should examine both the content validity (the degree to which a measure indexes all components of the construct being measured) and the construct validity (the degree to which the theoretical construct being assessed was actually measured) of a measure. A particularly good measure will also show evidence of incremental validity, that is, evidence that the measure adds unique information over and above other assessment methods. Furthermore, the EBA framework suggests that a measure should give evidence of validity generalization, which supports the use of that measure across age, gender, socioeconomic status, ethnic groups, and differing contexts – home, school, primary care, and inpatient settings.

Using the EBA framework, a competent clinician must also decide if an assessment measure demonstrates *clinical utility*. When the practical aspects of the measure are taken into account – and these include costs, administration difficulty, duration, availability of the measure, and norms – are the data gained from this measure going to demonstrate satisfactory clinical benefit? In particular, is there published evidence that the measure in question is able to detect clinical change? Table 7.1 provides therapists with a list of evidence-based assessment measures that are commonly utilized in the assessment of anxiety, depression, and related self-harm and suicide and can be used within a multi-method, multi-informant EBA.

Table 7.1 Examples of evidence-based measures for anxiety, depression, and self-harm/suicide.[a]

Measure	Delivery method	Reporter	Age group	Length
Anxiety				
ADIS C/P-IV (Silverman and Albano 1996)	Semi-structured interview	C/P	All	1–3 hours
SPAI-C (Beidel, Turner, and Morris 1995)	Self-report scale	C	8–14 years	20–30 minutes
SASC–R (la Greca and Stone 1993)	Self-report scale	C	7–13 years	10 minutes
MASC (March, Parker, Sullivan, Stallings, and Conners 1997)	Self-report scale	C	8–19 years	15 minutes
SCAS (Spence 1998)	Self-report scale	C/P	6–18 years	10 minutes
SCARED (Birmaher et al. 1997)	Self-report scale	C/P	8–18 years	10 minutes
PAS (Edwards, Rapee, Kennedy, and Spence 2010)	Self-report scale	P/T	3–5 years	10 minutes
Depression				
K-SADS (Puig-Antich and Chambers 1978)	Semi-structured interview	C/P	6–18 years	20–60 minutes
CDRS-R (Poznanski and Mokros 1999)	Self-report scale	C/P	6–12 years	15–20 minutes
CDI (Kovacs 1992)	Self-report scale	C	7–17 years	15–20 minutes
SMFQ (Angold, Costello, Messer, and Pickles 1995)	Self-report scale	C/P	8–18 years	5–10 minutes
RADS (Reynolds 1987)	Self-report scale	C	12 years +	5–10 minutes
Self-harm and suicide				
SITBI (Nock, Holmberg, Photos, and Michel 2007)	Structured interview	C/P	12–19 years	3–15 minutes
BSI (Beck and Steer 1991)	Self-report scale	C	12–17 years	5–10 minutes
SIQ (Reynolds 1988)	Self-report scale	C	12–18 years	10 minutes

[a]*Equivalences:*
C = Child;
P = Parent;
T = Teacher;
ADIS C/P-IV = Anxiety Disorders Interview Schedule for Children for DSM-IV;
SPAI-C = Social Phobia and Anxiety Inventory for Children;
SASC-R = Social Anxiety Scale for Children-Revised;

Multi-method assessment

The above criteria can be used to select high-quality assessment tools, including interviews, questionnaires, and observational methods. It is generally agreed that a competent assessment is one in which multiple methods of data collection are conducted (Kazdin 2003; Silverman and Ollendick 2005). Selecting which combination of measures to use for assessment should be guided by a consideration of the strengths and limitations of each method.

STRUCTURED OR SEMI-STRUCTURED INTERVIEWS: Structured or semi-structured interviews are considered the gold standard of assessment for internalizing disorders (Morris and Greco 2002). Research has shown that clinicians conducting unstructured interviews will often not ask about all-important elements of the relevant psychopathology and will make fewer diagnoses than in a semi-structured interview (Zimmerman 2003). A semi-structured interview ensures that a clinician covers the relevant disorder they are assessing, while also allowing for clinical judgment on differential diagnoses. During the interview the clinician is required to make an assessment of the frequency, severity, and duration of symptoms, as well as of the situations in which the child's symptoms occur. In addition, the therapist must also assess functional impairment as a consequence of the child's symptoms.

SELF-REPORT QUESTIONNAIRES: Although questionnaire methods typically don't provide enough information for making a diagnosis in isolation, they are useful tools to quickly gain information on a client's current symptoms. Due to the standardization of such measures, self-report measures are also useful for tracking changes in these symptoms over time. Therapist training for the administration and interpretation of self-report measures is less than is required for structured interviews. These factors, together, make self-reports particularly valuable in clinical settings.

OBSERVATIONAL METHODS: Observational methods are an under-utilized method for the diagnosis of anxiety disorders or depressive disorders. However, they possess clinical utility and can be useful for examining the level of fear and anxiety displayed by a client when exposed to threatening stimuli. Behavioral approach tests (i.e., client-led steps of increasing difficulty toward a feared object or situation, in a controlled

---

Table 7.1 *(cont'd)*

MASC = Multidimensional Anxiety Scale for Children;
SCAS = Spence Children's Anxiety Scale;
PAS = Preschool Anxiety Scale-Revised;
SCARED: Screen for Child Anxiety-Related Emotional Disorders;
K-SADS = Schedule for Affective Disorders and Schizophrenia for School-Age Children;
CDRS-R = Children's Depression Rating Scale-Revised;
CDI = Children's Depression Inventory;
SMFQ = Short Mood and Feelings Questionnaire;
RADS = Reynolds Adolescent Depression Scale;
SITBI = Self-Injurious Thoughts and Behaviors Interview;
BSI = Beck Scale for Suicide Ideation;
SIQ = Suicidal Ideation Questionnaire.

environment) for fears such as of dogs, needles, talking in front of others, and separation from caregivers can be conducted in clinical settings (Ollendick, Lewis, Cowart, and Davis 2012). Observational methods can also be useful for understanding specific factors – such as parental over-involvement – that may be maintaining the child's anxiety (Hudson and Rapee 2001).

Multi-informant assessment

Competent clinicians should utilize a multi-informant approach to assess for internalizing disorders in children and adolescents (Kazdin 2003; Silverman and Ollendick 2005). It is standard to assess the child and at least one parent or caregiver. This is because children may have a limited repertoire in their vocabulary to fully articulate the extent of their internalizing difficulties, or may exhibit reluctance to discuss the functional impairments related to their internalizing problems. Parents are often very helpful when filling in the narrative gaps of the child's ongoing problems across situations and across time. They are also sometimes the only source of information for certain assessment queries, such as first onset of the disorder – which may have occurred very early in the child's life, before the child was able to remember it. There are also certain diagnoses that can only be established through parent report; these include oppositional defiant disorder and conduct disorder.

Teachers and other health care providers can give additional information, though it is not always practical – or even possible – to access this information. Sending a questionnaire and consent form to parents to release information to the teacher or other health care workers can be a practical method. Engaging a child's teacher is particularly helpful in determining whether problems are context-specific to the home. This can be important for case formulation and sometimes diagnosis, in disorders such as attention deficit/hyperactivity disorder.

It is important that therapists not disregard the importance of gaining the child's perspective on the problem. Internalizing disorders, by nature, are not always observable. A child's report is sometimes more critical than those gleaned from parents and teachers, as the child often reports lower levels of internalizing symptoms (Jensen et al. 1999). Also, depressed parents may have a lower threshold for detecting depression in their children (Klein et al. 2005). Taken together with reports from other sources, such as parent and teachers, the child's perspective can provide important information, which may not be accessible if one consults only those other sources.

Integrating different sources of data

When undertaking a multi-method, multi-informant approach to assessment, data from all sources need to be integrated to generate a well-informed diagnostic profile. However, this is often a challenge for clinicians. Therapists are encouraged to be aware that some children may not be comfortable with revealing sensitive information in a face-to-face setting. In such cases self-report measures can be incrementally useful for filling in the gaps from the structured interview.

There is an extensive body of literature showing discordance between parent and child reports for anxiety and depression (Comer and Kendall 2004; De Los Reyes and Kazdin 2005). There are a number of different possible options for clinicians to decide how best to combine multi-informant reports. These include adopting the "and" rule, which requires several informants to corroborate the diagnosis, and the "or" rule, which assumes that a diagnosis is present if any informant reports it (Comer and Kendall 2004). De Los Reyes and Kazdin (2005) promote the use of the attributional bias contextual model, which suggests that informants are discrepant because of their discrepant attributions of the child's problems. The authors provide useful guidelines for clinicians as to how to best conceptualize informant discrepancies. Another procedure, referred to as the "best estimate" procedure, most closely mimics clinical practice and requires the competent clinician to use his or her best judgment on how best to combine the information (Klein et al. 2005).

As part of the "best estimate" procedure, it is important to take into account the age of the child and the symptoms being assessed. For example, a child's anxiety problems may not be observable to parents, or may manifest differently at school and at home. Symptoms may also have differing impacts for the child and the parents. For instance, parents will often report a higher level of interference for separation anxiety than will children. As a general guide, a child's report will tend to carry more weight the older she or he is. However, even very young children provide valid information and should not be ignored in a competent assessment.

Consideration of differential diagnosis

There is a high degree of comorbidity between childhood psychopathologies (Costello, Mustillo, Erkanli, Keeler, and Angold 2003). In particular, the majority of children diagnosed with an anxiety disorder will meet criteria for at least one other anxiety disorder (Benjamin, Costello, and Warren 1990; Kashani and Orvaschel 1990). There is also a high degree of overlap between anxiety and depression, anxious children being 8 to 29 times more likely to have a co-occurring depressive disorder (Costello et al. 2003; Ford, Goodman, and Meltzer 2003; Seligman and Ollendick 1998). Children with anxiety and depressive disorders also have an increased risk of externalizing disorders (Ford et al. 2003). A competent clinician will need to carefully consider the likely comorbid patterns that often occur with anxiety and mood disorders in children and adolescents. A structured or semi-structured interview covering all internalizing disorders is considered the best method for differential diagnosis in children and adolescents.

It is important to gather information on the full spectrum of child and youth psychopathology in order to make differential diagnoses, including developmental disorders and externalizing disorders. Sometimes there is a significant degree of confusion regarding child symptoms that frequently leads to misdiagnosis. For instance, children with generalized anxiety disorder (GAD) may appear inattentive in some situations (e.g., the classroom) due to high-degree engagement with worried thoughts, which results in an inability to concentrate on the task. Such symptoms should be considered as related to the diagnosis of GAD rather than to attention deficit hyperactivity disorder – inattentive type. Similarly, children with separation anxiety disorder who refuse to participate in activities requiring separation from their caregiver should not be given an additional diagnosis of oppositional defiant disorder purely on the basis of their opposition during feared situations. Such behaviors should be conceptualized as fearful avoidance rather than as a true behavior disorder.

Given the high occurrence of somatic symptoms in anxiety and depressive disorders, a clinician should also ensure that the child has received a medical work-up, to rule out any medical conditions that could explain the child's somatic symptoms. Further, there is a high degree of comorbidity between internalizing disorders and physical conditions – for instance asthma (Katon, Richardson, Lozano, and McCauley 2004). A medical examination will also allow the potential detection of comorbid physical conditions.

Assessment of current functioning, family functioning, peer relationships, developmental history and stage, and suitability for the intervention

A thorough assessment should consider broader factors that have important clinical implications for child and adolescent clients. These factors include the child's developmental level and functioning within systems such as the family unit, peers, and schools.

Developmental factors
It is important for the clinician to gain information about the child's developmental history and stage in order to ensure that the assessment methods selected are appropriate. A child's developmental level refers to his or her cognitive, biological, emotional, and social functioning, and how it compares against predictable age-related functioning in his or her developmental cohort. The therapist needs to consider not only the child's difficulties with internalizing problems, but also the normative skills, present or absent, that could impact on how well the child responds to the model of treatment selected. For instance, studies have shown that the effect of cognitive behavioral therapy (CBT) depends on age (e.g., Durlak, Furnham, and Lampman 1991), which suggests that some children may not have the developmental ability needed for cognitive therapy to be successful (Reinecke, Dattilio, and Freeman 1996).

While the child's chronological age provides a guideline regarding his or her developmental abilities, children differ in terms of their developmental profile. Hence the therapist should not use age as the only determinant of the child's abilities, but rather should be informally assessing for the child's abilities irrespective of age. This requires knowledge of child development research (seen in Chapter 5) and the ability to assess for this feature during the assessment session. The therapist who is able to take into account the child's developmental abilities at assessment stage will be able to select the most appropriate model of intervention for that child.

At assessment, the therapist must also have a sound knowledge base of developmental norms in order to make reliable diagnostic judgments (Holmbeck, Devine, and Bruno 2010). For instance, very young children, around the 24 months of age, will peak in behaviors that mimic obsessive–compulsive symptoms (Zohar and Felz 2001). However, these "compulsive" behaviors can be a part of normal development when they do not significantly interfere with daily functioning and when there is no family history of obsessive–compulsive disorder (Leckman, Bloch, and King 2009). Similarly, cognitive biases observed in children may be a reflection of a normal developmental progression rather than a symptom of an internalizing disorder. For instance, young non-anxious children have been found to endorse catastrophic and personalizing biases more than older non-anxious children (Leitenberg, Yost, and Carroll-Wilson 1986), which suggests that these biases are a reflection of developmental progression rather than symptomatic of a childhood anxiety disorder. More broadly, it is also worth noting that fear, anxiety, and sadness are normal human emotions, experienced universally. Young children experience a large number of fears (fear of separation, fear of the dark), and this is characterized as a *normal* developmental process (Gullone 2000).

A competent therapist will need to be able to extract from assessment how many of these child characteristics are indicative of normal development and how many represent more serious symptoms of an internalizing disorder. For parents, and for clinicians, it can be difficult to determine the point at which the frequency, severity, and duration of these emotions and behaviors are abnormal and require intervention. A semi-structured interview such as the ADIS-C/P is a useful guide, given that it takes into account the level of interference as a way of determining disorder diagnosis in clinical judgments. Beyond the semi-structured interview, the clinician can also determine the specific degree to which life is altered as a result of the symptoms: What is the child missing out on? How would life be different if these symptoms were removed? Determining the degree of interference is crucial in deciding on the clinical nature of the problem. A multi-informant assessment will also make this decision easier, as the clinician can determine whether the behaviors are observable to others outside the home. However, regardless of the technique used at assessment, a competent therapist should stay abreast of the developmental literature, to help guide his or her diagnostic judgment and case formulation at assessment (Holmbeck et al. 2010).

Finally, not only is developmental sensitivity integral to determining diagnoses, it is also important in choosing the format for the assessment. For preschool children, clinicians may choose to rely solely on parent report (e.g., Hudson, Dodd, and Bovopoulos 2011; Rapee, Kennedy, Ingram, Edwards, and Sweeney 2005). In contrast, for adolescents, self-report is given more weight in deciding on the diagnostic profile.

Multi-systemic approach: Family, peers, and school

Given the importance of a child's or adolescent's family and social environment, the therapist needs to fully appreciate systemic issues surrounding the child or the adolescent in order to accurately assess his or her ongoing difficulties and devise a treatment plan that takes into account these important factors (Friedberg and McClure 2002). Within the family unit, consideration should be given to family functioning, parent behaviors (e.g., overprotection, lack of autonomy granting, critical parenting), and parent psychopathology, since these factors can function as maintaining influences on the internalizing problems, or as potential obstacles or strengths during intervention. For instance, parental mental health problems pose a risk for childhood internalizing problems (Gravener et al. 2012) that can limit optimal treatment outcomes for the child (Cobham, Dadds, and Spence 1998; Hudson et al. 2013), and are linked to parent attrition from treatment (Lyneham and Rapee 2006; Waters, Wharton, and Cobham 2009).

A therapist who takes current or past parental anxiety or depression into account at assessment may devote more time to establish rapport, trust, and psycho-education around anxiety and depression with the parent. This may be especially important for young children, given that parents play a more influential role in younger children's lives than in that of adolescents, when peers become the dominant social influence. Although some of the research suggests that treatment of parental mental health disorder may have limited impact on the child's treatment outcomes (Cobham et al. 1998), providing the parent with the appropriate rationale for each intervention technique and with psycho-education about childhood internalizing disorders may increase parental engagement and willingness to allow the child to participate in certain treatment techniques that are anxiety-provoking for the parent (e.g., exposure therapy), thus preventing attrition from the program.

Taking into account a multi-informant approach at assessment across various settings – for instance, paying heed to whether the child exhibits problems at school, or to the teacher's perspective – also allows the therapist to evaluate whether the child's internalizing problems manifest themselves across contexts. This approach is particularly informative, given that, if the problems only arise in a specific setting, there may be situationally based factors that maintain them – such as bullying at school, parent disciplining styles, family dispute, or stress at home. Therefore, when assessing the child, a therapist who has thoroughly assessed familial, school, and peer factors can also plan to target these maintaining factors during treatment (e.g., address the issue of bullying with the child, the parents, and the teachers). Teachers may also be a unique source of information about the child's social development and peer engagement, given that they are more likely than parents to observe the child with other children. For instance, a teacher's report of poor social skills suggests that some of the child's anxious thoughts about social evaluation are not distorted and that treatment may need to prioritize the development of social skills in the course of the intervention.

Assessing the risk of self-harm and suicide

Children and adolescents with internalizing disorders are at an elevated risk of self-harm and suicide (Dougherty, Klein, Olino, and Laptook 2008; Hill, Castellanos, and Pettit 2011). Although self-injurious behaviors are more common in adolescents, it is important for the clinician to be aware that young children can also experience self-injurious thoughts and behaviors, and can attempt suicide. Therefore it is essential to routinely assess for the presence and severity of these problems in children of all ages. There is a number of structured and semi-structured interviews developed for the purpose of assessing self-injurious thoughts and behaviors – interviews that are suitable for use with children and adolescents (see Table 7.1). Before beginning an assessment for self-harm and suicide, a competent clinician should have a pre-existing framework for dealing effectively with self-harm/suicidal thoughts and behaviors if they are disclosed. It is vital to provide information to families about referral options, including access to emergency treatment and out-of-hours assistance. Also, when discussing these issues with the child, it is important to provide age-appropriate information about a clinician's duty of care and the limits of confidentiality. This is needed so as to not damage the therapeutic alliance in case it is necessary to inform the parent about previously undisclosed risk. A clinician will take into consideration the age of the child and the relevant legislation that may guide his or her decisions in this area.

In addition to assessing for self-harm and suicide, clinicians should be mindful of other forms of risk to children and adolescents, such as domestic violence in the home and abuse or neglect of children and adolescents. A clinician is to be mindful that, when assessing parental disciplining techniques, there is no risk to the child or adolescent. There are also considerations specific to children with internalizing disorders. For instance, there have been cases where parents were so protective of their anxious child that these children would log extensive absenteeism from school. This is considered borderline abuse and can be subject to mandatory reporting. Alternatively, a clinician may find out that the child's excessive anxiety is coming from considerable violence occurring at home between the parents. It is important to be aware that one of the best predictors of child physical abuse is domestic violence between the parents.

A competent therapist will need to have knowledge of his or her national and local guidelines for mandatory reporting. Clinicians must keep themselves updated in the matter of child protection policies in their country and always seek supervision from experienced colleagues when assessing the risk of harm.

Competence in Assessing the Anxiety Disorders and Depression

As mentioned above, anxiety and depressive disorders are frequently comorbid, particularly during adolescence, after the emergence of puberty (King, Gullone, and Ollendick 1990; Seligman and Ollendick 1998). Thus, when a child is displaying either anxiety or depression, a competent clinician needs to assess for both conditions. Recent evidence has also emerged showing that anxiety-disordered children with comorbid mood disorders have worse end-point outcomes after treatment (Rapee et al., 2013). Thus determining the degree of comorbidity between anxiety and depression is useful at the outset of treatment.

The domains of anxiety and mood disorders also overlap somewhat. For example, children with either disorder frequently report somatic and concentration problems. Even the best EBA self-report measures cannot perfectly distinguish between different disorders. Good assessment measures will converge most with the domains they are meant to be tapping, but some overlap is expected. This means that children who have one condition might be more likely to score higher on measures assessing the other condition, even if only one condition is "purely" present.

Common Obstacles to Competent Assessment

Parent and child disagreement

Novice clinicians often find it difficult to determine a diagnostic profile when the child and the parent have completely different views on the problem. For example, the adolescent may report that he or she has no fear or anxiety, while the parents report excessive fear and avoidance of numerous situations. Some children and adolescents may be unwilling participants in the assessment process, and this can be caused by a number of factors – such as stigma associated with mental health problems, not being told about the assessment, or conflict with the parents (to name just a few). Children and adolescents rarely seek treatment on their own and, as a result, the assessment process is likely to create some discomfort for the child. It can be useful for clinicians to determine the child's perspective on seeking treatment and whether he or she has an understanding of why he or she had been referred to the clinic at the *beginning* of the child clinical interview.

Disagreement between reporters is a common problem when assessing internalizing disorders in children and adolescents. In the section on integrating sources of the data we have identified a number of methods that have been proposed in the literature and that can be useful in determining the final diagnostic profile.

Developmentally sensitive pitch

A frequent problem experienced by clinicians is determining the appropriate level at which to pitch interview questions. Novice therapists often "talk down" to older children or adolescents, or they do the opposite – they "pitch too high" in the case of younger children. A key to this is to use a tone of voice that is respectful to the child as an individual and to avoid patronizing tones or childish voices. The first assessment is a critical period for developing an alliance with the child (see Chapter 6), so accurately determining the level at which to pitch your questions is important.

For many children and adolescents who are already fearful or sad, attending an assessment can be an extremely overwhelming and terrifying experience. Use the skills identified in Chapter 6 to allay the child's concerns by engaging in non-threatening activities (play, games, drawing) at the start of the assessment. Normalizing fear and sadness is also a critical part of the assessment, designed to reduce the child's concerns about being "weird" and to increase the chances that the child will disclose his or her own fears and sadness.

Conclusion

Adopting an evidence-based approach to guide the assessment of child and adolescent anxiety and depression is the key to a competent and thorough assessment. A multimethod (e.g., interviews, questionnaires), multiple-informant (e.g., child, parent, teacher) approach is likely to result in the most thorough assessment of the child's problem, allowing the clinician to accurately determine the child's clinical diagnosis and to differentiate specific disorders. This can be a challenging task for the clinician who assesses child and adolescent internalizing disorders, due to the high degree of comorbidity and to the higher levels of informant discrepancy. Finally, the clinician should consider the child's difficulties in the context of that child's environment (e.g., cultural background, school, family, peers) and of his or her developmental level and stage.

References

Angold, Adrian, Elizabeth J. Costello, Stephen C. Messer, and Andrew Pickles. 1995. "Development of a Short Questionnaire for Use in Epidemiological Studies of Depression in Children and Adolescents." *International Journal of Methods in Psychiatric Research*, 5: 237–49.

Beck, Aaron T., and Robert A. Steer. 1991. *Manual for the Beck Scale for Suicide Ideation*. San Antonio, TX: The Psychological Corporation.

Beidel, Deboarh C., and Candice A. Alfano. 2011. *Child Anxiety Disorders*. New York: Routledge.

Beidel, Deborah C., Samuel M. Turner, and Tracy L. Morris. 1995. "A New Inventory to Assess Childhood Social Anxiety and Phobia: The Social Phobia and Anxiety Inventory for Children." *Psychological Assessment*, 7: 73–9.

Benjamin, Richardean S., Elizabeth J. Costello, and Marcia Warren. 1990. "Anxiety Disorders in a Pediatric Sample." *Journal of Anxiety Disorders*, 4: 293–16.

Birmaher, Boris, Suneeta Khetarpal, David Brent, Marlane Cully, Lisa Balach, Joan Kaufman, and Sandra Mckenzie Neer. 1997. "The Screen for Child Anxiety Related Emotional Disorders (SCARED): Scale Construction and Psychometric Characteristics." *Journal of the American Academy of Child and Adolescent Psychiatry*, 36: 545–53. DOI: 10.1097/00004583-199704000-00018

Brown-Jacobsen, Amy M., Dustin P. Wallace, and Stephen P. H. Whiteside. 2011. "Multi-method, Multi-Informant Agreement, and Positive Predictive Value in the Identification of Child Anxiety Disorders Using the SCAS and ADIS-C." *Assessment*, 18: 382–92. DOI: 10.1177/1073191110375792

Chambless, Dianne L., and Steven D. Hollon. 1998. "Defining Empirically Supported Therapies." *Journal of Consulting and Clinical Psychology*, 66: 7–18.

Cobham, Vanessa E., Mark R. Dadds, and Susan H. Spence. 1998. "The Role of Parental Anxiety in the Treatment of Childhood Anxiety." *Journal of Consulting and Clinical Psychology*, 66: 893–905.

Comer, Jonathan S., and Philip C. Kendall. 2004. "A Symptom-Level Examination of Parent–Child Agreement in the Diagnosis of Anxious Youths." *Journal of the American Academy of Child & Adolescent Psychiatry*, 43: 878–886. DOI: 10.1097/01.chi.0000125092.35109.c5

Costello, Elizabeth J., Sarah Mustillo, Alaattin Erkanli, Gordon Keeler, and Adrian Angold. 2003. "Prevalence and Development of Psychiatric Disorders in Childhood and Adolescence." *Archives of General Psychiatry*, 60: 837–44. DOI: 10.1001/archpsyc.60.8.837

De Los Reyes, Andres, and Alan E. Kazdin. 2005. "Informant Discrepancies in the Assessment of Childhood Psychopathology: A Critical Review, Theoretical Framework, and Recommendations for Further Study." *Psychological Bulletin*, 131: 483–509. DOI: 10.1037/0033-2909.131.4.483

Dougherty, Lea R., Daniel N. Klein, Thomas M. Olino, and Rebecca S. Laptook. 2008. "Depression in Children and Adolescents." In *A guide to assessments that work*, edited by John Hunsley and Eric J. Mash (pp. 69–95). New York: Oxford University Press.

Durlak, Joseph A., Teresa Furnham, and Claudia Lampman. 1991. "Effectiveness of Cognitive Behaviour Therapy for Maladapting Children: A Meta-Analysis." *Psychological Bulletin*, 110: 204–14.

Edwards, Susan L., Ronald M. Rapee, Susan J. Kennedy, and Susan H. Spence. 2010. "The Assessment of Anxiety Symptoms in Preschool-Aged Children: The Revised Preschool Anxiety Scale." *Journal of Clinical Child and Adolescent Psychology*, 39: 400–9. DOI: 10.1080/15374411003691701

Ford, Tamsin, Robert Goodman, and Howard Meltzer. 2003. "The British Child and Adolescent Mental Health Survey 1999: The Prevalence of DSM-IV Disorders." *Journal of the American Academy of Child and Adolescent Psychiatry*, 42: 1203–11. DOI: 10.1097/00004583-200310000-00011

Friedberg, Robert D., and Jessica M. McClure. 2002. *Clinical Practice of Cognitive Therapy with Children and Adolescents*. New York: Guilford Press.

Gravener, Julie A., Fred A. Rogosch, Assaf Oshri, Angela J. Narayan, Dante Cicchetti, and Sheree L. Toth. 2012. "The Relations among Maternal Depressive Disorder, Maternal

Expressed Emotion, and Toddler Behavior Problems and Attachment." *Journal of Abnormal Child Psychology*, 40: 803–13. DOI: 10.1007/s10802-011-9598-z

Gullone, Eleonora. 2000. "The Development of Normal Fear: A Century of Research." *Clinical Psychology Review*, 20: 429–51.

Hill, Ryan M., Daniel Castellanos, and Jeremy W. Pettit. 2011. "Suicide-Related Behaviors and Anxiety in Children and Adolescents: A Review." *Clinical Psychology Review*, 31: 1133–44. DOI: 10.1016/j.cpr.2011.07.008

Holmbeck, Grayson N., Katie A. Devine, and Elizabeth F. Bruno. 2010. "Developmental Issues and Considerations in Research and Practice." In Alan E. Kazdin and John R. Weisz (Eds.), *Evidence-Based Psychotherapies for Children and Adolescents* (pp. 28–44). New York: Guilford Press.

Hudson, Jennifer L., and Ronald M. Rapee. 2001. "Parent–Child Interactions and Anxiety Disorders: An Observational Study." *Behaviour Research and Therapy*, 39: 1411–27. DOI: 10.1016/S0005-7967(00)00107-8

Hudson, Jennifer L., Helen Dodd, and Nataly Bovopoulos. 2011. "Temperament, Family Environment and Anxiety in Preschool Children." *Journal of Abnormal Child Psychology*, 39: 939–51. DOI: 10.1007/s10802-011-9502-x. DOI: 10.1007/s10802-011-9502-x

Hudson, Jennifer L., Carol Newall, Ronald M. Rapee, Heidi J. Lyneham, Carolyn A. Schneiring, Viviana M. Wuthrich, … Natalie S. Gar. 2013. "The Impact of Parental Anxiety Management on Child Anxiety Treatment Outcomes: A Controlled Trial." *Journal of Clinical Child & Adolescent Psychology*. DOI: 10.1080/15374416.2013.807734

Hunsley, John, and Eric J. Mash. 2007. "Evidence-Based Assessment." *Annual Review of Clinical Psychology*, 3: 29–51. DOI: 10.1146/annurev.clinpsy.3.022806.091419.

Jensen, Peter S., Maritza Rubio-Stipec, Glorisa Canino, Hector R. Bird, Mina K. Dulcan, Mary E. Schwab-Stone, and Benjamin B. Lahey. 1999. "Parent and Child Contributions to Diagnosis of Mental Disorder: Are Both Informants Always Necessary?" *Journal of the American Academy of Child and Adolescent Psychiatry*, 38: 1569–79.

Kashani, Javad H., and Helen Orvaschel. 1990. "A Community Study of Anxiety in Children and Adolescents." *American Journal of Psychiatry*, 147: 313–18.

Katon, Wayne J., Laura Richardson, Paula Lozano, and Elizabeth McCauley. 2004. "The Relationship of Asthma and Anxiety Disorders." *Psychosomatic Medicine*, 66: 349–55. DOI: 10.1097/01.psy.0000126202.89941.ea

Kazdin, Alan E. 2003. *Methodological Issues and Strategies in Clinical Research* (3rd ed.). Washington, DC: American Psychological Association.

King, Neville J., Eleonora Gullone, and Thomas H. Ollendick. 1990. "Childhood Anxiety Disorders and Depression: Phenomenology, Comorbidity, and Intervention Issues." *Scandinavian Journal of Behaviour Therapy*, 19: 59–70.

Klein, Daniel N., Lea R. Dougherty, and Thomas M. Olino. 2005. "Toward Guidelines for Evidence-Based Assessment of Depression in Children and Adolescents." *Journal of Clinical Child & Adolescent Psychology*, 34: 412–32. DOI: 10.1207/s15374424jccp3403_3

Kovacs, Maria. 1992. *Children's Depression Inventory Manual*. North Tonawanda, NY: Multi-Health Systems.

la Greca, Annette M., and Wendy L. Stone. 1993. "Social Anxiety Scale for Children –Revised: Factor Structure and Concurrent Validity." *Journal of Clinical Child Psychology*, 22: 17–27.

Leckman, James F., Michael H. Bloch, and Robert A. King. 2009. "Symptom Dimensions and Subtypes of Obsessive–Compulsive Disorder: A Developmental Perspective." *Dialogues in Clinical Neuroscience*, 11: 21–33.

Leitenberg, Harold, Leonard W. Yost, and Marilyn Carroll-Wilson. 1986. "Negative Cognitive Errors in Children: Questionnaire Development, Normative Cognitive Errors, and Comparisons between Children with and without Self-Reported Symptoms of Depression, Low

Self-Esteem and Evaluation Anxiety." *Journal of Consulting and Clinical Practice*, 54: 528–36. DOI: 10.1037/0022-006X.54.4.528

Lyneham, Heidi J., and Ronald M. Rapee. 2006. "Evaluation of Therapist-Supported Parent-Implemented CBT for Anxiety Disorders in Rural Children." *Behaviour Research and Therapy*, 44: 1287–300. DOI: 10.1016/j.brat.2005.09.009

March, John S., James D. Parker, Kevin Sullivan, Patricia Stallings, and C. Keith Conners. 1997. "The Multidimensional Anxiety Scale for Children (MASC): Factor Structure, Reliability, and Validity." *Journal of the American Academy of Child & Adolescent Psychiatry*, 36: 554–65. DOI: 10.1097/00004583-199704000-00019

Merikangas, Kathleen Ries, Jian-ping He, Marcy Burstein, Sonja A. Swanson, Shelli Avenevoli, Lihong Cui, … Joel Swendsen. 2010. "Lifetime Prevalence of Mental Disorders in US Adolescents: Results from the National Comorbidity Survey Replication–Adolescent Supplement (NCS-A)." *Journal of The American Academy of Child & Adolescent Psychiatry*, 49: 980–9. DOI: 10.1016/j.jaac.2010.05.017

Morris, Tracy L., and Laurie A. Greco. 2002. "Assessment and Treatment of Childhood Anxiety Disorders." In Leon VandeCreek (Ed.), *Innovations in Clinical Practice: A Source Book*, vol. 20. Sarasota, FL: Professional Resource Press, pp. 76–86.

Nock, Matthew K., Elizabeth B. Holmberg, Valerie I. Photos, and Bethany D. Michel. 2007. "Self-Injurious Thoughts and Behaviors Interview: Development, Reliability, and Validity in an Adolescent Sample." *Psychological Assessment*, 19: 309–17. DOI: 10.1037/1040-3590.19.3.309

Ollendick, Thomas H., Krystal M. Lewis, Maria J. W. Cowart, and Thompson Davis. 2012. "Prediction of Child Performance on a Parent–Child Behavioral Approach Test with Animal Phobic Children." *Behavior Modification*, 36: 509–24. DOI: 10.1177/0145445512448191

Poznanski, Elva O., and Hartmut B. Mokros. 1999. *Children Depression Rating Scale – Revised (CDRS-R)*. Los Angeles, CA: Western Psychological Services.

Puig-Antich, Joaquim, and William Chambers. 1978. *The Schedule for Affective Disorders and Schizophrenia for School-Age Children*. NY: New York State Psychiatric Institute.

Rapee, Ronald M., Carolyn A. Schniering, and Jennifer L. Hudson. 2009. "Anxiety Disorders during Childhood and Adolescence: Origins and Treatment." *Annual Review of Clinical Psychology*, 5: 335–65. DOI: 10.1146/annurev.clinpsy.032408.153628

Rapee, Ronald M., Susan Kennedy, Michelle Ingram, Susan Edwards, and Lynne Sweeney. 2005. "Prevention and Early Intervention of Anxiety Disorders in Inhibited Preschool Children." *Journal of Consulting and Clinical Psychology*, 73: 488–97. DOI: 10.1037/0022-006X.73.3.488

Rapee, Ronald M., Heidi J. Lyneham, Jennifer L. Hudson, Maria Kangas, Viviana M. Wuthrich, and Carolyn A. Schniering. 2013. "Effect of Comorbidity on Treatment of Anxious Children and Adolescents: Results from a Large, Combined Sample." *Journal of the American Academy of Child and Adolescent Psychiatry*, 52: 47–56. DOI: 10.1016/j.jaac.2012.10.002

Reinecke, Mark A., Frank M. Dattilio, and Arthur Freeman. 1996. *Cognitive Therapy with Children: A Casebook for Clinical Practice*. New York: Guilford.

Reynolds, William M. 1987. *Reynolds Adolescent Depression Scale: Professional Manual*. Odessa, FL: Psychological Assessment Resources.

Reynolds, William M. 1988. *Suicide Ideation Questionnaire: Professional Manual*. Odessa, FL: Psychological Assessment Resources.

Sburlati, Elizabeth S., Carolyn A. Schniering, Heidi J. Lyneham., and Ronald M. Rapee. 2011. "A Model of Therapist Competencies for the Empirically Supported Cognitive Behavioral

Treatment of Child and Adolescent Anxiety and Depressive Disorders." *Clinical Child and Family Psychology Review*, 14: 89–109. DOI: 10.1007/s10567-011-0083-6

Schniering, Carolyn A., Jennifer L. Hudson, and Ronald M. Rapee. 2000. "Issues in the Diagnosis and Assessment of Anxiety Disorders in Children and Adolescents." *Clinical Psychology Review*, 20: 453–478. DOI: 10.1016/S0272-7358(99)00037-9

Seligman, Laura D., and Thomas H. Ollendick. 1998. "Comorbidity of Anxiety and Depression in Children and Adolescents: An Integrative Review." *Clinical Child and Family Psychology Review*, 1: 125–44.

Silverman, Wendy K., and Anne Marie Albano. 1996. *The Anxiety Disorders Interview Schedule for Children for DSM-IV: Child and Parent Versions.* San Antonio, TX: Psychological Corporation.

Silverman, Wendy K., and Thomas H. Ollendick. 2005. "Evidence-Based Assessment of Anxiety and Its Disorders in Children and Adolescents." *Journal of Clinical Child & Adolescent Psychology*, 34: 380–411. DOI: 10.1207/s15374424jccp3403_2

Spence, Susan H. 1998. "A Measure of Anxiety Symptoms among Children." *Behaviour Research and Therapy*, 36: 545–66.

Waters, Allison M., Louise A. Ford, Trisha A. Wharton, and Vanessa E. Cobham. 2009. "Cognitive–Behavioural Therapy for Young Children with Anxiety Disorders: Comparisons of a Child + Parent Condition versus a Parent Only Condition." *Behaviour Research and Therapy*, 47: 654–62. DOI: 10.1016/j.brat.2009.04.008

Zimmerman, Mark. 2003. "What Should the Standard of Care for Psychiatric Diagnostic Evaluations Be?" *The Journal of Nervous and Mental Disease*, 191, 281–6.

Zohar, Ada H., and Levia Felz. 2001. "Ritualistic behavior in young children." *Journal of Abnormal Child Psychology*, 29: 121–8. DOI: 10.1023/A:1005231912747

Part II
CBT Competencies

8

Theoretical Foundations of CBT for Anxious and Depressed Youth

Sarah J. Perini and Ronald M. Rapee

Introduction

A therapist wishing to implement cognitive behavior therapy with depressed and anxious youth should be familiar with the theories that underpin the treatment protocols (Sburlati, Schniering, Lyneham, and Rapee, 2011). The present chapter will introduce the factors that, according to research and theory, play a role in the maintenance of these disorders; and this will lead to separate integrated models for anxiety and for depression in youth. The similarities between the two models will be highlighted by way of a conclusion.

The Cognitive Behavioral Theoretical Framework

Cognitive behavior therapy is a structured, present-focused and time-limited psychotherapy that emphasizes the role of cognitions and behaviors in the development and maintenance of psychological difficulties. It is based on the cognitive model, which highlights the interaction between a person's cognitive processes, his/her emotional experience and his/her behavioral response. While cognitive behavior therapy was originally developed for the treatment of adults, numerous controlled-outcome studies have demonstrated its effectiveness for children and adolescents with affective and anxiety disorders (Cartwright-Hatton, Roberts, Chitsabesan, Fothergill and Harrington 2004; Harrington, Whittaker, Shoebridge, and Campbell 1998).

Evidence-Based CBT for Anxiety and Depression in Children and Adolescents: A Competencies-Based Approach,
First Edition. Edited by Elizabeth S. Sburlati, Heidi J. Lyneham, Carolyn A. Schniering, and Ronald M. Rapee.
© 2014 John Wiley & Sons, Ltd. Published 2014 by John Wiley & Sons, Ltd.

Maintaining Factors in Childhood and Adolescent Depression

Family factors

Attachment theory

Attachment theorists propose that an individual's earliest relationships are crucially linked to their emotional experiences later in life. Bowlby (1980) argues that a child's bonds to his/her primary caregivers form the basis of his/her internal working model (IWM) of attachment figures and, on that basis, of the child's complementary model of him-/herself – that is, of his/her own self. A child who has experienced consistent sensitive and responsive caregiving is likely to become *securely* attached and will consequently develop an expectation that important others are available, accessible, and supportive of their needs. The child's complementary view of his/her self will be as someone valuable, lovable, and worthy of consistent support. Conversely, a child who has experienced caregiving that is inconsistent and largely determined by the caregiver's own needs is likely to develop an *anxious* attachment, whereby they feel they have little control over the others' responsiveness and become preoccupied with the attachment figures' availability. Bowlby (1980) postulates that anxiously attached children are likely to doubt their own efficacy and worth and are therefore particularly vulnerable to depression. This vulnerability is especially acute when they are faced with the loss of a close relationship, no matter whether through illness, death, or some other form of separation.

Parenting style

The role of caregivers, particularly in infancy but also in later childhood, is seen as crucial to the development of a child's sense of self (Bowlby 1980) or schemas (Beck 1967), and theories of youth depression consistently identify the important role of a child's earliest relationships. There is extensive evidence linking parental factors to depressed youth, including the vastly higher rates of depression among children of depressed parents (Weissman, Warner, Wickramaratne, Moreau, and Olfson, 1997) and a well-established relationship between parenting style and child depression. In particular, parenting that is characterized by high levels of psychological control (overprotectiveness, guilt induction, shaming, intrusiveness) combined with low warmth has, in several studies, been linked to child depression (Alloy, Abramson, Smith, Gibb, and Neeren 2006; McLeod, Weisz, and Wood 2007; Rapee 1997). Parents of depressed children have been observed to be more critical (McCarty, Lau, Valeri, and Weisz 2004); so, unsurprisingly, depressed youth have been found to have less supportive and more conflicted relationships with their parents (Sheeber and Sorensen 1998; Sheeber, Davis, Leve, Hops, and Tildesley 2007). Additionally, parental marital conflict has been strongly associated with child depression, although it must be noted that this association applies to child psychopathology in general, not just to depression (Cummings 1994). Readers interested in the family factors relating to youth depression are referred to the comprehensive review by Restifo and Bögels (2009).

Cognitive factors

Cognitive theories of depression posit that some individuals have particular ways of thinking and processing information, which leave them vulnerable to becoming depressed when they encounter particular external stressors. Essentially, cognitive theories identify two factors – cognitive vulnerability and stress – which interact to produce a third factor – depression. Each of these three factors exists on a continuum (Abramson, Metalsky, and Alloy 1989). The more extreme the stress, the less cognitive vulnerability will be necessary to trigger the onset of depressive symptoms. Conversely, the more cognitively vulnerable an individual is, the less severe a stressor need be for depressive symptoms to emerge. Finally, the severity of the depressive symptoms themselves will depend on the severity of both these causal factors, in addition to the content of the thought processes that follow the stressful event. Content that is situation-specific is posited to lead to less severe depression than content that is generalized.

Beck's cognitive theory
Beck's cognitive theory centers on the construct of schemas (Beck 1983), which are defined as stored bodies of knowledge that affect the encoding, comprehension, and retrieval of information. According to Beck, some individuals have depressogenic schemas, which encompass a range of dysfunctional attitudes relating to themes of loss, failure, inadequacy, and worthlessness. Beck postulates that such schemas lie dormant until the individual encounters a negative life event, at which point they are activated and trigger a pattern of negatively biased, self-referencing information processing. The individual makes errors in thinking (such as overgeneralization) that lead to negative cognitive patterns about three areas: the world, the self, and the future. Beck refers to this as the negative cognitive triad and argues that, once the triad develops, depressive symptoms inevitably ensue.

Hopelessness theory
Hopelessness theory (Abramson et al. 1989) is a revision of the reformulated helplessness theory of depression (Abramson, Seligman, and Teasdale, 1978). Like Beck's theory, hopelessness theory proposes that some individuals exhibit a depressogenic cognitive style that leaves them vulnerable to depression when a negative event occurs. However, hopelessness theory identifies a specific subtype of depression, called hopelessness depression. Hopelessness is defined as having the expectation that negative events will occur, that positive events will not occur, and that one is powerless to change this situation. The theory identifies the inferential styles that make one vulnerable to becoming hopeless. These are tendencies (1) to attribute negative events to global and stable causes; (2) to perceive negative events as having many disastrous consequences; and (3) to view the self as flawed and deficient following negative events. According to hopelessness theory, each of these inferential styles increases the chances of the occurrence of hopelessness. Hopelessness then leads to hopelessness depression.

Cognitive factors in children and adolescents
There is evidence that depressed youth exhibit a negative distortion in self-perception (Asarnow and Bates 1988; Hammen 1988; Kendall, Stark, and Adam 1990); but there have been some questions raised about the utility of cognitive theories when

applied to child and adolescent populations. For example, Cole and Turner (1993) have argued that depression at younger ages results most directly from encountering negative life events and from subsequent environmental feedback rather than from the interaction of negative attributional style with stress. In a review of the literature regarding cognitive theories of depression in children and adolescents, Lakdawalla, Hankin, and Mermelstein (2007) concluded that the magnitude of effect for the cognitive vulnerability–stress interaction is in the small range in child populations and moderately larger in adolescent populations. More recently, however, evidence suggests that cognitive vulnerability theories may emerge as being more applicable to child populations when researchers statistically control for cognitive development (Weitlauf and Cole 2012).

Behavioral factors

Interpersonal skills

Interpersonal theories of depression emphasize the role of social relationships in the maintenance of depression. Theorists such as Coyne (1976) and Joiner (2002) argue that depressed individuals unintentionally generate interpersonal stress and conflict. Depressed individuals may generate this conflict both by selecting unsuitable relationships and by behaving in ways that cause relational difficulties. Interpersonal conflicts then serve to prolong or intensify depressive symptoms and result in the future recurrence of depression.

Rudolph, Flynn, and Abaied (2008), present an interpersonal model of youth depression that integrates traditional interpersonal theories with a developmental psychology perspective. They propose that early family disruption – such as insecure attachment or parental depression – interferes with the development of social competencies, resulting in social–behavioral deficits. Examples of such deficits are excessive reassurance seeking, social disengagement, social helplessness, aggression, and ineffective interpersonal problem solving. These social–behavioral deficits lead to relationship disturbances and cause youth to select maladaptive relationships, which add to the ongoing difficulties that may already exist within their family. Rudolph and colleagues (2008) argue that such relationship disturbances create a vulnerability to depression, and that this vulnerability is especially marked in youth whose personalities and sociocognitive styles make them particularly reactive to interpersonal stress. As youth move into adolescence, they are faced with a number of challenges such as the changes of puberty, the emergence of romantic relation-ships, and the growing complexity of peer relationships. Any interpersonal vulnera-bility to depression is therefore amplified at this time; this is particularly true of girls, who are more likely to rely on relationships as a source of self-definition. Depressive symptoms then interfere with young people's interpersonal functioning and long-term social development, increasing their chances of further depressive episodes.

In a longitudinal study of young adolescents over two years, Flynn and Rudolph (2011) found that avoidance and denial in response to stress predicted subsequent self-generated interpersonal stress, and that this type of stress predicted, in turn, depression. There is also evidence that particular interpersonal behaviors are predictive of subsequent stress and conflict within child and adolescent relationships. These maladaptive behaviors include excessive reassurance seeking about one's worth (Prinstein, Borelli, Cheah, Simon, and Aikins 2005; Shih, Abela, and Starrs, 2009), being unassertive or overly dependent on others (Shih and Eberhart, 2008), and negative feedback seeking (Borelli and Prinstein 2006).

Rumination
Response styles theory (Nolen-Hoeksema 1991) proposes that the way an individual responds to his/her own depressive symptoms impacts the severity and duration of these symptoms. In particular, Nolen-Hoeksema (1991) identifies rumination (as opposed to distraction or problem solving) as a response style that intensifies the depressive experience. It is argued that ruminative coping worsens depression in three ways. First, rumination impacts negatively on cognitions and information processing, as it increases the recall of negative events and reduces the individual's perception of control. Second, rumination reduces the likelihood that the individual will engage in helpful, mood enhancing behaviors; and, finally, rumination impairs problem-solving abilities. Nolen-Hoeksema and Girgus (1994) have argued that response styles theory may help to explain why, although depression is equally common among boys and girls before puberty, adolescent females develop depression at a far higher rate than adolescent males. Women are known to ruminate more than men, and this sex difference has been replicated in adolescent populations (Rose and Rudolph 2006).

Environmental factors

Stressors
The role of stressors is another key feature that overlaps across models of youth depression. It is commonly argued that depressive symptoms arise when a child's or an adolescent's underlying vulnerabilities interact with one or more stressful events. The ecological transactional model discussed below notes that stressors may arise from the family, from the community, and from the broader culture. Additionally, this model draws attention to the role of developmental adaptation and to the cumulative consequences of developmental challenges that are not adequately resolved. An especially important developmental period for girls appears to be adolescence, when rates of depression rise dramatically (Wade, Cairney, and Pevalin 2002). This may be, at least in part, due to greater exposure to total stress, particularly interpersonal episodic stress, for adolescent girls (Shih, 2006).

A community study of over 400 seventh graders by Ge, Conger, Lorenz, and Simons (1994) demonstrates the role of stress in youth depression within a family context. Stressful events experienced by the students' parents were found to be related to parental depressed mood. This low mood was found to impact parenting practices negatively, which in turn placed the children of these parents at increased risk of developing depressive symptoms. This relationship between stress and parenting also featured in a meta-analytic study by Grant and colleagues (2003), which found that negative parenting mediates the relationship between a particular stressor – poverty – and psychological symptoms in children and adolescents.

Transactional/developmental theories

Cicchetti and Toth (1998) have argued for the importance of a developmental psychopathology conceptualization of childhood depression. Their ecological transactional model identifies a range of psychological, social, and biological factors, each of which influence a child's capacity to meet new developmental challenges. It is argued that, when children are able to positively adapt to a developmental challenge, this leads to competence and better preparedness for the next developmental demand. Conversely, inadequate resolution of a stage-salient developmental challenge is likely to compromise the resolution of future developmental tasks. Cicchetti and Toth (1998) postulate that the occurrence of childhood depression depends not only on the presence or absence of specific vulnerability or protective factors, but also on the interplay between these factors and current and previous levels of developmental adaptation, as well as on the developmental period during which risk factors are experienced. In addition to this transactional complexity, they argue that risk and protective factors exist not only within the individual child, but also within his/her family (microsystem), the community in which the family lives (exosystem), and the broader culture of which the community is part (macrosystem).

Other models that emphasize the complex transactional nature of youth depression include those outlined by Restifo and Bögels (2009) and Shortt and Spence (2006). Some of the numerous risk factors identified by transactional models are genetic factors; parental psychopathology; low socioeconomic status; parental death, divorce, or separation; child maltreatment; parenting style; marital discord; low perceived academic confidence; poor adjustment to school; low availability of treatment services; rapid cultural changes and erosion of traditional cultural practices. Central to these models is the notion that none of these single risk factors will result in a depressive outcome, but rather that they interact with one another across all stages of the child's development.

An Integrated Model of Youth Depression

Across all the models of depression there are common factors that consistently implicate the impact of early experiences and of the subsequent sense of self on the way children process information and behave. Cognitive theories emphasize the impact of early experiences on cognitive style, whereas interpersonal theories emphasize their impact on relational and social skills. These are not independent: a child's perception of him-/ herself and others will impact on his/her social behavior, and conversely a child's social relationships will impact on his/her beliefs and attributions. Attachment, cognitive, and interpersonal theories all stress the transactional nature of their specific components. Depressive symptoms are noted to be both a cause and a consequence of difficult relationships and negative thinking styles.

An integrated model of child and adolescent depression is shown in Figure 8.1. Caregiver characteristics such as parental insensitivity, absence, or inconsistency interact with the child's own characteristics, for instance their genetic makeup and temperament. This interaction leads to an insecure attachment relationship, which manifests in the child's negative schemas about themselves, others, and the world.

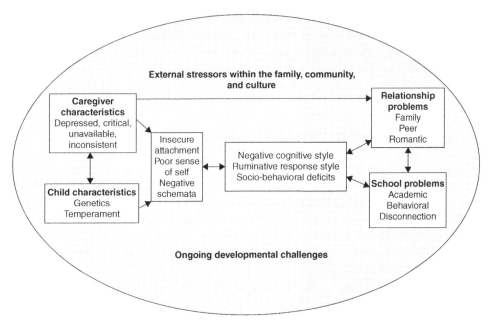

Figure 8.1 An integrated model of child and adolescent depression.

These negative schemas impact on the way in which the child processes information, interacts with others, and behaves in response to periods of low mood. The child's negative cognitive style and socio-behavioral deficits result in relationship difficulties with peers, with family members, and, in adolescence, with romantic relationships. These relationship difficulties may also be a result of conflicts within the family and of poor modeling of interpersonal skills from caregivers. Additionally, the child's or adolescent's negative cognitions and socio-behavioral deficits result in compromised performance at school – academically, behaviorally and in his/her general engagement with school life. Difficulties at school and in relationships reinforce the child's negative beliefs about him-/herself and others and exacerbate socio-behavioral deficits, perpetuating a vicious cycle of depressive thoughts, interactions, and behaviors. All of this occurs against a background of dynamic stressors and developmental challenges, which may interact with existing vulnerabilities to trigger depressive symptoms.

Clinical Implications

First, treatment should consider the family of the child or adolescent, with a view to increasing parental warmth, reducing parental criticism and psychological control, and generally improving the parent–child relationship where possible. Cognitive restructuring interventions may be used to target depressive cognitive distortions, although clinicians must keep in mind the cognitive development of their young client when doing this work. Behavioral interventions should be utilized to promote healthy and effective responses to stress and to reduce unhelpful and avoidant coping strategies that the depressed child or adolescent may use. Skills for dealing with relationships and conflict may be particularly useful for adolescent girls, who experience greater exposure to interpersonal stress. Finally, clinicians working with this population should remain alert to ongoing developmental challenges faced by their growing client and to the impact of stressors on the young person and his/her family.

Maintaining Factors in Child and Adolescent Anxiety

Several models have been proposed describing key factors and their interactions that lead to the development of anxiety disorders (Chorpita and Barlow 1998; Hudson and Rapee 2004; Manassis and Bradley 1994). Few of these models tend to differentiate between anxiety disorders; and they typically refer to anxiety disorders in childhood generically. As for theories of depression, most theories of anxiety tend to refer to relatively similar constructs, although the emphasis has varied between models.

Internal factors

Avoidant coping style
At a behavioral level, the core feature of anxiety is avoidance. A fundamentally avoidant style of dealing with the world seems to be characteristic of anxiety and marks temperamental styles that have been shown to precede anxiety disorders. Extensive evidence has shown that fearful or inhibited styles of temperament displayed very early in a child's life dramatically increase the likelihood that they will later develop anxiety disorders (Chronis-Tuscano et al. 2009; Hudson and Dodd 2012; Schwartz, Snidman, and Kagan 1999). Interestingly, there appears to be some specificity, and it seems that interpersonal withdrawal early in life tends to predict only social anxiety later on (Hirshfeld-Becker et al. 2007). It is likely that physical fearfulness early in life would be a better predictor of nonsocial anxiety disorders, but the evidence for this is less extensive.

Emotional lability
In landmark research, Kagan and Snidman (1991) showed that infants who were more emotional and physically aroused at 3 months of age were more likely to become inhibited children by the age of 2. Consequently, high levels of physiological arousal and difficulties with emotion regulation are fundamental characteristics of anxiety across the lifespan and are likely to reflect core maintaining processes.

Among the poor emotional regulation strategies shown by anxious individuals are cognitive processes and content that play a key role in anxious reactivity. In the adult field there is extensive research of the hypothesis that a cognitive style that pays excessive attention to threat and interprets ambiguous cues as threatening is associated with anxiety disorders, and is even causally linked to them (MacLeod and Mathews, 1988). It now appears that the same types of relationships are also evident among young people with anxiety disorders (Hadwin, Garner, and Perez-Olivas 2006). Anxious children are characterized by the allocation of excessive attention to threat, biases toward interpreting ambiguous material in a threat-consistent manner, and high levels of automatic thoughts related to social and physical threat (Britton, Lissek, Grillon, Norcross, and Pine 2011; Muris and Field 2008; Schniering and Rapee 2004). These processes help to maintain a sense of present threat for the anxious young person, and it is this sense of current danger that directly increases the experience of anxiousness.

Family and environmental factors

Role of the family

In contrast to the situation encountered in depression, in anxiety there is very little empirical evidence supporting a key role for broader family factors in its genesis or maintenance (Rapee 2012). However, a wealth of evidence supports the importance of the parent–child relationship. In several models this has been discussed in terms of both attachment (Chorpita and Barlow 1998; Manassis and Bradley 1994) and parenting (Chorpita and Barlow 1998; Hudson and Rapee 2004; Rapee 2001), the empirical evidence being particularly focused on the parenting factors of over-protection and criticism. Parental overprotection is likely to increase anxiety by teaching the child that the world is a dangerous place and that he or she has little control (Rapee 1997; Drake and Ginsburg 2012). Similarly, a critical parent can reinforce the message that the child is not capable of coping or of controlling potential risks in the world. Several reviews have described the evidence that supports these parenting factors and their association with childhood anxiety (Bögels and Brechman-Toussaint 2006; McLeod et al. 2007; Rapee 1997). Naturally, there is less evidence to indicate whether these parenting styles precede anxiety. However, at least some research with both younger children and teenagers has shown that overprotective parenting at one time can predict increases in anxiety at a later time (Edwards, Rapee, and Kennedy 2010; Hudson and Dodd 2012).

In addition to the parent–child relationship, parental psychopathology has also been implicated as a factor important to the development and maintenance of anxiety. There is little question that anxious children are more likely to have anxious parents, and a large part of this relationship is clearly genetic (Gregory and Eley 2007). However, it is also likely that anxious parents will be more overprotective of their child and will model more avoidant coping styles (see below).

Conditioning and learning

Probably the most fundamental theory in psychology is the proposal that phobic fear and avoidance have their origins in conditioning. Over the years, the theory that clinical phobias could develop through conditioning experiences has been variously criticized and resurrected (e.g., Menzies and Clarke 1995; Rachman 1977; Seligman 1971). Perhaps surprisingly, then, few recent models of the development of anxiety disorders have included a strong focus on conditioning (notwithstanding some notable exceptions; e.g., Bouton, Mineka, and Barlow 2001).

In a paper considering the role of conditioning in the development of children's anxieties, Field (2006) pointed to recent developments in the understanding of conditioning and argued that this better understanding could help explain some of the apparent anomalies in the application of the theory to clinical phenomena. For example, Field pointed out that a variety of experiences that involve a feared cue and occur before an aversive association – experiences such as prior irrelevant associations or prior non-aversive exposures – can affect the strength, duration, and nature of the learned association. Perhaps most importantly, he reviewed current conceptualizations of conditioning that view this phenomenon as a form of acquiring information about stimuli and their predictive relationships, and in this way utilize the same mechanisms as in learning through observation or verbal information. Thus a very wide variety of experiences early in life may produce associations between a set of stimuli and aversive outcomes. In addition to learning from specific negative experiences, learning via ongoing environmental influences (like parents or peers) is highly likely and has received some evidence. For example, several studies have shown that very young children can learn about novel fears by observing their mothers acting in a fearful or avoidant manner (de Rosnay, Cooper, Tsigaras, and Murray 2006; Gerull and Rapee 2002). Similarly, a series of studies by Field and his colleagues has shown that children can learn to become fearful of previously unknown stimuli following the verbal delivery of threatening information about the stimulus (Muris and Field 2010). As noted above, these displays (fearful reactions or verbalizations) are more likely to come from parents who are themselves anxious.

It should be noted that, regardless of views about the role of conditioning in the onset of anxiety disorders, there is little doubt that principles of conditioning are extremely relevant to some of the key methods of anxiety reduction, exposure, and cognitive restructuring. Therapists therefore need a good understanding of current conceptualizations of conditioning and extinction (Craske et al. 2008; Lovibond 2004) in order to better understand the principles behind their own techniques. In particular, understanding that extinction involves learning new information about a stimulus and its predicted relationships can help a great deal in applying exposure in complex cases.

Life events

Although the relationship between negative life events and anxiety disorders is not as strong as it is in several other disorders, including depression, it is clear that anxious children do experience a greater number of negative events in their lives than do non-clinical controls (Allen and Rapee 2009; Goodyer and Altham 1991). Interestingly, this difference appears to be primarily produced by a greater number of so-called "dependent" life events – in other words, life events that could potentially be a product of the child's own actions (Allen and Rapee 2009). This would suggest that negative life events are more likely to be a result of having an anxiety disorder, although they, in turn, may be responsible for the maintenance of that disorder. Nonetheless, at least some evidence suggests that a slightly higher proportion of independent life events (events that could not be caused by the child) immediately precede the onset of anxiety disorders, which suggests that negative life events might also trigger anxiety disorders among vulnerable youth (Allen, Rapee, and Sandberg 2008). Several specific events have also been associated with anxiety disorders (although generally less strongly than in other disorders). For example, both sexual and physical abuse appear to increase the risk of anxiety disorders (Hudson and Rapee 2009), as do teasing and peer victimization (Hudson and Rapee 2009). Socially anxious children appear to display poorer interaction skills (Spence, Donovan, and Brechman-Toussaint 1999), and they are commonly excluded or ignored by peers (Hudson and Rapee 2009).

An Integrated Model of Anxiety in Young People

Extensive research has pointed to aspects of cognitions and behavior as both initiating and maintaining factors in anxiety among young people. Several overlapping factors are highlighted by the various models of child anxiety and by the accompanying evidence. These common factors are largely summarized in a model of the development of generalized anxiety disorder proposed by Rapee (2001) and later modified by Hudson and Rapee (2004). Although the models were said to be focused on generalized anxiety, the authors argued that the described factors were relevant to all anxiety disorders.

In brief, the model draws on the evidence that shows that one of the strongest predictors of later anxiety disorder is early temperamental vulnerability (inhibition, withdrawal). This temperamental style is partly a result of inherited characteristics. The temperamental style is composed of several factors; foremost among them is a basic avoidant style of dealing with perceived threat. However, a general emotionality (including heightened arousal and information-processing biases) is also likely to be important. The model further emphasizes the importance of specific styles of parenting, especially a tendency for parents to support the child's avoidant coping (overprotection). However, it is clearly argued that this process is a reciprocal one, where the child's distress elicits parental protection that, in turn, strengthens the avoidance. The parent's own anxiety is also a key in the theory, naturally influencing genetic factors, but also moderating the parent support of avoidance as well as modeling anxious responding (as argued by conditioning theories). Finally, the influence of negative environmental experiences is described: these experiences influence the onset of anxiety disorder through their interaction with the child's temperament. A new development that has become apparent from more recent empirical evidence and was not clear when the model was originally proposed is the likely influence of the child's temperament in eliciting negative life events. In other words, the process is reciprocal: a withdrawn and inhibited child is more likely to experience negative life events (e.g., being bullied) and these life events interact with the vulnerability to increase the experience of anxiety. Finally, the concept of disorder also depends on a degree of life interference, and this construct is in turn influenced by several additional factors. In light of this more recent evidence, a slightly revised model is shown in Figure 8.2.

Clinical Implications

The model shown in Figure 8.2 suggests a number of clear predictions for potentially relevant intervention strategies. Most directly, the avoidant style of coping needs to be directly addressed by teaching the child to approach rather than avoid feared cues (exposure). The emotional arousal that characterizes the underlying temperament also

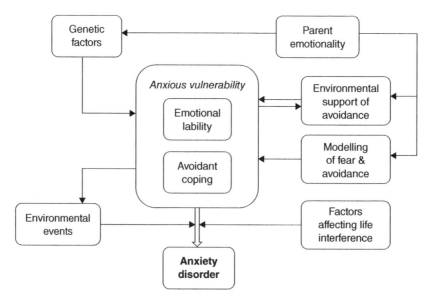

Figure 8.2 A model of the development of anxiety disorders in children. Adapted from Rapee (2001) and Hudson and Rapee (2004).

needs to be addressed through arousal reduction strategies. Several such strategies exist, including cognitive restructuring, relaxation, or attention-focusing techniques (such as mindfulness), and all have been shown to be of value in the management of anxiety. A fundamental difference between anxiety in young people and anxiety in adults, which has been highlighted by most models, is the presence of an overprotective or overly controlling parenting style. Thus the model suggests that teaching the parents methods to reduce their own protectiveness, and also to reduce the modeling of anxious or avoidant coping, should help to cut the cycle and to improve the longer-term maintenance of anxiety reduction. A component of the anxious parenting style is the parent's own anxiety, and the model therefore predicts that helping the parent to manage his/ her own anxiety should increase the efficacy of the treatment for the child's anxiety. Somewhat surprisingly, evidence for this component has met with relatively little success (Cobham, Dadds, and Spence 1998; Hudson et al. 2013), but this may reflect practical difficulties of implementing parent anxiety management rather than its lack of value, in case it could be achieved. Finally, the model suggests that directly reducing the impact of negative life events should further reduce anxiousness and help to maintain gains. This might be achieved by teaching a variety of social, problem-solving, or coping skills designed to help the child better deal with real-world stressors.

References

Abramson, Lyn Y., Gerald I. Metalsky, and Lauren B. Alloy. 1989. "Hopelessness Depression: A Theory-Based Subtype of Depression." *Psychological Review*, 96: 358–72. DOI: 10.1037/0033-295x.96.2.358

Abramson, Lyn Y., Martin E. P. Seligman, and John D. Teasdale. 1978. "Learned Helplessness in Humans: Critique and Reformulation." *Journal of Abnormal Psychology*, 87: 49–74. DOI: 10.1037/0021-843x.87.1.49

Allen, Jennifer L., and Ronald M. Rapee. 2009. "Are Reported Differences in Life Events for Anxious Children Due to Comorbid Disorders?" *Journal of Anxiety Disorders*, 23: 511–18. DOI: 10.1016/j.janxdis.2008.10.005

Allen, Jennifer L., Ronald M. Rapee, and Seija Sandberg. 2008. "Severe Life Events and Chronic Adversities as Antecedents to Anxiety in Children: A Matched Control Study." *Journal of Abnormal Child Psychology*, 36: 1047–56. DOI: 10.1007/s10802-008-9240-x

Alloy, Lauren B., Lyn Y. Abramson, Jeannette M. Smith, Brandon E. Gibb, and A. M. Neeren. M. 2006. "Role of Parenting and Maltreatment Histories in Unipolar and Bipolar Mood Disorders: Mediation by Cognitive Vulnerability to Depression." *Clinical Child and Family Psychology Review*, 9: 23–64.

Asarnow, Joan R., and Susan Bates. 1988. "Depression in Child Psychiatric Inpatients: Cognitive and Attributional Patterns." *Journal of Abnormal Child Psychology*, 16: 601–15.

Beck, Aaron T. 1967. *Depression: Clinical, Experimental, and Theoretical Aspects*. New York: Harper & Row.

Beck, Aaron T. 1983. "Cognitive Therapy of Depression: New Perspectives." In P. J. Clayton and J. E. Barrett (Eds.), *Treatment of Depression: Old Controversies and New Approaches* (pp. 256–84). New York: Raven Press.

Bögels, Susan M., and Brechman-Toussaint, Margaret L. 2006. "Family Issues in Child Anxiety: Attachment, Family Functioning, Parental Rearing and Beliefs." *Clinical Psychology Review*, 26 (7): 834–56.

Borelli, Jessica L., and Mitchell J. Prinstein. 2006. "Reciprocal, Longitudinal Associations among Adolescents' Negative Feedback-seeking, Depressive Symptoms, and Peer Relations." *Journal of Abnormal Child Psychology*, 34: 159–69. DOI: 10.1007/s10802-005-9010-y.

Bouton, Mark E., Susan Mineka, and David H. Barlow. 2001. "A Modern Learning Perspective on the Etiology of Panic Disorder." *Psychological Review*, 108: 4–32.

Bowlby, John. 1980. *Attachment and Loss*. Volume 3: *Loss: Sadness and Depression*. New York: Basic Books.

Britton, Jennifer C., Shmuel Lissek, Christian Grillon, Maxine A Norcross, and Daniel S Pine. 2011. "Development of Anxiety: The Role of Threat Appraisal and Fear Learning." *Depression and Anxiety*, 28: 5–17. DOI: 10.1002/da.20733.

Cartwright-Hatton, Sam, Chris Roberts, Prathiba Chitsabesan, Claire Fothergill, and Richard Harrington. 2004. "Systematic Review of the Efficacy of Cognitive Behaviour Therapies for Childhood and Adolescent Anxiety Disorders." *British Journal of Clinical Psychology*, 43: 421–36.

Chorpita, Bruce F., and David H. Barlow. 1998. "The Development of Anxiety: The Role of Control in the Early Environment." *Psychological Bulletin*, 124: 3–21.

Chronis-Tuscano, Andrea, Kathryn A. Degnan, Daniel S. Pine, Koraly Perez-Edgar, Heather A. Henderson, Yamalis Diaz, Veronica L. Raggi, and Nathan A. Fox. 2009. "Stable Early Maternal Report of Behavioral Inhibition Predicts Lifetime Social Anxiety Disorder in Adolescence." *Journal of the American Academy of Child & Adolescent Psychiatry*, 48: 928–35. DOI: 10.1097/CHI.0b013e3181ae09df

Cicchetti, Dante, and Sheree L. Toth. 1998. "The Development of Depression in Children and Adolescents." *The American Psychologist*, 53: 221–41.

Cobham, Vanessa E., Mark R. Dadds, and Susan. H. Spence. 1998. The Role of Parental Anxiety in the Treatment of Childhood Anxiety. *Journal of Consulting and Clinical Psychology*, 66 (6): 893–905.

Cole, David A., and Jackson E Turner, Jr. 1993. "Models of Cognitive Mediation and Moderation in Self-Reported Child Depression." *Journal of Abnormal Psychology*, 102: 271–81. DOI: 10.1037//0021-843X.102.2.271

Coyne, James C. 1976. Depression and the Response of Others. *Journal of Abnormal Psychology*, 85: 186–93.

Craske, Michelle G., Katharina Kircanski, Moriel Zelikowsk, Jason Mystkowski, Najwa Chowdhury, and A. Baker. 2008. "Optimizing Inhibitory Learning during Exposure Therapy." *Behaviour Research and Therapy*, 46: 5–27.

Cummings, E. Mark. 1994. "Marital Conflict and Children's Functioning." *Social Development*, 3 (1): 16–36. DOI: 10.1111/j.1467-9507.1994.tb00021.x

de Rosnay, Mark, Peter J. Cooper, Nicholas Tsigaras, and Lynne Murray. 2006. "Transmission of Social Anxiety from Mother to Infant: An Experimental Study Using a Social Referencing Paradigm." *Behaviour Research and Therapy*, 44: 1165–75. DOI: 10.1016/j.brat.2005.09.003

Drake, Kelly L., and Golda S. Ginsburg. 2012. "Family Factors in the Development, Treatment, and Prevention of Childhood Anxiety Disorders." *Clinical child and Family Psychology Review*, 15: 144–62. DOI: 10.1007/s10567-011-0109-0

Edwards, Susan L., Ronald M. Rapee, and Susan Kennedy. 2010. "Prediction of Anxiety Symptoms in Preschool-Aged Children: Examination of Maternal and Paternal Perspectives." *Journal of Child Psychology & Psychiatry*, 51: 313–21. DOI: 10.1111/j.1469-7610.2009.02160.x

Field, Andy P. 2006. "Is Conditioning a Useful Framework for Understanding the Development and Treatment of Phobias?" *Clinical Psychology Review*, 26: 857–75. DOI: 10.1016/j.cpr.2005.05.010

Flynn, Megan, and Karen D. Rudolph. 2011. "Stress Generation and Adolescent Depression: Contribution of Interpersonal Stress Responses." *Journal of Abnormal Child Psychology*, 39: 1187–98. DOI: 10.1007/s10802-011-9527-1

Ge, Xiaojia, Rand D. Conger, Frederick O. Lorenz, and Ronald L. Simons. 1994. "Parents' Stressful Life Events and Adolescent Depressed Mood." *Journal of Health & Social Behavior*, 35: 28–44.

Gerull, Friedericke C., and Ronald M. Rapee. 2002. "Mother Knows Best: Effects of Maternal Modelling on the Acquisition of Fear and Avoidance Behaviour in Toddlers." *Behaviour Research and Therapy*, 40: 279–87. DOI: 10.1016/S0005-7967(01)00013-4

Goodyer, Ian M., and Patricia M. Altham. 1991. "Lifetime Exit Events and Recent Social and Family Adversities in Anxious and Depressed School-Age Children and Adolescents." *Journal of Affective Disorders*, 21: 229–38.

Grant, Kathryn E., Bruce E. Compas, Alice F. Stuhlmacher, Audrey E. Thurm, Susan D. McMahon, and Jane A. Halpert. 2003. "Stressors and Child and Adolescent Psychopathology: Moving from Markers to Mechanisms of Risk." *Psychological Bulletin*, 129: 447–66. DOI: 10.1037/0033-2909.129.3.447

Gregory, Alice M., and Thalia C. Eley. 2007. "Genetic Influences on Anxiety in Children: What We've Learned and Where We're Heading." *Clinical Child and Family Psychology Review*, 10: 199–212. DOI: 10.1007/s10567-007-0022-8

Hadwin, Julie A., Matthew Garner, and Gisela Perez-Olivas. 2006. "The Development of Information Processing Biases in Childhood Anxiety: A Review and Exploration of Its Origins in Parenting." *Clinical Psychology Review*, 26: 876–94. DOI: 10.1016/j.cpr.2005.09.004

Hammen, Constance. 1988. "Self-Cognitions, Stressful Events, and the Prediction of Depression in Children of Depressed Mothers." *Journal of Abnormal Child Psychology*, 16: 347–60.

Harrington, Richard, Jane Whittaker, Philip Shoebridge, and Fiona Campbell. 1998. "Systematic Review of Efficacy of Cognitive Behaviour Therapies in Childhood and Adolescent Depressive Disorder." *British Medical Journal*, 316: 1559–63. DOI: 10.1136/bmj.316.7144.1559

Hirshfeld-Becker, Dina R., Joseph Biederman, Aude. Henin, Stephen V. Faraone, Stephanie Davis, Kara Harrington, Jerrold F. Rosenboum. 2007. "Behavioral Inhibition in Preschool Children at Risk Is a Specific Predictor of Middle Childhood Social Anxiety: A Five-Year Follow-up." *Journal of Developmental & Behavioral Pediatrics*, 28: 225–33.

Hudson, Jennifer L., and Helen F. Dodd. 2012. "Informing Early Intervention: Preschool Predictors of Anxiety Disorders in Middle Childhood." *PLoS ONE*, 7, e42359.

Hudson, Jennifer L., Carol Newall, Ronald M. Rapee, Heidi J. Lyneham, Carolyn C. Schniering, Viviana M. Wuthrich, … Natalie S. Gar. 2013. The Impact of Brief Parental Anxiety Management on Child Anxiety Treatment Outcomes: A Controlled Trial. *Journal of Clinical Child & Adolescent Psychology*, 1–11. DOI: 10.1080/15374416.2013.807734

Hudson, Jennifer L., and Ronald M. Rapee. 2004. "From Anxious Temperament to Disorder: An Etiological Model of Generalized Anxiety Disorder. In Richard G. Heimberg, Cynthia L. Turk, and Douglas S. Mennin (Eds.), *Generalized Anxiety Disorder: Advances in Research and Practice* (pp. 51–76). New York: Guilford Publications.

Hudson, Jennifer L., and Ronald M. Rapee. 2009. "Familial and Social Environments in the Etiology and Maintenance of Anxiety Disorders." In Martin M. Antony and Murray B. Stein (Eds.), *Oxford Handbook of Anxiety and Anxiety Disorders* (pp. 173–89). New York: Oxford University Press.

Joiner, Thomas E. 2002. "Depression in Its Interpersonal Context." In Ian H. Gotlib and Constance L. Hammen (Eds.), *Handbook of Depression* (pp. 295–313). New York: Guilford Press.

Kagan, Jerome, and Nancy Snidman. 1991. "Infant Predictors of Inhibited and Uninhibited Profiles." *Psychological Science*, 2: 40–4. DOI: 10.1111/j.1467-9280.1991.tb00094.x

Kendall, Philip C., Kevin D. Stark, and Therese Adam. 1990. "Cognitive Deficit or Cognitive Distortion in Childhood Depression." *Journal of Abnormal Child Psychology*, 18: 255–70.

Lakdawalla, Zia, Benjamin L. Hankin, and Robin Mermelstein. 2007. "Cognitive Theories of Depression in Children and Adolescents: A Conceptual and Quantitative Review." *Clinical Child and Family Psychology Review*, 10: 1–24. DOI: 10.1007/s10567-006-0013-1

Lovibond, Peter F. 2004. "Cognitive Processes in Extinction." *Learning & Memory*, 11: 495–500. DOI: 10.1101/lm.79604

MacLeod, Colin, and Andrew Mathews. 1988. "Anxiety and the Allocation of Attention to Threat." *The Quarterly Journal of Experimental Psychology*, 40A: 653–70. DOI: 10.1080/14640748808402292

Manassis, Katharina, and Susan J. Bradley. 1994. "The Development of Childhood Anxiety Disorders: Toward an Integrated Model." *Journal of Applied Developmental Psychology*, 15: 345–66. DOI: 10.1016/0193-3973(94)90037-X

McCarty, Carolyn A., Anna S. Lau, Sylvia M. Valeri, and John R. Weisz. 2004. "Parent–Child Interactions in Relation to Critical and Emotionally Overinvolved Expressed Emotion (EE): Is EE a Proxy for Behavior?" *Journal of Abnormal Child Psychology*, 32: 83–93.

McLeod, Bryce D., John R. Weisz, and Jeffrey J. Wood. 2007. "Examining the Association between Parenting and Childhood Depression: A Meta-Analysis." *Clinical Psychology Review*, 27: 987–1003.

Menzies, Ross G., and J. Christopher Clarke. 1995. "The Etiology of Phobias: A Nonassociative Account." *Clinical Psychology Review*, 15: 23–48. DOI: 10.1016/0272-7358(94)00039-5

Muris, Peter, and Andy P. Field. 2008. "Distorted Cognition and Pathological Anxiety in Children and Adolescents." *Cognition and Emotion*, 22: 395–421. DOI: 10.1080/02699930701843450

Muris, Peter, and Andy P. Field. 2010. "The Role of Verbal Threat Information in the Development of Childhood Fear. 'Beware the Jabberwock!'" *Clinical Child and Family Psychology Review*, 13: 129–50. DOI: 10.1007/s10567-010-0064-1

Nolen-Hoeksema, Susan. 1991. "Responses to Depression and Their Effects on the Duration of Depressive Episodes." *Journal of Abnormal Psychology*, 100: 569–82.

Nolen-Hoeksema, Susan, and Joan S. Girgus. 1994. "The Emergence of Gender Differences in Depression during Adolescence." *Psychological Bulletin*, 115: 424–43.

Prinstein, Mitchell J., Jessica C. Borelli, Charissa S. L. Cheah, Valerie A. Simon, and Julie W. Aikins. 2005. "Adolescent Girls' Interpersonal Vulnerability to Depressive Symptoms: A Longitudinal Examination of Reassurance-Seeking and Peer Relationships." *Journal of Abnormal Psychology*, 114: 676–88. DOI: 10.1037/0021-843X.114.4.676

Rachman, S. 1977. "The Conditioning Theory of Fear Acquisition: A Critical Examination." *Behaviour Research and Therapy*, 15: 375–87. DOI: 10.1016/0005-7967(77)90041-9

Rapee, Ronald M. 1997. "Potential Role of Childrearing Practices in the Development of Anxiety and Depression." *Clinical Psychology Review*, 17: 47–67.

Rapee, Ronald M. 2001. The Development of Generalised Anxiety. In Michael W. Vasey and Mark R. Dadds (Eds.), *The Developmental Psychopathology of Anxiety* (pp. 481–504). New York: Oxford University Press.

Rapee, Ronald M. 2012. "Family Factors in the Development and Management of Anxiety Disorders." *Clinical Child and Family Psychology Review*, 15: 69–80. DOI: 10.1007/s10567-011-0106-3

Restifo, Kathleen, and Susan Bögels. 2009. Family Processes in the Development of Youth Depression: Translating the Evidence to Treatment. *Clinical Psychology Review*, 29: 294–316. DOI: 10.1016/j.cpr.2009.02.005

Rose, Amanda J., and Karen D. Rudolph. 2006. "A Review of Sex Differences in Peer Relationship Processes: Potential Trade-offs for the Emotional and Behavioral Development of Girls and Boys." *Psychological Bulletin*, 132: 98–131. DOI: 10.1037/0033-2909.132.1.98

Rudolph, Karen D., Megan Flynn, and Jaimie L. Abaied. 2008. A Developmental Perspective on Interpersonal Theories of Youth Depression. In John R. Z. Abela and Benjamin L. Hankin (Eds.), *Handbook of Depression in Children and Adolescents* (pp. 79–102). New York: Guilford Press.

Sburlati, Elizabeth S., Carolyn A. Schniering, Heidi J. Lyneham, and Ronald M. Rapee. 2011. "A Model of Therapist Competencies for the Empirically Supported Cognitive Behavioral Treatment of Child and Adolescent Anxiety and Depressive Disorders." *Clinical Child and Family Psychology Review*, 14: 89–109. DOI: 10.1007/s10567-011-0083-6

Schniering, Carolyn A., and Ronald M. Rapee. 2004. "The Relationship between Automatic Thoughts and Negative Emotions in Children and Adolescents: A Test of the Cognitive Content-Specificity Hypothesis." *Journal of Abnormal Psychology*, 113: 464–70.

Schwartz, Carl E., Nancy Snidman, and Jerome Kagan. 1999. "Adolescent Social Anxiety as an Outcome of Inhibited Temperament in Childhood." *Journal of the American Academy of Child and Adolescent Psychiatry*, 38: 1008–15. DOI: 10.1097/00004583-199908000-00017

Seligman, Martin E. P. 1971. "Phobias and Preparedness." *Behavior Therapy*, 2: 307–20.

Sheeber, Lisa B., and Eric Sorensen. 1998. "Family Relationships of Depressed Adolescents: A Multimethod Assessment." *Journal of Clinical Child Psychology*, 27: 268–77. DOI: 10.1207/s15374424jccp2703_4

Sheeber, Lisa B., Betsy Davis, Craig Leve, Hyman Hops, and Elizabeth Tildesley. 2007. "Adolescents' Relationships with their Mothers and Fathers: Associations with Depressive Disorder and Subdiagnostic Symptomatology." *Journal of Abnormal Psychology*, 116: 144–54. DOI: 10.1037/0021-843X.116.1.144

Shih, Josephine H. 2006. "Sex Differences in Stress Generation: An Examination of Sociotropy/Autonomy, Stress, and Depressive Symptoms." *Personality and Social Psychology Bulletin*, 32: 434–46. DOI: 10.1177/0146167205282739

Shih, Josephine H., and Nicole Eberhart. 2008. "Understanding the Impact of Prior Depression on Stress Generations: Examining the Roles of Current Depressive Symptoms and Interpersonal Behaviours." *British Journal of Psychology*, 99: 413–26. DOI: 0.1348/000712607X243341

Shih, Josephine H., John R. Z. Abela, and Claire Starrs. 2009. "Cognitive and Interpersonal Predictors of Stress Generation in Children of Affectively Ill Parents." *Journal of Abnormal Child Psychology*, 37: 195–208. DOI: 10.1007/s10802-008-9267-z

Shortt, Alison L., and Susan H. Spence. 2006. "Risk and Protective Factors for Depression in Youth." *Behaviour Change*, 23: 1–30. DOI: 10.1375/bech.23.1.1

Spence, Susan H., Caroline Donovan, and Margeret Brechman-Toussaint. 1999. "Social Skills, Social Outcomes, and Cognitive Features of Childhood Social Phobia." *Journal of Abnormal Psychology*, 108: 211–21. DOI: 10.1037/0021-843X.108.2.211

Wade, Terrance J., John Cairney, and David J. Pevalin. 2002. "Emergence of Gender Differences in Depression during Adolescence: National Panel Results from Three Countries." *Journal of the American Academy of Child & Adolescent Psychiatry*, 41: 190–8. DOI: 10.1097/00004583-200202000-00013

Weissman, Myrna, Virginia Warner, Priya Wickramaratne, Donna Moreau, and Mark Olfson. 1997. "Offspring of Depressed Parents: 10 Years Later." *Archives of General Psychiatry*, 54: 932–40. DOI: 10.1001/archpsyc.1997.01830220054009

Weitlauf, Amy S., and David A. Cole. 2012. "Cognitive Development Masks Support for Attributional Style Models of Depression in Children and Adolescents." *Journal of Abnormal Child Psychology*, 40: 1–14. DOI: 10.1007/s10802-012-9617-8

9

Case Formulation and Treatment Planning for Anxiety and Depression in Children and Adolescents

Heidi J. Lyneham

Introduction

Case formulation is the process of identifying the causes, antecedents, and maintaining factors related to a client's emotional, interpersonal, and behavioral problems. It provides a template from which an individualized treatment plan can be derived. Importantly, case formulations are flexible. They account for all the information gathered at any point in time, and they are updated to reflect new information as it arises. The models of anxiety and depression presented in Chapter 8 are *nomothetic*, that is, they describe the general "laws" of how these problems arise. The purpose of the case formulation is to create an *idiographic* model relevant only to a specific case. Persons (1989) identifies numerous other functions of a case formulation. First, by ensuring that the therapist understands and communicates the presenting problems within the client's personal context, it conveys hope that these problem(s) can be addressed. Second, it guides the development of a treatment plan that deliberately targets causal and maintaining factors that underlie the problems, increasing the likelihood of appropriate response to treatment. Third, it can pre-empt potential barriers that may undermine treatment progress or engagement. The treatment plan can subsequently be adjusted to proactively address these potential barriers, decreasing the likelihood that the barrier will interfere with progress.

Several different approaches have been devised to guide the production of case formulations (Boschen and Oei 2008; Macneil, Hasty, Conus, and Berk 2012; Persons 1989). Surprisingly, though, there has been minimal research on the clinical utility and accuracy of case formulations and subsequent treatment plans, particularly with regard to child and adolescent populations. Inter-rater reliability of

Evidence-Based CBT for Anxiety and Depression in Children and Adolescents: A Competencies-Based Approach,
First Edition. Edited by Elizabeth S. Sburlati, Heidi J. Lyneham, Carolyn A. Schniering, and Ronald M. Rapee.
© 2014 John Wiley & Sons, Ltd. Published 2014 by John Wiley & Sons, Ltd.

case formulations has been found to be adequate (Kuyken, Fothergill, Musa, and Chadwick 2005), the quality of case formulations improving with therapist experience and training (Eells et al. 2011). The clinical utility of case formulation as used in a community setting with adult anxiety and depression has been examined, case-formulated treatment leading to statistically and clinically significant change, comparable to that seen in randomized controlled trials of empirically supported treatments (Persons, Roberts, Zalecki, and Brechwald 2006). Direct comparison of case-formulated treatment and standardized treatment has shown slight superiority for the former (Persons and Tompkins 1997).

Cognitive behavioral therapy (CBT) for child anxiety has been shown to be maximally effective when CBT interventions are matched to the specific anxiety symptoms experienced by the individual (Eisen and Silverman 1993, 1998), and long-term efficacy has been established for a majority of individuals after a CBT program for adolescent depression that incorporated use of case formulation (Treatment of Adolescent Depression [TADS] Team 2009). The case-formulation approach has also been shown to improve some aspects of the therapeutic alliance (Chadwick, Williams, and Mackenzie 2003); and client acceptance of a treatment rationale – one aspect of the case formulation – is related to good treatment outcome (see, e.g., Addis and Jacobson 2000). Despite the small amount of research to date, existing results are promising and case formulation is considered by organizations such as the APA to be fundamental to evidence-based practice (APA 2006). The distinct advantage of case formulation for the therapist in community practice is the flexibility it provides in determining a treatment plan for individuals who may or may not fit the criteria on which manual-based approaches were evaluated.

Devising a Case Formulation and a Treatment Plan

Theoretically driven, context-aware case formulation

For the purposes of this chapter, it will be assumed that the therapist has established, through appropriate assessment, that the targeted child or adolescent has an anxiety and/or a depressive disorder that is the basis for presentation to treatment (see Chapter 7 for more details on conducting an assessment). To devise a case formulation, a competent therapist will need to add, to the standard diagnostic and symptom severity assessment tools, a targeted assessment of the typical cognitions, behaviors, and emotions that relate to the presenting problem for the individual, as well as an evaluation of interpersonal processes between the individual and other people (e.g., parents, peers) during periods of high anxiety or low mood. This can be achieved by eliciting detailed descriptions of one or two recent events that highlight the presenting concerns and by enquiring about cognitions and behavioral choices during the chosen event(s) from both the perspective of the parent and that of the child or adolescent. Information on comorbidity, family history, current anxiety or depression in immediate family, the client's developmental and academic functioning, and the family's socio-demographic and cultural environment are also needed for a comprehensive case formulation.

Following thorough assessment, the therapist should select the nomothetic model that is appropriate for the presenting individual, his/her family, and the organizational setting in which treatment is being offered. The chosen model will either reflect a particular manualized program or should be drawn from general models of anxiety or depression, such as those provided in Chapter 8. Once the model has been selected, the therapist should attach relevant evidence gathered during assessment to each aspect of the model. For example, Figure 9.1 applies the anxiety model presented in Chapter 8 to the case of an 11-year-old boy assessed as meeting criteria for generalized anxiety disorder and social phobia. As can be seen, a picture emerges from the idiographic model of what is causing and maintaining the presenting problem for the individual.

In addition to developing the idiographic representation of the chosen model, the potential impact that socio-demographics, culture, comorbidity, and development will have on engagement with treatment and on the likelihood of experiencing common obstacles during treatment should be considered. These influences can be described within a written case formulation or, if a visual representation of the case formulation is preferred, displayed on the idiographic model as contextual layers that surround the issues identified in the model. Finally, the formulation should consider the strengths of the individual and family, as recognition of these factors not only facilitates an optimistic view of the future, but can provide the therapist with a basis on which (s)he can build resilience (Macneil et al. 2012). These strengths should be added to any written or visual representation of the case formulation in a way that emphasizes their importance – for example they can be added to the outer layer of the contextual–idiographic model.

Dynamic Treatment Planning

Once an initial case formulation is established, the therapist needs to convert it into a treatment plan. Each child or adolescent will have a unique mix of factors implicated in the development of his/her anxiety and/or depressive disorder. Each factor will also vary on the strength of its association with current problems. Consequently the amount of emphasis given to a particular skill within a treatment plan must also vary. The treatment plan must therefore *select* the specific CBT techniques that will best address the identified problems, *sequence* the techniques in such a way that progress toward goals is optimized, and implement each technique at an appropriate *dose*, to ensure that the targeted problem is effectively overcome or managed. Each of these processes is described below.

Selecting specific CBT techniques

The competent therapist must ensure that (s)he has a thorough understanding of the purpose of each specific CBT technique, so that (s)he can appropriately link it to the causal or maintaining factor(s) that it is designed to address. Specific CBT techniques may focus on a single factor or may deliberately target multiple factors. Treatment manuals will provide guidance on the selection of appropriate techniques or, through design,

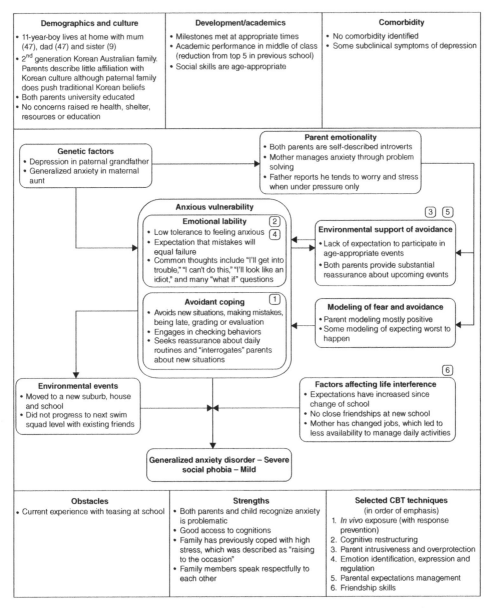

Figure 9.1 Example of idiographic application of the anxiety model to the case of an 11-year-old boy. Chosen specific CBT skills are indicated by numerical indicators. Adapted from Figure 8.2, which was adapted from Rapee (2001) and Hudson and Rapee (2004).

will have made assumptions about the selection of techniques on the basis of the chosen nomothetic model and the target population. Where a therapist is using a module-based treatment manual, the clinical algorithms provided by the manual should be followed. In situations where treatment is guided by CBT theory and the therapist's clinical judgment, the sections on clinical implication in Chapter 8 here, together with the reviews provided of each specific CBT technique in Chapters 12 through 19, should be used to guide the selection of appropriate techniques. On the basis of the case formulation, the therapist can overlay what specific CBT techniques will be used to address each component of the case formulation. (For an example of this, see Figure 9.1, where each numerical indicator provides the chosen specific CBT technique that will form the treatment plan.)

The competent therapist must remain flexible throughout treatment. The initial case formulation, and consequently the treatment plan, must be updated as new information is discovered and as a result of the experience implementing each specific CBT technique with the client. For example, during the implementation of in-session exposure, it may become apparent that the parent encourages flight from challenging situations at the first sign of the child's distress, despite having been presented with psycho-education regarding the role of overprotection in child anxiety. The flexible therapist will revise the case formulation or the treatment plan to work directly on the parent's reactions during exposure, through one-on-one work on his/her beliefs regarding the child's ability to cope with risk and/or by incorporating reduction of parent involvement directly into the child's exposure hierarchy.

Sequencing selected specific CBT techniques

Depending on the manual selected, the therapist may have limited or substantial control on the order of presentation of specific CBT techniques. In manuals where there is limited flexibility in the sequencing of techniques, the presented order reflects the nomothetic understanding of the targeted disorder(s). Therapist flexibility in this case focuses more on the tailoring of the technique to the specific cognitions, behaviors, or situations that the client experiences. In module-based manuals that provide greater flexibility, or in situations where the therapist is working within a general CBT framework, the sequence of selected techniques will be guided by the manual's clinical algorithms (e.g., Chorpita 2007) or will be inferred from the direction and strength of relationships between factors identified in the case formulation.

Sequencing selected specific CBT techniques for anxiety disorders

Within CBT models and at the diagnostic level, avoidance is key to all forms of anxiety. The specific CBT technique that directly targets avoidance and the only skill that appears without exception in every evidence-based treatment manual for anxiety is exposure. Consequently, after basic psycho-education, exposure would be considered the most essential technique to implement with a child or adolescent who has an anxiety disorder. In determining the sequence of skills for the treatment plan, the therapist may do best to ask him-/herself what skills will be needed prior to implementing exposure and what skills may be developed concurrently with it. For example, successful exposure to social situations in the school playground may not be possible until an underlying deficit in social skills is addressed. Therefore the treatment plan should reflect an early focus on developing basic social skills *prior to* exposure, as implementation of the newly learnt social skills would improve the likelihood of early success in exposure to social situations. Alternatively, the case formulation may indicate that excessive reassurance from the parent undermines the child's ability to learn that (s)he can cope with challenging situations. In this case the treatment plan may reflect that, *concurrently with* the implementation of exposure, the parent would require (i) psycho-education concerning the role of excessive reassurance in his/her child's evaluation of a situation; (ii) therapist modeling of the appropriate parent management during in-session exposure exercises; and, ultimately, (iii) parent-led *in vivo* exposure.

Sequencing selected specific CBT techniques for depressive disorders
Core components of CBT models for child and adolescent depression relate to the negative cognitive styles and behavioral deficits that exist in the relationships and interactions that individuals have with society, family, and friends and with formal organizations. Change in the individual may be undermined by lack of change in his/her external interactions; consequently, a sequencing of skills needs to reflect pre-emptive or concurrent intervention on the external environment. For example, increasing an adolescent's engagement in enjoyable activities through the specific CBT technique of pleasant events scheduling may not be possible if a parent's expectations of commitment to school work is unrealistic and if that parent encourages the child or the adolescent to engage in school work and discourages socialization or relaxation. Ensuring that these parental beliefs are addressed concurrently will increase the likelihood that the client will be able to implement between-session homework that aims to increase the frequency of pleasant events. The competent therapist needs to carefully examine the relationships between each factor in the case formulation, in order to predict the most appropriate initial order of skill development. This initial sequencing may then be modified if a causal barrier is identified during treatment or if response to a planned technique is undermined by other difficulties.

Dosage of techniques

In an ideal world dosage would be determined by success in both the learning and the application of each specific skill. The therapist would follow the treatment plan until the client's goals were achieved and, with a view to ensuring gain maintenance, until the core specific CBT techniques were understood sufficiently to be successfully applied when future challenges arise. In reality, the available number of sessions will likely be determined by an organizational or funding limit or may be based on the chosen manual (which may suggest a fixed or flexible "dose" for each skill). Where the therapist is responsible for determining treatment length, the dosage of individual skills can be estimated by adding the average time required to teach the basics of the skill to the number of sessions estimated as necessary to successfully apply the skill to address current problems, given the severity and complexity of the factors present in the case formulation. For example, in a child who has a single diagnosis of separation anxiety with avoidance that becomes evident only during night-time separation, exposure may be planned over three or four sessions, one for teaching the skill and for developing an initial hierarchy and then two or three sessions (which may be held fortnightly) for reviewing and planning *in vivo* exposure. For a child who has severe social phobia and moderate generalized anxiety disorder where avoidance is extensive across all social situations and evident through a regular use of safety behaviors such as checking and reassurance seeking, exposure may be planned over six or seven sessions – two for teaching the basic skill and for extending knowledge of exposure to costs and response prevention approaches, and then four or five sessions for reviewing and planning *in vivo* exposure and for conducting in-session exposure. In CBT generally, early sessions will tend to be more heavily loaded with "teaching" of new skills. During later sessions more time will be spent on the application of skills, each session generally leaving sufficient time for the practice of multiple skills.

Initial treatment plans that reflect the dosage of each skill are *estimates*; where not restricted by a manual, the competent therapist should review the effectiveness of the intervention and the adequacy of the formulation in relation to progress toward goals. In the Treatment for Adolescents with Depression Study protocol (Rogers, Reinecke, and Curry 2005), for example, formal reviews of the formulation and treatment plan occur after six and 12 weeks of treatment. After the first six weeks, during which the client and the therapist have identified specific problematic thoughts, behaviors, and emotions and have introduced core coping strategies, the therapist reviews the case material and constructs a case formulation that decides on whether the next five sessions will be spent on consolidating skills already introduced or on developing further skills (which may be individual or focused on the family). At the 12-week mark, a case review occurs. If the client is identified as a "full responder," a further six weeks of treatment focuses on rehearsal and consolidation of the skills that have led to improvement. If a partial response has occurred, the clinician reevaluates the case formulation to identify if (i) the initial formulation was inaccurate and consequently inappropriate modules were selected; (ii) an inadequate formulation was designed, leading to omission of needed modules; or (iii) an accurate formulation and treatment plan exists but more time for skill acquisition is required. This cyclic process of formulation, plan, and review at set points encourages the therapist to deliberately evaluate and reflect on his/her practice at the individual client level. The timing of the reviews may be varied according to the severity of the initial and ongoing problems and the degree of engagement with treatment. A maximum of six weeks between deliberate reflections on the case formulation and treatment plan is, however, an appropriate guide for the competent therapist.

Communicating and Negotiating with Children, Adolescents, and Parents

Initiating treatment through effective communication

In the first treatment session it is crucial that the therapist provide appropriate psycho-education about the nature of the disorder(s), the case formulation, and the treatment plan to both the parent and the child or adolescent. To begin this process, the therapist should present information on how (s)he has conceptualized the problem, using the terminology that best fits with the chosen nomothetic model (that is, choosing between concepts like anxiety, depression, low mood, social phobia, and the like) and the common factors that cause or maintain that problem. The language of this explanation needs to be appropriate for the age of the client and for his/her ability to understand the information provided. For children, such an explanation might amount to a simple listing of two to three reasons why they experience feelings of worry or sadness more often and/or more severely than others. For adolescents and parents, a more sophisticated explanation can be provided. During this explanation, the case formulation can be conveyed by way of showing how the client's experiences relate to the nomothetic model. Using a diagram that illustrates the case formulation can often assist this explanation. The therapist should assist the adolescent or the parent to apply the formulation to his/her own situation by using examples gathered during assessment and by eliciting examples from his/her own experience that fit with the case formulation. During this discussion it is important that fault for current problems is not attributed to a single behavior, cognition or individual. The emphasis should be on understanding how the identified factors have interacted to trigger the problematic anxiety and/or depression.

After case formulation, the treatment techniques designed to address each component of the formulated case should be presented. Care must be taken not to overwhelm the clients with information and not to induce excessive fear about the tasks that will be undertaken. The primary goal of presenting the treatment plan is to explain that this plan covers the factors related to the current problem comprehensively and, in doing so, to instill a sense of hope that change is possible and that you, as the therapist, are confident that the treatment plan can lead to that change. A brief overview of typical outcomes and a description of the usual course of improvement (for example that change is not linear, that some problems respond quicker than others, that setbacks may occur) can assist in creating realistic expectations of progress and of the likely outcomes. In addition, ensuring that the client's and the family's strengths – which have been incorporated into the case formulation and treatment plan – are emphasized during the psycho-education process will assist in building a sense of hope and encourage engagement with the coming sessions.

Setting Treatment Goals

After the presentation of the case formulation and treatment plan, the focus should move to the negotiation of treatment goals. To ensure that both the child or adolescent and the parents are engaged in the treatment process, both parties should be asked to suggest potential goals. The therapist will need to guide collaboration on the combination and selection of individual goals, and will be best served by encouraging the selection of goals that will allow focus on the child's or adolescent's primary diagnosis or on the issues that best reflect the reason(s) for seeking help. The therapist should be wary of setting goals that, although reflecting a real problem, do not address the core presenting problem. For example, in an adolescent who has a principal diagnosis of social phobia and secondary diagnoses of dysthymia and specific phobia (other type – dentists), the treatment may become side-tracked from dealing with the core issues related to the social phobia if a major goal of the treatment is to make the client go to the dentist. The therapist will need to negotiate with the family to select two or three treatment goals. Where there is major disagreement between parent and child or adolescent, allowing each party to select and develop a goal can avoid reaching an impasse from the first session. Such a course would be taken with a view to fostering collaboration and the two parties' engagement with each other's goal as sessions progress. It should also be noted that, where parents are to have a role in the treatment, it is appropriate to set a goal related to changes in their parenting. This procedure can also be used to spread the focus away from a child or adolescent who feels unfairly targeted – which is achieved by highlighting that it is not only his/her behavior that will be targeted, but also that of his/her parents. A final goal to consider is the addition of a therapist goal that reflects the CBT approach of "skilling up" vulnerable individuals to make them able to manage independently their experiences with anxiety and depression. Adding a therapist goal that states that the client should become "able to independently use [core skills from the treatment plan] to manage [worries/fears/low mood]" reminds families that one of the purposes of the CBT approach is to learn new skills. Reflection on the achievement of this goal can provide evidence that the client may be ready to terminate treatment, since, if the goal is achieved, the likelihood of relapse should be lessoned.

Once the general goals have been selected, the therapist should work with the child or adolescent or with the family to refine these goals, so that each one is sufficiently detailed. It is preferable for goals to be stated in a positive way, that is, to express what the client will do rather than what (s)he will not do. In particular, the therapist should focus on ensuring that written goals can be measured and/or that it will be clear when the goal is achieved. "Spend a minimum of one hour, six days a week, socializing with family or friends" may be an appropriate way to quantify success in achieving an initially suggested goal of "Spend less time alone," for example. The therapist should also collaborate with families to ensure that goals are realistic in terms of what will be achieved in relation to current functioning, that they are achievable within the time frame allowed for the treatment plan, and that, as stated earlier, they are relevant to the primary presenting problem(s). "Attend gymnastics class independently," where *independently* is defined as being dropped off and picked up at the front of the building, for a child who currently needs a parent to be in the gym during the lesson, is an example of a goal that appropriately focuses on the presenting problem and is realistic in relation to current functioning and time available for therapy.

At times a therapist may find that the child's or adolescent's mood and expectations of change are not sufficiently positive to make him/her able to imagine ever reaching the desired goals. The therapist may also find that a child or adolescent is unwilling to commit to any long-term goals, particularly where (s)he is attending therapy unwillingly or does not believe that (s)he has a "problem." In this situation the therapist may choose to set goals that are relevant to only the next one or two weeks, or to delay setting goals until work on motivation and engagement has been completed. After this, therapy goals can be revisited.

Progress, Obstacles, and Termination during Treatment

The role of assessment during treatment

As has been mentioned several times, case formulations and treatment plans are flexible guides that need to be reviewed and updated on the basis of the client's progress, as a result of increased understanding of the client's causal and maintaining factors, and as new information is discovered. This process can be facilitated through the use of formal and informal assessment. The most obvious assessment will be in the form of reflection on goal attainment. Rating each goal on achievement by using percentages, a rating out of 10, or a pictorial sequence of sad to happy faces (depending on the age of the client) helps to maintain session focus on the overall goals and prompts regular reflection on progress and on how close the client is to therapy termination. In addition, therapists should consider the administration of self-report and parent report symptom measures, in order to track change over time. Ideally the full measures, selected from those reviewed in Chapter 7, that were administered before treatment should be administered prior to making a decision to terminate treatment. While these measures are often utilized to track treatment outcome for quality assurance or for research purposes, they also have their place in determining whether a child or adolescent has improved sufficiently to warrant treatment termination. Preferably a therapist would not terminate treatment unless there had been a return to the nonclinical range on these independent measures or, alternatively, if a marked improvement in symptom severity and functioning has occurred.

Symptom severity tracking can also be conducted on a more regular basis. As the burden on clients and therapists would be unrealistic for full measures to be used and scored on a regular basis, individualized measures that focus on the most concerning symptoms can be developed for each client. The therapist could either choose to use the most relevant subscale of a full measure or select the top three symptoms from a measure to be completed by the client regularly. The therapist can determine how often this monitoring is conducted. Where the projected treatment length is of fewer than 10 sessions, rating goal attainment and the top three symptoms could easily be completed at the beginning of every session. Alternatively, if the projected treatment duration will be of three or more months, the therapist might find fortnightly or monthly ratings of progress sufficient. The advantage of such regular monitoring is two-fold. First, results can be quantified and graphed as an illustration of progress to the client and family. Second, the therapist can use the results to flag lack of progress, which may then initiate reflection and review of the case formulation and treatment plan.

Managing obstacles during treatment

Obstacles in the treatment may have been anticipated within the case formulation (see discussion in the section on deriving a case formulation), may be discovered during treatment, or may arise unexpectedly. The competent therapist needs to respond appropriately to ensure that therapy is not undermined or side-tracked by obstacles. If the obstacle to treatment is a newly identified factor that is causing or maintaining the presenting problem or represents a lack of response to a planned treatment technique, the therapist should review the case formulation and modify the treatment plan so as to incorporate new techniques or to adjust the presentation, order, or length of focus on the existing techniques. This "review and modify" approach would also be appropriate when the obstacle relates to lack of motivation, lack of belief in treatment utility, or lack of effective collaboration between parents and child or adolescent or between client and therapist.

Another form of obstacle is the occurrence of a "crisis" – that is, an event that is all-encompassing for the individual or the family and prevents work on therapy-related tasks; or an event that is more important than the initial treatment goals. These crises may be a consequence of the child's or adolescent's presenting problem, or they may be unexpected and unrelated to it. In either case, they can be harnessed as teaching material on which planned specific CBT techniques can be practiced. The competent therapist will allow the client to briefly vent and will acknowledge the distress experienced, then will guide the client to apply a treatment technique to the situation. For example, an adolescent who is overwhelmed by an assignment's deadline (which (s)he has avoided working on for several weeks) might be guided either (i) through a cognitive restructuring exercise designed to make him/her address negative thoughts related to his/her likely achievement on the task; or (ii) through a problem-solving exercise designed to enable him/her to initiate productive work on completing the assignment. For a situation not directly caused by the child's symptoms, such as having a substitute teacher for the next week, the therapist can either use a previously introduced technique to illustrate how to cope with challenging situations, or (s)he can use the incident itself to illustrate how a new technique may be applied.

A final note: occasionally an event may occur in a family that fundamentally shifts the priorities for change, and sometimes even the resources that the family has to dedicate to the therapy. Events such as diagnosis of a family member with a terminal illness, defense force deployment, natural disasters, or parental separation inevitably interfere with the direction or timing of therapy. The therapist will need to evaluate with the family how to deal with the crisis without neglecting the existence of preexisting problems. An appropriate plan may be to take a hiatus from the treatment plan and either have a treatment break or use treatment sessions to provide support related to the crisis for a set period of time. In both cases provision should be made for a time when planned treatment sessions will be reinitiated, or at least for a "check-in" call from the therapist to evaluate the need for further intervention in case a "hiatus" is taken. In such circumstances the therapist will need to review the case formulation and treatment plan to ensure its adequacy, given the new situation.

Ending Therapy and Fostering Maintenance of Gains

The final skill that a competent therapist must demonstrate during the provision of CBT is the ability to plan for the end of the therapy and to proactively foster the long-term maintenance of treatment gains. Treatment termination should be prepared for, irrespective of whether this termination is determined by the end of a manualized program or the end of funded sessions or is based on the achievement of goals. One or two sessions prior to the anticipated end of therapy, the child or adolescent, the parent, and the therapist should review goal achievement. Depending on progress, this review may be used (i) to encourage a final, concerted effort to achieve goals through increased practice; (ii) to encourage discussion of how the achievement of the therapist's "skilling up" goal will allow the family to continue to make progress toward the remaining goals; or, (iii) in situations where progress toward goals has been poor, to suggest that therapy should be extended rather than terminated (with an accompanying review of the case formulation and treatment plan). If therapy is to be terminated, then the therapist should elicit any concerns that the child or adolescent or the parent has about ending the treatment and should address any unrealistic beliefs or expectations regarding the client's ability to cope independently. When moving toward termination of treatment, the therapist may also want to consider the utility of spacing sessions fortnightly or monthly, to allow the client to experience growing independence while still accessing support.

The majority of manuals have specific content that addresses expectations regarding the potential for relapse and proactivity in maintaining gains. If the therapist works according to CBT principles, (s)he should make sure that the client and family are provided with psycho-education on the risk of relapse and the methods of responding to relapse. Most importantly, given that one of the goals of CBT is to have "skilled up" a client to manage the symptoms independently despite a higher underlying vulnerability, the therapist should illustrate to the client how to maintain gains through the continued application of the newly learnt skills. A personalized plan should be developed for how the client will continue to be proactive in dealing with his/her anxiety and/or depression and what his/her individual "tool kit" includes for managing these emotions; the plan should list the emotions, cognitions, and behaviors that may signal the client's need to utilize his/her CBT skills. Within this plan there should be a section on help seeking that includes supports from family and community, and also how to seek further professional help. Therapists should dedicate session time to setting short and long-term goals for the client. These may relate to continued work toward the initial therapy goals or, for clients who have achieved all the set goals, toward the recognition of those situations that may be challenging in the future (such as first school camp, applying for a job, or moving to high school), where CBT skills may be used to prepare for the event and, by doing so, may decrease the likelihood of a relapse.

Conclusion

Case formulation and treatment planning are fundamental skills for competent practice. They are, however, highly challenging skills to learn. All therapists, but particularly those in the early stages of their career, should take advantage of supervision – either from senior therapists in the case of trainees or through peer supervision for independent practitioners. Discussion of assessment results, your case formulation, and the resultant treatment plan will assist you to identify "gaps" in your logic and will ensure that you can express that logic to the client and his/her family in a confident manner. Havighurst and Downey (2009: 256) warn that, without a "combination of humility, confidence and clarity" in designing case formulations, the clinician risks de-emphasizing his/her professional knowledge, may derive tentative and somewhat meaningless formulations, or may come to make judgments that are not carefully considered or based on the collected data. Case formulation is part science, part art, and it is consequently important to remember that, at times, you will create a formulation that does not work. However, if you adapt flexibly to contradictory or new information, you are still working in the best interests of your client.

References

Addis, Michael E., and Neil S. Jacobson. 2000. "A Closer Look at the Treatment Rationale and Homework Compliance in Cognitive–Behavioral Therapy for Depression." *Cognitive Therapy and Research*, 24: 313–26. DOI: 10.1023/A:1005563304265

APA, Presidential Task Force on Evidence-Based Practice. 2006. "Evidence-Based Practice in Psychology." *American Psychologist*, 61: 271–85. DOI: 10.1037/0003-066X.61.4.271

Boschen, Mark J., and Tian P. S. Oei. 2008. "A Cognitive Behavioral Case Formulation Framework for Treatment Planning in Anxiety Disorders." *Depression and Anxiety*, 25: 811–23. DOI: 10.1002/da.20301

Chadwick, Paul, Clare Williams, and Joanna Mackenzie. 2003. "Impact of Case Formulation in Cognitive Behaviour Therapy for Psychosis." *Behaviour Research and Therapy*, 41: 671–80.

Chorpita, Bruce F. 2007. *Modular Cognitive–Behavioral Therapy for Childhood Anxiety Disorders*. New York: Guilford Press.

Eells, Tracy D., Kenneth G. Lombart, Nicholas Salsman, Edward M. Kendjelic, Carolyn T. Schneiderman, and Cynthia P. Lucas. 2011. "Expert Reasoning in Psychotherapy Case Formulation." *Psychotherapy Research*, 21: 385–99. DOI: 10.1080/10503307.2010.539284

Eisen, Andrew R., and Wendy K. Silverman. 1993. "Should I Relax or Change My Thoughts? A Preliminary Examination of Cognitive Therapy, Relaxation Training, and Their Combination with Overanxious Children." *Journal of Cognitive Psychotherapy*, 7: 265–79.

Eisen, Andrew R., and Wendy K. Silverman. 1998. "Prescriptive Treatment for Generalized Anxiety Disorder in Children." *Behavior Therapy*, 29: 105–21. DOI: 10.1016/S0005-7894(98)80034-8

Havighurst, Sophie S., and Laurel Downey. 2009. "Clinical Reasoning for Child and Adolescent Mental Health Practitioners: The Mindful Formulation." *Clinical Child Psychology and Psychiatry*, 14: 251–71. DOI: 10.1177/1359104508100888

Hudson, Jennifer L., and Ronald M. Rapee. 2004. "From Anxious Temperament to Disorder: An Etiological Model of Generalized Anxiety Disorder. In Richard G. Heimberg, Cynthia L. Turk, and Douglas S. Mennin (Eds.), *Generalized Anxiety Disorder: Advances in Research and Practice* (pp. 51–76). New York: Guilford Publications.

Kuyken, Willem, Claire D. Fothergill, Meyrem Musa, and Paul Chadwick. 2005. "The Reliability and Quality of Cognitive Case Formulation." *Behaviour Research and Therapy*, 43: 1187–201. DOI: 10.1016/j.brat.2004.08.007

Macneil, Craig A., Melissa K. Hasty, Philippe Conus, and Michael Berk. 2012. "Is Diagnosis Enough to Guide Interventions in Mental Health? Using Case Formulation in Clinical Practice." *BMC Medicine*, 10: 111. DOI: 10.1186/1741-7015-10-111

Persons, Jacqueline B. 1989. *Cognitive Therapy in Practice: A Case Formulation Approach* New York: W. W. Norton.

Persons, Jacqueline B, and Michael A. Tompkins. 1997. "Cognitive–Behavioral Case Formulation." In Tracy D. Eells (Ed.), *Handbook of Psychotherapy Case Formulation* (pp. 314–39). New York: Guildford Press.

Persons, Jacqueline B., Nicole A. Roberts, Christine A. Zalecki, and Whitney A. G. Brechwald. 2006. "Naturalistic Outcome of Case Formulation-Driven Cognitive-Behavior Therapy for Anxious Depressed Outpatients." *Behaviour Research and Therapy*, 44: 1041–51. DOI: 10.1016/j.brat.2005.08.005 DOI:10.1016/j.brat.2005.08.005

Rapee, Ronald M. 2001. "The Development of Generalised Anxiety." In Michael W. Vasey and Mark R. Dadds (Eds.), *The Developmental Psychopathology of Anxiety* (pp. 481–504). New York: Oxford University Press.

Rogers, Gregory M., Mark A. Reinecke, and John F. Curry. 2005. "Case Formulation in TADS CBT." *Cognitive and Behavioral Practice*, 12: 198–208. DOI: 10.1016/S1077-7229(05)80025-2

Treatment for Adolescents with Depression Study (TADS) Team. 2009. "The Treatment for Adolescents With Depression Study (TADS): Outcomes over 1 Year of Naturalistic Follow-Up." *American Journal of Psychiatry*, 166: 1141–9. DOI: 10.1176/appi.ajp.2009.08111620

10

Effectively Engaging and Collaborating with Children and Adolescents in Cognitive Behavioral Therapy Sessions

Jeremy S. Peterman, Cara A. Settipani, and Philip C. Kendall

Introduction

Cognitive behavioral therapy (CBT) is a collaborative undertaking that presupposes participant engagement, "collaboration" being seen to consist of working together toward a common goal, and "engagement" referring to one's investment and involvement in the treatment. Collaboration is central to therapy with youth. It has been associated with less attrition, positive treatment outcomes, and a more favorable therapeutic alliance (Chu et al. 2004; Creed and Kendall 2005). Collaboration can be said to create the foundation of the alliance, fostering trust and increasing the child's motivation. Engagement, or involvement, is of particular importance because youth typically do not refer themselves to treatment and may not see their situation as problematic. Accordingly, CBT therapists working with youth engage the child with a goal of making therapy both relevant and enjoyable. Often the CBT therapist uses engagement strategies such as rewards, stories, metaphors, drawings, games, and other interactive methods. Strategies of engagement are also tailored for adolescents.

Key Features of Competencies and Behavioral Markers

Ability to collaboratively set and adhere to the session goals or agenda

Agenda and goals are potentially influenced by the parent, the youth, the therapist, and the treatment manual. Thus a negotiation regarding the goals and the agenda is needed between the involved parties, including the youth. Importantly, collaboratively

Evidence-Based CBT for Anxiety and Depression in Children and Adolescents: A Competencies-Based Approach, First Edition. Edited by Elizabeth S. Sburlati, Heidi J. Lyneham, Carolyn A. Schniering, and Ronald M. Rapee. © 2014 John Wiley & Sons, Ltd. Published 2014 by John Wiley & Sons, Ltd.

setting goals has been found to relate to a stronger therapeutic alliance, as perceived by the child (Creed and Kendall 2005). Within this collaborative model, the therapist takes the role of a "coach" (Kendall 2012). As a coach, the therapist explains to the child that her role includes some teaching, some practice, as well as providing encouragement and support throughout. The coach is equipped with specialized knowledge about ways to treat the presenting concern and to reach set goals. Equally relevantly, the therapist emphasizes that the child contributes important knowledge about himself, his family, and his experiences and that parents may contribute complementary knowledge. Within collaboration, the therapist highlights that she, the child, and (depending on the treatment manual or the circumstances) the parents work together as a team, each bringing valuable expertise that can be integrated. It is important to keep in mind these complementary roles when setting the agenda and determining goals, and to ensure that each party has a balanced influence on goals and tasks. For example, the therapist can check in with all parties at the end of each session to discuss opinions on progress toward goals.

When using an empirically supported treatment for youth internalizing disorders (Kendall and Hedtke 2006; Stark et al. 2007), much of the therapy agenda will be outlined in the treatment manual. Adherence to the core components of the manual is important, but treatment is also tailored to the individual child; the principle for this is "flexibility within fidelity" (Kendall and Beidas 2007; Kendall, Gosch, Furr, and Sood 2008). Manuals are not to be used in "cookie cutter" fashion, but rather as guides. For example, implementing exposure, behavioral activation, and cognitive restructuring is central to the treatment of anxiety and depression, yet the content and application of these tasks will vary depending on the child's idiosyncratic presentation. By allowing a child to influence the choice of the topic from which he is to learn or practice a new skill, the therapist can ensure that the session is engaging and, through a judicial selection of the options offered by the child, that each session contributes to the overall goals.

Ability to communicate the rationale for each specific CBT technique

Taking the time to explain CBT activities conveys the message that the therapist wants the youth to understand the importance of the intervention rather than blindly follow an authority's orders. Discussing the rationale exemplifies collaboration and motivates the child to "buy in," thereby increasing compliance during in-session and homework tasks. When discussing CBT with youth, it is important to avoid jargon and to use developmentally appropriate language. The use of metaphors can make CBT accessible to young children and provides a simple way to understand complex concepts (Friedberg and Wilt 2010). For example, when introducing mood-regulating strategies – such as relaxation, coping thoughts, or behavioral activation – the therapist could say: "In the upcoming sessions we're going to go through a tool box with lots of different tools you can use when you are feeling upset. Different tools can be used for different situations, just as a screwdriver and a hammer are used for different things. I can help provide you with several possible tools, and then we can decide what works best for you."

In the Coping Cat treatment for youth anxiety (Kendall and Hedtke 2006), the therapist uses the metaphor of a fire alarm to explain somatic reactions in anxiety. For example, the therapist may say:

> When we feel really anxious, it's like our bodies have their own fire alarms. They provide cues when danger may be present. For example, when your body's fire alarm goes off, your heart beats fast, your palms get sweaty, and you may feel butterflies in your stomach. But sometimes a fire alarm goes off because it thinks there's a fire but there really isn't one. This is called a false alarm. Has that ever happened to you at school, when the school fire alarm goes off, but it's just a test … not a real fire? Your body can sometimes do the same thing. You may feel those bodily reactions, like there's a danger, but there is really no danger, it's just a false alarm.

Similarly, stories and appropriate therapist self-disclosure are other methods to explain the CBT rationale and to improve the therapeutic alliance. The therapist should determine if the rationale has been understood by asking youth, in a fun and nonconfrontational way, to explain it back to the therapist or to parents, or by eliciting feedback to assess whether the information was communicated clearly and effectively.

Prior to presenting a rationale to a child, a therapist needs to ensure her own comfort with explaining the relevant details. This can be achieved through practice, by explaining each rationale to people unfamiliar with the treatment, and through analysis of video recordings of sessions focused on a child's reactions and evidence of comprehension.

Ability to elicit and respond to feedback

Delivering feedback can be empowering for the child (Friedberg and McClure 2002) and can illustrate that the therapist and the child are working as a "team." Furthermore, eliciting feedback allows for a more individualized protocol. For example, when constructing a fear hierarchy, it is important to have the child contribute items to the list. Once the hierarchy is established, the therapist can elicit feedback about what makes each item harder or easier (for example social anxiety exposure tasks can involve girls or boys, younger or older children, large or small groups of people); and this will assist in a further application of the skill.

The timing of feedback is important. The end of a session provides a natural time to inquire about feedback, but feedback can also be elicited before, after, and during therapy tasks. The purpose of this feedback is to gather objective evidence regarding what can be learnt from skill implementation, for example by contrasting anxiety before or during and after an exposure, and to compare the child's comprehension or experience of the skill with the intended goal. This latter feedback can be used to identify and address potential ruptures in the session before the agenda – or progress – is derailed. Therapists should also be cognizant of the child's nonverbal feedback. A sudden mood shift, change in body posture, cessation of regular eye contact, or eye-rolling are signals that the therapist should pause and check in with the child. Responding to these nonverbal cues with questions such as, "I noticed you've been looking away for the past minute or so, what's going on," or "what I just said seemed to upset you, tell me how you're feeling" makes the child feel attended to and provides the therapist with valuable information to guide the next therapeutic interaction. The therapist needs to adjust therapy tasks in response to feedback, in a way that guarantees continued progress toward skill development and goals, while also ensuring that the child remains engaged.

Ability to facilitate in-session collaboration

In addition to working on direct collaboration between child and therapist through goal or agenda setting, by communicating rationales, and by utilizing feedback, incorporating parents into the collaboration has benefits. These include improvement in the internalizing symptoms, greater family participation, and less frequent cancellations (Hawley and Weisz 2005; McLeod and Weisz 2005). The role taken by the parent is determined by the selected manual, the setting of the therapy, and that parent's willingness to be a part of it. All collaboration may occur with the direct involvement of the child or through parent–therapist discussions, conducted independently of the child. The latter are crucial when the matters discussed may be embarrassing or punitive for the child. When working with the parent independently, it is crucial to frame for the child how you will protect his privacy, what the purposes of the discussions are, and how you will use the information you gather.

Kendall (2012) proposed three ways in which parents can contribute to therapy for youth. Parents can be consultants, collaborators, or co-clients. The "consultant" parent provides input on treatment concerns and goals and on progress over time, as well as a different point of view on the success (or otherwise) of skill practice and generalization. "Collaborative" parents help facilitate a "transfer of control" (Silverman, Ginsburg, and Kurtines 1995): for children, the therapist is gradually phased out and parents take charge, to help their child cope (e.g., a parent responds to a child's apparent worry about a school performance by guiding the child to use coping self-talk). With adolescents, the therapist transfers her control to the adolescents themselves, allowing the parents to take a supportive role on request (e.g., when the adolescent requests the parent to facilitate a pleasant event by providing transport). To enable a successful transfer of control, the therapist may include the parent in some sessions during the treatment: in this way she can exchange therapist knowledge and skills with that parent. For instance, at the end of a relaxation training session, the youth would teach the parent, under the therapist's guidance, how to do deep breathing and progressive muscle relaxation; or the therapist would dedicate session time to teach the parent relevant skills, independently. Finally, the parent may be a "co-client" in situations where the direct targeting of parenting behavior is necessitated by a manual (e.g., training in family conflict resolution) or by the fact that the parent's behavior impacts on the child's progress (e.g., the parent's anxiety discourages the child's completion of exposure tasks). Each of these roles can be used to facilitate collaboration with the therapist and child to support treatment progress.

Ability to implement specific CBT techniques flexibly

"Flexibility within fidelity" represents another competency. CBT procedures are optimal when presented flexibly and in sync with the youth's presenting problem, needs, preferences, cultural background, level of emotional and cognitive development, and current mood. For example, Friedberg and Gorman (2007) proposed that clients who are older, motivated, high in hopelessness, afraid of negative evaluation, and more stable (e.g., not in crisis) or who have a high tolerance for frustration may benefit from increased collaboration and less direction and structure. All CBT strategies can be tailored to the needs of the client. For example, therapists may personalize relaxation recordings to reflect visualizations that are meaningful to the client; they may present "thinking traps" and other cognitive restructuring methods via visual or verbal methods in response to the client's preferred learning style; they may adjust the content in problem solving to reflect issues salient to the child's recent experience; and they may introduce visual aids, such as a fear hierarchy or a mood thermometer, which can be decorated according to the child's interests (e.g., Harry Potter themed visual aids). A discussion of modifications recommended for specific disorders and for the developmental level appears later in the chapter.

Although there is no single framework for adapting interventions designed for culturally diverse youth (Crawley, Podell, Beidas, Braswell, and Kendall 2010), culture does impact notions of etiology, treatment, compliance, and goals. Broadly speaking, the therapist benefits from having an awareness of the child's cultural context. For example, a family whose cultural beliefs emphasize respect for the knowledge of experts (as seen in many Asian cultures) may prefer a therapist to be directive rather than collaborative, or may need additional explanations of why collaboration is crucial to progress. Awareness of the child's environmental context is also crucial. For example, during cognitive restructuring, a therapist might test a negative belief by asking: "How likely is it for a feared outcome to occur?" (e.g., fear of being hurt). If the child is living in a dangerous environment, then the concern may not be irrational. Testing its likelihood would be both unproductive and insensitive, given the child's context. Under these circumstances it would be preferable to use problem solving or to evaluate the worst case scenario and devise ways to cope.

Ability to make use of experiential strategies

The ability to make use of experiential strategies so as to implement specific CBT techniques is worth a brief discussion; however, specific examples are provided in each of the CBT technique chapters. Experiential strategies – such as reinforcement, role-play, and modeling – make CBT content accessible to children. Implementation of the more "adult," discussion-based model of CBT may elicit disengagement, boredom, and poor understanding of the concepts of therapy. Reinforcement is particularly important for increasing the factors of motivation and compliance in youth. Unlike adults, most youth do not volunteer to come to therapy and, accordingly, may require external incentives. For example, anxious youth can receive "brave bucks" for completing exposure tasks, and then they can choose how to spend their "bucks" on available rewards and privileges. Importantly, rewards do not have to cost money and can include privileges – like choosing the family dinner, watching a movie with a parent, or being excused from a disliked chore. Therapists can evaluate the effectiveness of the reinforcement by determining whether it increases the targeted behavior. Modeling and role-play are active tasks that engage a youth in understanding therapy content and in practicing newly learnt skills. For example, a therapist can illustrate the application of a skill by modeling its use in an imagined scenario; the youth then proceeds to roleplay use of that skill. The process may also pull on additional resources, such as watching videos in which others are using a skill, or recording videos to obtain feedback on skill use. The effectiveness of these approaches is evaluated through the child's engagement in the task and the child's ability to complete the behavior, initially with the therapist's assistance, then independently.

Ability to end sessions in a planned manner

A successful therapist aims to accomplish all the session goals without feeling rushed. A therapist can work toward this aim by utilizing a manual's checklist or the agenda set collaboratively at the start of the session to actively keep track of progress during the session. When planning sessions, therapists need to ensure that sufficient time is allowed for any consultation with the parents and for reward activities promised to the child. Sometimes therapists will realize that they still have too much session material to cover in the remaining time and may hurry through the remaining tasks, sacrificing depth of content. Other times therapists may end the session abruptly, without allowing time for crucial feedback processes. In situations where the therapist does not have time to complete the tasks, it is recommended to leave content for the next session rather than rush through material. In the next session the therapist should reorient the child to the material from the prior week. If the therapist promised the child a game at the end, it is important for the therapist to follow through regardless of the amount of uncovered content, so that the therapy relationship is not undermined.

Competence in Treating Specific Disorders

The treatment of specific youth internalizing disorders often requires the use of specialized therapy techniques. Flexibility to adapt standard protocols to meet the particular presentation of an individual child is a highly valuable therapist skill. Ways in which the aforementioned competencies may vary for particular disorders are discussed below.

Youth with generalized anxiety disorder (GAD) or obsessive–compulsive disorder (OCD) are often rigid in their style of thinking and behaving. They commonly have low tolerance for uncertainty. Explicitly structuring the sessions in a predictable manner helps such a child to focus on session content rather than fixate on what will happen next. Noticing that an anxious youth is overly rigid in adhering to a session agenda is an important therapeutic observation, which can be used to inform exposure sessions. In addition, therapists should consider how disruption to a session's routine (e.g., the need to end a session before covering previously planned session content) may affect such youth and proactively address any concerns. Experiential techniques may be difficult to implement with youth who have rigid thinking styles or who prefer to follow set rules. Rationales may need to be explained in more depth. Therapists may need to encourage these youth to be creative and to remind them that therapy does not have rules, like school (e.g., spelling does not matter) and that there is no "grade." Finally, youth with GAD or OCD may be particularly resistant to change. They may interpret their anxious symptoms as "helpful," which can impact the collaboration between therapist and child. Therapists should be prepared to elicit and respond to negative feedback from the child in order to maintain collaboration.

The impact that social anxiety has on the therapist–client relationship can present a particular challenge to effectively engaging youth in therapy. Youth with social phobia may be inclined to try to please the therapist. This social desirability bias can be problematic for the creation of a therapist–child collaboration, as difficult and at times unflattering situations or events need to be discussed in the session. Sessions, in and of themselves, may be exposures for youth with social phobia, given that speaking with adults is typically anxiety provoking for youth with the disorder. Compounded with the focus on the child's own anxiety symptoms, youth with social phobia may feel quite vulnerable in session. To effectively engage such youth, therapists should be cognizant of the child's potential discomfort and should structure the sessions such that rapport can be built without placing too much burden on the child to initiate conversation. For example, playing a "getting to know you" game or ice-breaker provides more structure than an open-ended conversation and can be less intimidating for socially anxious youth. Therapists may also wish to consider focusing on the experience of anxiety more broadly to begin with – for example, they could start by asking the child to imagine what it's like for a family member or a friend to experience anxiety – thereby normalizing the experience of anxiety. When they obtain feedback, therapists could have the child write or draw rather than carry an oral discussion. Resorting to yes/no and forced choice options or drawing on the parent to provide responses may also be helpful, particularly during the early period of building trust and comfort. Early sessions will likely need to be more heavily guided by the therapist, who can encourage the child's participation and gradually work toward increasing his leadership of the sessions. Engaging in experiential strategies and exposures may prove difficult for youth who fear negative evaluation from the therapist and others. In such instances, the therapist can model "messing up" in front of the child (e.g., by dropping a book in a crowded area), to show the child that even the therapist does embarrassing things at times, which may help the child feel more at ease. Socially anxious youth may also be particularly sensitive to corrective feedback, a point that therapists should be mindful of when they respond to a child's attempts to engage in therapy.

Facilitating collaboration can also be difficult when treating youth with post-traumatic stress disorder (PTSD), particularly if the child is distrustful of adults as a result of the traumatic event, or if feelings of shame and guilt are present. Furthermore, the child may not have shared all the details of the trauma with his parents. The therapist is faced with the challenge of getting the child to feel comfortable about disclosing this information while respecting the child's privacy and at the same time maintaining collaboration with both the child and parents. Though challenging, building a strong collaboration with the child at the beginning of therapy may be particularly important in treating youth with PTSD.

Youth with separation anxiety disorder (SAD) may present logistical challenges to collaboratively conducting CBT. For example, youth with severe separation anxiety are reluctant to separate from a parent in order to meet with a therapist individually. Therapists can build collaboration by initially allowing the parent to be in the room, or just outside the door, and by rewarding the child for any efforts to increase the amount of separation from the parent. Establishing set breaks from therapy in which the child is allowed to see the parent can get the child to be more engaged in the session and less focused on reunification. Communicating the rationale for exposures may be difficult and upsetting for youth with SAD. They may not be interested in improving their ability to cope with being away from their parent, but rather view always being near the parent as the only solution to their anxiety. Thus, in the exposure phase of the treatment, therapists may encounter difficulties setting a session agenda in a collaborative manner. Allowing these youth to have greater control over other aspects of the session may reduce frustration and maintain the collaborative, team approach.

Special considerations are necessary when treating youth with depressive disorders. These youth may have low levels of motivation, or they may lack the energy needed to change their current functioning. Youth who feel hopeless and have an external locus of control may be difficult to engage in the therapeutic process if they feel they have limited ability to change their situation. Thus, setting session goals may have to be more therapist-guided. In addition, getting a depressed child to implement CBT techniques such as behavioral activation in their daily lives may be particularly challenging. Even if the rationale is clearly communicated, therapists will also need to explicitly hook into factors that may motivate the child to change. The usual luster associated with tangible or social rewards may be lacking among youth who are depressed. Drawing on family members' support to facilitate activity scheduling may be necessary. Furthermore, depressed youth may believe that their feedback is not important and unlikely to bring about change; the therapist can demonstrate that the youth has the ability to effect change by being persistent in eliciting feedback and by responding to such feedback clearly, with corresponding adjustments to therapy.

Developmental Considerations: Competence in Treating Children and Adolescents

The competent implementation of empirically supported treatments requires appropriate responsiveness to the developmental level of the child or adolescent. In terms of setting session goals, younger children may be unable to articulate goals and may require the therapist to keep it simple and take the lead. However, as sessions progress and become more predictable, therapists can have youth draw on their experiences in past sessions to say what they think should be part of the agenda. Adolescents, on the other hand, may have from the very beginning different goals for therapy from those of the therapist and of parents. It is important for the therapist to identify right from start particular "treatment deliverables" for the adolescent and parents and to balance each person's goals, which may be quite divergent. Issues with peers and family may be particularly important from the adolescents' point of view, and incorporating these topics will increase the likelihood that the youth will be engaged in session.

Similarly, building rapport and collaboration with adolescents looks very different from building rapport and collaboration with children. Younger children often enjoy playing games with the therapist, whereas adolescents find such activities too child-like and prefer getting to know the therapist by simply having a conversation. With adolescents, taking a walk while talking, so that the focus is not on direct eye contact, can often help break down barriers. Finding ways to connect with teens – and ways that are not forced: for example, the therapist could share how she feels after she has a misunderstanding with a friend, when the adolescent recounts a similar event – can enhance the collaboration and demonstrate understanding of the adolescent's perspective. Importantly, therapists need to convey that their sharing with adolescents is genuine, even if this means admitting to a lack of knowledge of, or to a (respectful) dislike for, something the adolescent loves; for adolescents rarely engage positively when they sense deceit or condescension.

Communicating the rationale for specific CBT strategies will also vary with the developmental stage. With children, the goal is to use language that is comprehensible – no jargon or technical terms. Using metaphors, cartoons, and real-life examples can increase the accessibility of concepts. Breaking concepts into smaller, more digestible parts and linking themes across sessions can be helpful. Adolescents, on the other hand, prefer being treated like adults and may be turned off by language or activities that seem child-like in nature. Conveying ideas in a relaxed manner, without seeming overly formal or trying too hard to be like the teen (e.g., avoiding the use of phrases that are popular with teens but sound odd coming from an adult) is appropriate. Eliciting feedback varies according to the client's age: younger children may not have the vocabulary to give detailed feedback. They may be intimidated by the perceived authority of the adult therapist or erroneously concerned that such information will be shared with their parents, who will reprimand them for negative feedback. Specifically asking for feedback on something they enjoyed and something they thought "boring" can help elicit negative feedback. To elicit feedback from adolescents, the therapist can frame giving feedback as an opportunity for the youth to be the boss and decide whether the therapist is meeting expectations.

Experiential strategies require tailoring to developmental level. With younger children, reinforcement may consist in concrete, short-term rewards. Therapists can be creative with visually displaying sticker charts, to make the experience of earning rewards even more enjoyable and interactive. Any handouts should be age-appropriate and may involve cartoons or depictions of concepts and less written material. To keep the child engaged while modeling skills such as relaxation techniques, the therapist and the child can imagine what a superhero would look like if he were taking deep breaths before embarking on a brave adventure. Art projects, acting, and creating videos tend to be more appealing to children than the discussion of concepts, and techniques that require the child to generate the material can also reinforce learning.

Though reinforcements still play an important role when treating adolescents, adolescents may have a more difficult time identifying meaningful rewards or may feel bashful about earning rewards. Coming to session prepared with adolescent-friendly reward options (e.g., gift certificates to the movies or to restaurants) and normalizing the process of earning rewards for hard work (e.g., likening it to earning a paycheck at work) can help adolescents feel at ease. Adolescents' reluctance can show when they are engaging in strategies such as relaxation, which may be perceived as strange, or in experiential strategies such as role-play, which requires them to be creative. Therapists can normalize the youth's concern and be collaborative (e.g., by saying, "I know this might seem strange … I thought it was the first time I did it, too)" and praise adolescents for their efforts to try new things.

Common Obstacles to Competent Practice and Methods to Overcome Them

Much to the chagrin of therapists, obstacles to treatment can be more the rule than the exception. In general, the test of a therapist's competence is not solely in knowledge of the treatment protocol, but also in the reactions needed when challenges arise.

When behavioral disorders such as attention-deficit/hyperactivity disorder (ADHD) and oppositional defiant behavior (ODD) co-occur with internalizing disorders, therapists must draw on skills to maintain fidelity to treatment protocols. Youth with these comorbidities may exhibit more behavioral difficulties in session, and often have difficulty staying on task and complying with directions. When setting session goals, therapists who work with these youth may wish to explicitly note when goals are achieved and to reward the child for on-task behavior. Breaking goals down into more manageable chunks, allowing the child frequent breaks, and incorporating physical activities (such as building an exposure stepladder on the floor) can also be beneficial. When noncompliant or defiant behavior is exhibited by the child, collaboration can be difficult to maintain. Such youth may test the therapist's authority. Maintaining firm expectations and following through with consequences for noncompliance is important in the context of a warm, supportive relationship. Covering session content and ending sessions in a planned manner may be challenging when one is working with youth with attention difficulties. Setting realistic expectations for the session in the basis of the child's presentation is important for maintaining structure and for ensuring that sessions are not rushed at the end.

There are many potential obstacles that have the capacity to undermine collaborative engagement with youth, including the ability to set and adhere to the session goals and agenda. In addition to the challenges presented by ADHD/ODD, at the other extreme are internalizing and detail-oriented children who get too preoccupied with the agenda. For example, anxious youth with high intolerance of uncertainty may ask excessive questions about the details of the session plan. Addressing every question is unproductive and may reinforce reassurance-seeking behavior. Therapists need to redirect the child to the activity at hand and note that some issues will be addressed at a later time. Importantly, there may be times when issues or crises arise that are not part of the planned agenda. The therapist should respond appropriately to the nature of the issue but also needs to be alert that the child or parent is not introducing issues in an attempt to derail the agenda. This may occur as a strategy to avoid particular therapy components, or it may reflect ambivalence about treatment goals.

The ability to respond to feedback is susceptible to obstacles. The therapist must balance sensitivity with compliance to therapy, particularly when children note that they do not want to participate in a therapeutic task. Disregarding the feedback makes the therapist appear flippant and may detract from the sense of collaboration; yet acquiescence can be counterproductive, and it can even reinforce avoidance. The therapist can validate the child's feelings and thank him for providing their feedback. For example, the therapist could say: "I understand why you think that this might not work for you. Other kids have thought that too, but with practice they saw it differently and became more confident ..." Ultimately, the therapist remains resolute that the child will at least attempt the activity. When children are stubborn, therapists can motivate them through rewards for task completion or problem-solving ways to make the activity more acceptable. For example, the therapist can present the choice of two or three tasks of comparable difficulty, from which the child must choose. This choice empowers the child and illustrates that therapy is a collaborative process. Other times, children may refuse to provide verbal feedback but may find alternative methods, such as writing, drawing, texting, or using an anonymous feedback form acceptable.

Difficulties can also arise when one is attempting to facilitate collaboration with parents. Suveg and colleagues (2006) outline several important issues when working with parents. Parents may hinder therapy by being under- or overinvolved. With regard to the former, therapists can try to understand the parent's reasons for being minimally involved. The use of motivational interviewing (e.g., "How do you see your child in five years if nothing changes?") – as well as psycho-education about the treatment model and individual treatment components – can get parents on board with the treatment. A therapist can also invite parents to sessions, to learn concurrently with their children. For parents who are too involved, a discussion of boundaries and an explicit conversation about their role in therapy may be warranted. Regardless of the parents' presentation, goals and expectations should be outlined early in therapy. The therapist may need to provide corrective feedback for unrealistic expectations and goals, particularly within the context of what is developmentally appropriate.

Finally, it is worth noting that therapists need to be cognizant of their own reactions to a youth's engagement, feedback, and cooperativeness during therapy. Some children and adolescents are difficult to work with and can challenge a therapist's confidence. In these situations seeking supervision to discuss concerns and to receive guidance on appropriate management strategies is crucial.

Conclusion

The dissemination of empirically supported treatments has been advanced with the delineation of therapist competencies required to conduct CBT with youth (Sburlati et al. 2011). The competencies can be challenging, given the complexity and individual variation of children and adolescents. Developmental level, motivation for treatment, and presentation of internalizing disorders can influence a therapist's ability to effectively engage and collaborate with youth. The therapist should have an understanding of the behavioral markers of these competencies, of the ways in which they often need to be tailored to a particular child's presentation, and of the obstacles that are likely to arise; at the same time the therapist should keep an eye on creativity and flexibility. Maintaining this balance puts a therapist in a strong position to engage a child in therapy most effectively and to bring about the success of the treatment.

References

Chu, Brian C., Muniya S. Choudhury, Alison L. Shortt, Donna B. Pincus, Torrey A. Creed, Philip C. Kendall. 2004. "Alliance, Technology, and Outcome in the Treatment of Anxious Youth." *Cognitive And Behavioral Practice*, 11: 44–55. DOI: 10.1016/S1077-7229(04)80006-3

Crawley, Sarah A., Jennifer L. Podell, Rinad S. Beidas, Lauren Braswell, and Philip C. Kendall. 2010. "Cognitive–Behavioral Therapy with Youth." In Keith S. Dobson (Ed.), *Handbook of Cognitive–Behavioral Therapies* (3rd ed., pp. 375–410). New York: Guilford Press.

Creed, Torrey A., and Philip C. Kendall. 2005. "Therapist Alliance-Building Behavior within a Cognitive–Behavioral Treatment for Anxiety in Youth." *Journal of Consulting and Clinical Psychology*, 73: 498–505. DOI: 10.1037/0022-006X.73.3.498

Friedberg, Robert D., and Angela A. Gorman. 2007. "Integrating Psychotherapeutic Processes with Cognitive Behavioral Procedures." *Journal Of Contemporary Psychotherapy*, 37: 185–93. DOI: 10.1007/s10879-007-9053-1

Friedberg, Robert D., and Jessica M. McClure. 2002. *Clinical Practice of Cognitive Therapy with Children and Adolescents: The Nuts and Bolts.* New York: Guilford.

Friedberg, Robert D., and Laura H. Wilt. 2010. "Metaphors and Stories in Cognitive Behavioral Therapy with Children." *Journal of Rational–Emotive & Cognitive Behavior Therapy*, 28: 100–13. DOI: 10.1007/s10942-009-0103-3

Hawley, Kristin M., and John R. Weisz. 2005. "Youth versus Parent Working Alliance in Usual Clinical Care: Distinctive Associations with Retention, Satisfaction, and Treatment Outcome." *Journal of Clinical Child and Adolescent Psychology*, 34: 117–28. DOI: 10.1207/s15374424jccp3401_11

Kendall, Philip C. 2012. "Guiding Theory for Therapy with Children and Adolescents." In Philip C. Kendall (Ed.), *Child and Adolescent Therapy: Cognitive Behavioral Procedures* (4th ed., pp. 3–24). New York: Guilford Press.

Kendall, Philip C., and Rinad S. Beidas. 2007. "Smoothing the Trail for Dissemination of Evidence-Based Practices for Youth: Flexibility within Fidelity." *Professional Psychology: Research and Practice*, 38: 13–20. DOI: 0.1037/0735-7028.38.1.13

Kendall, Philip C., and Kristina Hedtke. 2006. "Cognitive–Behavioral Therapy for Anxious Children: Therapist Manual" (3rd ed.). Ardmore, PA: Workbook Publishing.

Kendall, Philip C., Elizabeth Gosch, Jami M. Furr, and Erica Sood. 2008. "Flexibility within Fidelity." *Journal of the American Academy of Child and Adolescent Psychiatry*, 47: 987–93. DOI: 10.1097/CHI.0b013e31817eed2f

McLeod, Bryce D., and John R. Weisz. 2005. "The Therapy Process Observational Coding System-Alliance Scale: Measure Characteristics and Prediction of Outcome in Usual Clinical Practice." *Journal of Consulting and Clinical Psychology*, 73: 323–33. DOI: 10.1037/0022-006X.73.2.323

Sburlati, Elizabeth S., Carolyn A. Schniering, Heidi J. Lyneham, and Ronald M. Rapee. 2011. "A Model of Therapist Competencies for the Empirically Supported Cognitive–Behavioral Treatment of Child and Adolescent Anxiety and Depressive Disorders." *Clinical Child and Family Psychology Review*, 14: 89–109. DOI: 10.1007/s10567-011-0083-6

Silverman, Wendy K., Golda S. Ginsburg, and William M. Kurtines. 1995. "Clinical Issues in Treating Children with Anxiety and Phobic Disorders." *Cognitive and Behavioral Practice*, 2: 93–117.

Stark, Kevin D., Jane Simpson, Sarah Schnoebelen, Jennifer Hargrave, Johanna Molnar, and R. Glen. 2007. *Treating Depressed Youth: Therapist Manual for "ACTION."* Ardmore, PA: Workbook Publishing.

Suveg, Cynthia, Tami L. Roblek, Joanna Robin, Amy Krain, Sasha Aschenbrand, and Golda S. Ginsburg. 2006. "Parental Involvement when Conducting Cognitive–Behavioral Therapy for Children with Anxiety Disorders." *Journal of Cognitive Psychotherapy*, 20: 287–99.

11

Facilitating Homework and Generalization of Skills to the Real World

Colleen M. Cummings, Nikolaos Kazantzis, and Philip C. Kendall

Introduction

Homework is one of the fundamental components of cognitive behavioral therapy (CBT) for youth anxiety and depressive disorders. Practicing CBT therapists report widespread use of therapeutic homework (Kazantzis, Lampropoulos, and Deane 2005), but they also acknowledge variations in how it is used (Houlding, Schmidt, and Walker 2010). Theoretically, homework tasks are important because they (i) encourage opportunities to practice skills learned in session; (ii) give the therapist a chance to determine the youth's understanding of skills; (iii) allow the youth to generalize therapeutic skills to real-life situations; and (iv), in anxiety, help the youth gradually face feared situations in his/her own environment (Hudson and Kendall 2002). CBT homework is typically discussed and assigned during each session and reviewed at the beginning of the next session. Therapy homework for anxiety initially includes skills practice and eventually out-of-session exposure tasks: in both, the youth practices skills learned in therapy by engaging in real-life situations (Kendall and Hedtke 2006a). Therapy homework for youth suffering from depression entails keeping a mood diary or log, skills practice (e.g., challenging depressogenic thinking), and pleasant activity scheduling through behavioral activation (Clarke, Lewinsohn, and Hops 1990; Curry et al. 2005; Stark et al. 1996).

Among adults, homework assignments have shown small to moderate relationships with treatment outcome (see the meta-analysis by Kazantzis, Whittington, and Datilio 2010; also Mausbach, Moore, Roesch, Cardenas, and Patterson 2010). The same may be true for anxious youth: out-of-session exposure tasks are linked to improved treatment outcome. In one report (Puleo and Kendall 2011), out-of-session

Evidence-Based CBT for Anxiety and Depression in Children and Adolescents: A Competencies-Based Approach,
First Edition. Edited by Elizabeth S. Sburlati, Heidi J. Lyneham, Carolyn A. Schniering, and Ronald M. Rapee.
© 2014 John Wiley & Sons, Ltd. Published 2014 by John Wiley & Sons, Ltd.

homework was found to be critical to positive gains for youth with anxiety and comorbid moderate autism spectrum disorders (ASD; Puleo and Kendall 2011; and see also Simons et al. 2012). When working with youth, therapists can use a variety of strategies to encourage therapeutic homework completion. Popular strategies include praising the client for completion, trouble-shooting any difficulties the child may have had, aligning homework completion with therapy goals, targeting client strengths, choosing homework collaboratively, and problem solving around barriers (Houlding et al. 2010). Homework is tailored on the basis of the therapist's case conceptualiza-tion, and client beliefs about the homework can be explored. Determining homework tasks that facilitate real-world use of skills requires core therapeutic competencies (Weck, Richtberg, Esch, Höfling, and Stangier 2013). Non-compliance with home-work, in particular, can require therapist creativity and flexibility (Kazantzis, Datilio, Cummins, and Clayton 2013). Among depressed youth, for instance, homework compliance has been reported to be moderate (approximately 50 percent of assignments completed) and declining over time (Clarke et al. 1992; Gaynor, Lawrence, and Nelson-Gray 2006). Features of the specific anxiety and depressive disorders can complicate the use of homework. Adolescents in particular may have difficulty adhering to rec-ommendations for out-of-session practice. With youth, including caregivers (here-after referred to as "parents") in therapy homework tasks may be helpful. This chapter reviews these topics and considers some potential obstacles to therapy homework completion and real-world applications of skills.

Key Features of Competencies

Therapeutic homework is not an assignment that is always viewed favorably by children and adolescents. Unlike adults, youth are typically brought to therapy by their parents, as opposed to being self-referred. As a result, the youth may not be fully "on board" with the therapy, and the idea of therapy homework may be resisted. A key competency is the therapist's ability to present homework as beneficial, personally rel-evant to the youth, and potentially enjoyable. In the Coping Cat for anxious children (Kendall and Hedtke 2006a) and in the Cat Project for anxious adolescents (Kendall, Choudhury, Hudson, and Webb 2002), therapeutic homework assignments are referred to as "Show-That-I-Can" (STIC) tasks and "Take-Home Projects," respectively. Thus STIC tasks and take-home projects are conceptually distinct from school assignments, as the therapist will neither assign a grade on the basis of performance nor punish noncompletion. Rather, therapists provide a clear rationale for homework completion that is congruent with the youth's goals – for example: "You can practice applying the skills you learned in session to other areas in your life, like making new friends."

The competent therapist demonstrates the ability to collaboratively select and plan appropriate homework tasks with the youth. In brief, collaboration is teamwork, where the therapist and youth work together, the therapist encouraging the youth's involvement, providing helpful feedback, and offering contributions to the youth's goals (Lambert and Cattani 2012). Collaboration has been linked to successful treatment outcomes of anxious youth (Chu and Kendall 2004; see also Chapter 10 of this volume). Many CBT manuals offer assignments for the youth; some provide sample handouts or worksheets. Keep in mind that these can be flexibly applied, to take into account each youth's particular needs and goals (Kendall and Barmish 2007). When planning homework assignments, a collaborative therapist brainstorms with the youth possible ways to practice skills outside of session, while ultimately allowing the youth to decide. For example, when choosing an out-of-session exposure task for a socially anxious child, the therapist could say:

THERAPIST: Wow, we practiced talking to a lot of new people during our session today. Nice work by you. I remember that we decided one of your goals would be for you to talk to some kids at school. What do you think would be a good challenge to work on this week to help with that goal?

CHILD: Maybe I could talk to (my friend) Sam?

THERAPIST: Yeah that's a great idea! What do you think about, maybe, talking to Sam and talking to one new person? Would that be OK? Is there another kid you would like to get to know?

Depending on the child's responses, the therapist and the child would decide together whom the child could talk to and what the child might say. In planning the homework task, the therapist considers the child's ultimate goal: talking to other children at school.

Positive reinforcement, often in the form of rewards, facilitates homework completion. Environmental contingencies are essential in shaping behaviors (Skinner 1969), and positive reinforcement for homework is no different. Children in the Coping Cat program might earn stickers for each STIC task completed, and eventually stickers can be traded for a desirable reward of the child's choice. Rewards are best when immediate and effective for each child. Rewards can be tangible, like stickers, small toys, gift cards, or a favorite food or treat. Non-tangible activity rewards are inexpensive and may be preferred, including time spent playing a game with the therapist, staying up past bedtime at home, or spending one-on-one time with a parent. The therapist can speak with the youth and the parent regarding preferred and appropriate rewards for homework completion. Of course, follow-through and consistency are very important: reward the youth for his/her efforts. In the Coping Cat it is emphasized: "Rewards are not just for perfect work." Rather, rewards are given when the youth gives his/her best effort, for instance by facing a feared situation. Additionally, the therapist can emphasize the experimental nature of homework to the child; even if (s)he is unable to complete the homework task, the child may still learn something through his/her attempts. The therapist could illustrate this through the use of examples:

You know, even when we try our best, things don't always work out the way we hoped they would. Even with our best efforts, we may make mistakes. I can think of a time when I had to take a test at school and I was really nervous. I missed some of the questions. But, hey, I tried my best, so I still rewarded myself by watching a movie later. Remember, we can try our hardest, but no one is perfect!

Youth are encouraged to reward themselves with positive self-talk (e.g., "I did it ... I tried really hard!"). Tangible rewards may be phased out, as the youth experiences some of the nonmaterial benefits that come from completing homework tasks. These can include feeling proud, having fun, and feeling less anxious or sad.

The competent therapist strives to personalize homework tasks to the unique needs and goals for treatment of each child and adolescent (Houlding et al. 2010). Consider the child's diagnoses and developmental level, as well as any environmental factors that may impede or facilitate homework completion. Therapists can also explore each client's beliefs toward the homework: Does the client find the task relevant and doable? Appropriate levels of parental involvement will vary. For instance, Puleo and Kendall (2011) found that parental involvement in homework tasks was particularly valuable among anxious children with ASD. ASD has been associated with limited generalization across settings; this example illustrates the value of homework tasks for real-world applications of the skills learned. Some youth may have difficulty completing homework or grasping the skills, at which point homework assignments may need to be repeated or varied. Therapists strive for "flexibility within fidelity" (Kendall, Gosch, Furr, and Sood 2008) – maintaining fidelity to the important ingredients of CBT, but doing so with the flexibility needed to meet individual needs. Thus defined, therapist flexibility (that is, the therapist's effort of adapting the treatment to the needs of a particular youth) may increase youth involvement and promote positive outcomes (Chu and Kendall 2009).

Competence in Treating Anxiety and Depressive Disorders in Youth

Therapists can consider how homework tasks in CBT may vary across different anxiety and depressive disorders. Notably, homework tasks will also vary at an individual level, so we offer guidelines, not rules, for planning and conducting homework tasks for each disorder.

We have found homework tasks to be particularly salient among youth with social phobia (SoP). Although youth with SoP respond poorly to treatment by comparison with youth with other anxiety diagnoses, there are some data to suggest that SoP may be a predictor of non-remission on some outcome measures for CBT (Ginsburg et al. 2011). Additionally, youth with SoP may have more difficulties with the long-term maintenance of gains (Puleo et al. 2011). One possible reason for poor response rates is that exposure tasks conducted in the clinic may not generalize to the youth's real-world experiences with others, in particular his/her peers. Using the client's real peers when conducting exposure tasks in the clinic may not be possible (confidentiality concerns), in which case out-of-session exposure tasks with peers may be especially helpful. Youth with SoP may show initial reluctance to plan and engage in out-of-session exposure tasks with peers, and such fears can be targeted in treatment. The therapist may increase the youth's self-efficacy by role-playing such encounters with the youth during session. Imaginal exposures to real-life situations can also be a useful start. Social skills and assertiveness training is included in the *Stand Up, Speak Out* manual for SoP in adolescents (Albano and DiBartolo 2007) and may target skill deficits that would impede real-world applications. Examples of out-of-session exposure tasks for youth with SoP can include talking to a new peer, calling a friend, raising one's hand in class, or performing in front of others. Additionally, therapists can prepare the youth for the out-of-session challenge by practicing the "worst case scenario" during session. For example, the youth can make a speech in front of a group of confederates in the clinic and purposely make some errors. In doing so, the youth may discover that what is thought to be "errors" may go unnoticed, or that the worst outcome (e.g., "everyone will think I'm stupid") does not actually occur. Additionally, sharing feelings and thoughts when reviewing completed homework assignments can be in itself an exposure task for a youth with SoP. The therapist can provide a supportive environment by rewarding the youth for the effort and by normalizing anxiety through modeling of the homework tasks. For instance, the therapist can say:

> Let's see, as I recall, your take-home project was to write about a time you felt anxious this past week. Is that right? OK. You know, I remember feeling worried when I forgot my friend's birthday this past Tuesday. I worried that she would be disappointed in me, think that I forgot her, and never forgive me. But, you know, I realized that everyone forgets once in a while. When I called her the next day to say "Happy belated birthday" she actually understood and didn't seem angry. What about you? When were you nervous this week?

A diagnosis of generalized anxiety disorder (GAD) also calls for specific therapist competencies in planning homework tasks. Youth with GAD can be perfectionists around homework. The therapist may wish to place a time limit on homework completion (e.g., 10 minutes) and recruit the parents to help enforce this. The therapist takes particular care not to reinforce perfectionism during homework review; for instance, spelling and grammatical errors are not corrected. In fact the therapist may suggest that the youth purposefully makes mistakes on his/her homework and may reward the youth for his/her efforts. For instance, the youth can do the assignment with the non-dominant hand, or with the eyes closed. GAD is often associated with rigid thinking and an intolerance of uncertainty. The therapist can target this by varying the homework tasks or by providing incomplete or vague instructions. Youth with GAD may also experience more abstract worries, which require particular creativity in the planning of out-of-session exposure tasks. For instance, a youth who fears thunderstorms could engage in out-of-session exposure tasks, where (s)he views videos and/or recordings of thunderstorms. Sometimes, out-of-session exposure tasks focusing on school-related concerns may require the help of teachers. A teacher can be notified that the youth has been given the task of answering one question per class. If the child does not complete this task, the teacher may be asked to call on the child.

Children with obsessive–compulsive disorder (OCD), like those with GAD, often display rigidity and perfectionism concerns. Homework will include skills practice and planned out-of-session exposure and response prevention (Lewin, Peris, Bergman, McCracken, and Piacentini 2011). In their manual, March and Mulle (1998) emphasize that homework tasks are chosen by both the youth and the therapist. As with GAD, homework is time-limited. As OCD is characterized by recurrent obsessions and compulsions that cause impairment in a youth's daily life, homework assignments may need to be completed every day. Additionally, as family members often participate in a youth's rituals and routines, these family members may need to change their own behavior in the home. The therapist can gently explain to the youth, ahead of time, that (s)he will be asking the parent to avoid participating in the daily rituals, which will prepare the youth and may prevent arguments when the parents refrain. At the same time, children are not expected to immediately cease their daily rituals, as homework takes a gradual approach. March and Mulle (1998) suggest choosing a "too easy" task for the initial out-of-session practice, in order to promote positive views of homework and of the child's own self-efficacy. The therapist may wish to call the family between sessions to problem-solve the difficulties the youth may have in completing the exposure task.

Conducting homework assignment for youth with separation anxiety disorder (SAD) requires particular planning on the behalf of the therapist, child, and parent. Parental involvement is usually a necessity, not an option. The therapist can include the parents in the discussions surrounding out-of-session exposure, planning to ensure their feasibility and follow-through. The out-of-session challenges may require the parents to change their behavior: for example, a parent may agree to leave his/her child home with a baby-sitter and not answer calls or texts from the child who seeks reassurance.

Homework assignments for youth with post-traumatic stress disorder (PTSD) require sensitivity from the therapist. The youth may be distrustful of adults or may struggle with feelings of shame, guilt, or self-blame. The therapist can carefully take into account the youth's circumstances. In trauma-focused CBT, an evidence-based treatment for PTSD (TF-CBT Web 2012: Medical University of South Carolina 2005), some tasks are not assigned as homework; such as creating a trauma narrative, which can lead to distress for the caregiver and youth and therefore is best completed during session. Otherwise homework can include practicing appropriate feelings expression, relaxation techniques, cognitive coping, and challenging trauma-related dysfunctional cognitions. After the youth has created the trauma narrative, (s)he may be asked to listen to an audio recording of the narrative each night. Gradually the therapist, the parent, and the youth work together to decrease avoidance of trauma-related cues in the youth's environment. For example, a youth who has avoided going into a room in the house where a traumatic event occurred may be asked to spend increasing amounts of time per day in that room. At the same time, the therapist always takes into account the youth's safety when planning out-of-session exposure tasks.

Although not an official diagnosis in the *Diagnostic and Statistical Manual of Mental Disorders* (DSM-IV TR; American Psychological Association 2000), school refusal occurs when a youth is chronically tardy to school, has difficulty staying for a full day, is frequently absent from school, or engages in misbehaviors to avoid school. Such school refusal behaviors can result from anxiety and avoidance of fearful school-related stimuli or from difficulty with separating from the parents (Kearney and Albano 2007). For school refusal cases, homework assignments for parents may involve monitoring the youth's behaviors and resistance to school throughout the day. Children may be assigned the task of recording throughout the day their levels of anxiety associated with school. Behavioral homework assignments include gradually increasing the youth's school attendance and following an established contingency plan. As chronic absenteeism from school can have serious consequences for both the child and his/her family (see review by Kearney 2008), families and school staff often communicate a sense of urgency to the therapist. Nonetheless, homework assignments are carefully planned in the best interest of the youth. For instance, a child who is more fearful of attending school in the morning can arrive in the afternoon. Once this is achieved, the child can go earlier each day until (s)he is attending for the full day.

Pleasant activity scheduling or behavioral activation is an important competency for treating youth depressive disorders. When depressed, youth tend to decrease the time spent in enjoyable activities, which serves to maintain depression over time. The therapist works with the youth in session to identify and list naturally reinforcing and easily accessible activities. The youth can be encouraged to identify a range of activities that are fun, social, active, and/or helpful to others. It is recommended that the therapist and youth first engage in some of these activities during session, to demonstrate their impact on mood (Bearman and Weisz 2009). Continuing to practice and monitoring these activities at home can increase real-world practice and application of these skills.

Perhaps one of the greatest challenges is that youth with depression often experience low levels of motivation, accompanied by poor energy and diminished goal-directed behavior. As a result, youth may have difficulty completing their school assignments and may feel daunted by the concept of additional therapy homework. In the *Adolescent Coping with Depression Course*, Clarke and colleagues (1990) recommend four principles to emphasize with depressed adolescents: (i) homework can help you gain control over depression and is for you, not for the therapist; (ii) unlike school assignments, therapy homework has real-life significance by allowing reflection on things that are bothering you; (iii) homework is kept brief and easily fits into your schedule; (iv) homework is ultimately voluntary, and it is up to you to complete it. If homework is not finished, youth are encouraged to complete it at the beginning of each session. Pleasant activity scheduling can be linked to rewards to motivate the youth for change. Additionally, explaining the rationale of the homework can help the youth understand its importance. Curry and colleagues (2005) recommend reinforcing even partial completion. Maladaptive self-talk (e.g., "This isn't going to help me, so what's the point?") and behavioral skill deficits that may be associated with non-completion can be targeted directly in therapy. Likewise, youth are encouraged to make internal attributions when they succeed in completing their homework.

Developmental Considerations: Competence in Treating Children and Adolescents

When working with youth, therapists consider the developmental level of the youth when they collaboratively plan and assign homework tasks. The following illustrates some competencies to consider when utilizing CBT homework for children versus adolescents. At the same time, children and adolescents may vary greatly at the individual level, and comorbidities such as pervasive developmental, attention-deficit hyperactivity and conduct problems can require various degrees of the strategies described below.

In therapy with children, in most cases, parents are involved at least minimally in homework tasks. As described above, some anxious children may need time limits placed on their homework assignments to target perfectionism concerns, which can be monitored by the parents. Particularly young children may lack insight into their difficulties, and parents can help with goal setting and the selection of out-of-session tasks that may increase generalization to the real world. Often, meeting with the parents and the children at the beginning of the session to discuss progress made on homework tasks can be very rewarding, as the youth may have the opportunity to hear a parent "brag about" the child's accomplishments that week.

In many instances, parents are integral to the planning of more behaviorally oriented homework tasks. For example, in order for a child with SoP to practice talking to new people, the parent must provide the child with these opportunities between sessions. Parents may need to plan to bring their child to a new friend's house, or to attend a restaurant where the child can order for her-/himself a favorite food. The parent is encouraged to review coping strategies and role-play with the child prior to the task, and to provide immediate praise and rewards after the child has completed the task. Such behavior exemplifies transfer of control, where knowledge, skills, and techniques are gradually transferred from the therapist in the clinic to the parent and child in the real world (Kendall and Hedtke 2006a).

In many instances, parents may have homework tasks of their own. For young children, parents can collect data throughout the week: the particular situation, the child's behaviors, and the parent's response. As described earlier, for specific problems such as SAD, the parent may play the central role in an out-of-session exposure task, perhaps by leaving the child with a baby-sitter for increasing amounts of time, to run errands. Finally, the therapist may ask parents to monitor and reduce behaviors that unknowingly reinforce the child's anxious or depressive behaviors. Parents of children with GAD, for instance, are encouraged to decrease reassurance-giving behaviors, and parents of children with OCD may need to evaluate their own role in their child's compulsive routines. Therapists normalize this process and empathize with the parents around these maladaptive behaviors, as many parents may feel blamed and defensive. The therapist might say:

> You know, it's natural for parents to want to protect their child from harm and to provide comfort when he or she is distressed. In general, these seem like the right things to do. However, with overly anxious kids, parents who protect their children may be allowing them to *avoid* things, and the child may not get the chance to see that they can cope on their own. This week, I'd like you to be your own detective: pay attention to what you do that might allow your child to "avoid" … watch and write down any instances where you may be allowing your child to avoid distressful situations. We'll discuss them together.

Similarly, the therapist works with the child to select relevant homework tasks. Younger children may have difficulties completing homework with abstract concepts and may benefit from increased numbers of examples and exercises.

For instance, helping a young child understand the difference between a thought and a feeling could be illustrated through the use of "thought bubbles" that the child practices at home. Children could be sent home with specific tools to practice the skills learned in therapy, such as an audio recording of a relaxation script. Finally, material rewards are particularly useful for encouraging homework completion among young children, as more abstract rewards such as "feeling better" may be too vague.

Utilizing homework techniques in CBT with adolescents can require a very different approach on the part of the therapist (Jungbluth and Shirk 2012). Adolescents are the age group least adherent to a variety of treatment regimens (see, e.g., Hack and Chow 2001). Although the specific mechanisms underlying this finding are unknown, adolescents' aspiration of independence from parents and professionals, peer pressure and social demands, and negative attitudes toward treatment may play a role. In consequence, the therapist can approach CBT homework as the adolescent's own responsibility as a mature young adult (Clarke et al. 1990; Kendall and Barmish 2007). Actively collaborating with the adolescent to select effective homework assignments can help the adolescent feel empowered and claim ownership over his/her successes. The adolescent and the therapist can work together to identify goals that are personally relevant to the adolescent, and these goals can be directly targeted through homework tasks. For instance, an adolescent may wish to make more friends, learn to play the guitar, or simply "feel better" each day, and homework tasks can be framed to achieve these goals. The adolescent's fear of embarrassment in front of peers can be directly targeted in treatment by helping the adolescent identify maladaptive thinking patterns, such as the belief in an imaginary audience (Elkind and Bowen 1979). Parental involvement in homework tasks for adolescents can be varied, as some adolescents may wish to exercise independence. Finally, adolescents may feel self-conscious about identifying rewards for their homework completion. Activity rewards may be particularly reinforcing for adolescents, and parents can agree to allow the adolescent to earn extra time on the phone or computer, or to drive the adolescent to a favorite restaurant or sporting event.

Common Obstacles to Competent Practice and Methods to Overcome Them

Obstacles in the collaborative planning and completion of CBT homework can and do occur, and competent implementation needs to be prepared. Two common obstacles are: (i) non-compliance; and (ii) difficulty in generalizing skills.

Non-compliance is a common hurdle to homework assignments (Gaynor et al. 2006). To address it, the therapist begins with simple, nonthreatening homework tasks (shape homework compliance by starting with easy assignments). For example, in the *Coping Cat* (Kendall and Hedke 2006b, p. 4), the first STIC task is:

Describe a time this week when you felt really great – when you weren't upset or worried. Remember to describe the situation you were in, what you were thinking, and what you were feeling. You can write it in your workbook.

This initial task allows the child to elaborate on a positive experience, with minimal direction or requirements. This STIC task introduces the idea of homework in a nonthreatening way, while allowing the child to practice the skills learned in the first session: mainly the connection between thoughts, feelings, and situations.

Despite this, the youth may still be non-adherent to the homework, either by not doing the assignment or by doing a poor or incomplete job. First, the therapist adopts a non-punitive approach, and can offer the youth the opportunity to complete the homework in session. If the youth tries very hard in session, a partial reward could be offered, such as one sticker instead of two. Next, if non-compliance with the homework appears to be a pattern, the therapist may wish to explore with the youth specific reasons for non-compliance. This can vary from child to child, but common reasons can include forgetting, avoidance, faking good, or homework that is too challenging for the youth (Hudson and Kendall 2002). Additionally, a youth may refuse to complete homework as a way of acting out or rebelling against the therapy. Once these specific reasons have been identified, the therapist and the youth can identify either personal or environmental barriers to homework completion.

Once the potential barriers have been identified, the therapist, the youth, and the parent can find solutions to overcome these barriers. A youth may forget to complete the homework due to a busy schedule or to comorbid symptoms of attention deficit hyperactivity disorder. If so, the parent can gently remind the youth during the week, or the youth and the therapist can create a reminder note to be displayed in a noticeable place. Avoidance is a trademark symptom of anxiety in youth and can affect homework completion. A youth may be able to complete exposure tasks during session with the support and encouragement of the therapist, but completing them on his/her own may seem daunting. The therapist can target this avoidance through therapeutic techniques such as cognitive restructuring and setting realistic expectations for the youth. At-home practice of therapeutic skills and exposure tasks is typically gradual.

Additionally, the youth may complete homework inaccurately due to a desire to make a favorable impression on the therapist. For instance, the youth may be hesitant to report times (s)he felt anxious or depressed, for fear of disappointing the therapist. The therapist can normalize these feelings, while targeting anxiety about disappointing others. Hudson and Kendall (2002) suggest that it may be helpful to assign a task where the youth has to complete the homework incorrectly for one week. Thus the youth learns to cope with making mistakes and potentially disappointing the therapist. When tasks are overly difficult, the therapist, the youth, and the parent determine what level the youth is capable of achieving. While homework aims to challenge the youth, a seemingly impossible task will leave the youth feeling discouraged and hopeless. A collaborative, teamwork approach toward homework where the therapist, youth and parent work together to identify challenging yet achievable homework tasks for the youth to undertake will also reduce the possibility of this occurrence.

Finally, the therapist watches for any comorbid behavioral problems that may interfere with homework completion. An unwilling youth may go to therapy each week when taken by a parent, but homework completion may become a battle. If so, the therapist may wish to integrate parent training into the sessions. Further, homework assignments can be tailored to meet the youth halfway. For instance, a youth who does not wish to write a homework task can describe it to a parent, who can record it for the therapist. An artistically inclined youth can draw a picture or make a collage that achieves similar goals as the original homework task. Practicing a skill every day can be reduced to practicing it every other day. If the youth still does not complete the homework despite these efforts, extra time can be carved into the therapy session to allow the youth to complete the homework from the previous week. Finally, non-compliance may occur naturally over the course of therapy, particularly as a youth experiences symptom relief (Gaynor et al. 2006). The therapist can emphasize the importance of continued practice for reducing the probability of a relapse of the symptoms. Anxious children are often encouraged to adopt an "exposure lifestyle," where confronting instead of avoiding the feared stimuli becomes a way of life.

Effective CBT homework planning and completion are designed to facilitate the generalization of skills learned in therapy to the youth's environment. Despite the therapist's efforts, youth may not view homework as being relevant to everyday life. The youth may not plan to continue exposure tasks or pleasant activity scheduling once the therapy is terminated. To target this, the therapist encourages the youth to engage in homework tasks over a variety of settings and with a variety of people during treatment. For instance, an adolescent may find speaking to a new peer much more anxiety provoking than speaking to an unfamiliar store clerk, so both skills would be practiced outside of therapy. In doing so, these tasks are repeated until they become routine for the youth. Once routine, the youth will be more likely to continue these tasks after therapy termination.

Utilizing flexibility (as described above) when prescribing homework tasks is also important for promoting generalization. For instance, an adolescent may feel that relaxation is "embarrassing" but might enjoy engaging in activities that promote it, such as mindful meditation or yoga classes. Pleasant activity scheduling can include joining an afterschool sports team or club. The youth can create reminders of the skills learned in therapy that can be posted around the home environment, such as coping cards, where coping techniques can be easily accessed. Also, a final project that summarizes the youth's success in therapy can be helpful to reiterate the skills learned. In the Coping Cat, the child's last STIC task is to plan a commercial that describes accomplishments in therapy. During the last session, the therapist helps the child create this commercial, which allows the child the opportunity to "show off" with what (s)he has learned. Importantly, the child is provided with a copy of the commercial to take home for the future. Adolescents may also enjoy making a commercial; if not, they can write a story or a poem, draw a picture, perform a song, or keep a journal to record the progress made for future reference.

Conclusion

Homework is one of the valuable components of CBT, extending across a variety of manual-based CBTs for youth anxiety and depression. Several therapeutic competences can improve the value and effectiveness of CBT homework, such as: (i) framing homework positively and with personal relevance for the youth; (ii) collaborating with the youth in generating homework tasks; (iii) using appro-priate rewards; and (iv) being flexible in personalizing the homework to each client's

Box 11.1 Quick reference summary of homework competencies

- Provides a clear rationale for homework completion that is congruent with the youth's goals.
- Utilizes collaboration to select and plan homework tasks with the youth.
- Implements positive reinforcement to shape homework completion. Reinforcements are immediate, tailored to the child, and earned on the basis of effort, not performance.
- Personalizes homework tasks to the unique goals and needs of each youth, also considering the youth's own beliefs about the homework. Applies "flexibility within fidelity" to homework tasks.
- Considers how homework tasks may vary across differing anxiety, depressive, and comorbid disorders.
- Takes into account the developmental level of the youth when planning and assigning homework tasks.
- Encourages the involvement of parents and other family members in homework tasks as appropriate.
- Determines barriers to homework and solves problems around obstacles to completion.
- Takes time to discuss the youth's beliefs about the perceived difficulty of the homework. If necessary, practices homework in session through role-play or imaginal exposure.
- Designs homework to facilitate the generalization of skills learned in therapy to the youth's environment.

Source: Kazantzis, Deane, Ronan, and L'Abate (2005).

needs. Homework is personalized by taking into account each youth's individual needs including diagnosis, comorbidity, and developmental level. Because homework is not always well received, competent therapists are prepared to troubleshoot any difficulties related to homework compliance. When done collaboratively, CBT homework is a rewarding and effective way to lessen the gap between the therapy clinic and the youth's real world environment. It is our belief that an increased understanding and competent use of CBT homework tasks will play an active role in the dissemination of evidence-based treatment in the community (Sburlati, Schniering, Lyneham, and Rapee 2011).

References

Albano, Anne Marie, and Patricia DiBartolo. 2007. *Cognitive–Behavioral Therapy for Social Phobia in Adolescents: Stand Up, Speak Out Therapist Guide*. New York: Oxford University Press.

American Psychiatric Association (APA). 2000. *Diagnostic and Statistical Manual of Mental Disorders* (4th ed. rev.). Washington, DC: Author.

Bearman, Sarah K., and John R. Weisz. 2009. "Primary and Secondary Control Enhancement Training (PASCET): Applying the Deployment-Focused Model of Treatment Development and Testing." In Cecilia Essau (Ed.), *Treatments for Adolescent Depression: Theory and Practice* (pp. 97–121). New York: Oxford University Press.

Chu, Brian C., and Philip C. Kendall. 2004. "Positive Association of Child Involvement and Treatment Outcome within a Manual-Based Cognitive–Behavioral Treatment for Children with Anxiety." *Journal of Consulting and Clinical Psychology*, 72: 821–9. DOI: 10.1037/0022-006X.72.5.821

Chu, Brian C., and Philip C. Kendall. 2009. "Therapist Responses to Child Engagement: Flexibility within a Manual-Based CBT for Anxious Youth." *Journal of Clinical Psychology*, 65: 736–54. DOI: 10.1002/jclp.20582

Clarke, Gregory, Peter Lewinsohn, Judy Andrews, John R. Seeley, and Julie Williams. 1992. "Cognitive–Behavioral Group Treatment of Adolescent Depression : Prediction of Outcome." *Behavior Therapy*, 23: 341–54.

Clarke, Gregory, Peter Lewinsohn, and Hyman Hops. 1990. *Leader's Manual for Adolescent Groups: Adolescent Coping with Depression Course*. Portland, OR: Kaiser Permanente.

Curry, John F., Karen C. Wells, David A. Brent, Gregory N. Clarke, Paul Rohde, Anne Marie Albano, … John S. March. 2005. *Treatment for Adolescents with Depression Study (TADS) Cognitive Behavior Therapy Manual: Introduction, Rationale, and Adolescent Sessions*. Durham, NC: The TADS Team.

Elkind, David B., and Robert Bowen. 1979. "Imaginary Audience Behavior in Children and Adolescents." *Developmental Psychology*, 15: 38–44. DOI: 10.1037/0012-1649.15.1.38

Gaynor, Scott T., Scott Lawrence, and Rosemery O. Nelson-Gray. 2006. "Measuring Homework Compliance in Cognitive–Behavioral Therapy for Adolescent Depression: Review, Preliminary Findings, and Implications for Theory and Practice." *Behavior Modification*, 30: 647–72. DOI: 10.1177/0145445504272979

Ginsburg, Golda S., Philip C Kendall, Dara Sakolsky, Scott N. Compton, John Piacentini, Anne Marie M. Albano, … John March. 2011. "Remission after Acute Treatment in Children and Adolescents with Anxiety Disorders: Findings from the CAMS." *Journal of Consulting and Clinical Psychology*, 79: 806–13. DOI: 10.1037/a0025933

Hack, Sabine, and Byron Chow. 2001. "Pediatric Psychotropic Medication Compliance: A Literature Review and Research-Based Suggestions for Improving Treatment Compliance." *Journal of Child and Adolescent Psychopharmacology*, 11: 59–67. DOI: 10.1089/104454601750143465

Houlding, Carolyn, Fred Schmidt, and Diane Walker. 2010. "Youth Therapist Strategies to Enhance Client Homework Completion." *Child and Adolescent Mental Health*, 15: 103–9. DOI: 10.1111/j.1475-3588.2009.00533.x

Hudson, Jennifer L., and Philip C. Kendall. 2002. "Showing You Can Do It: Homework in Therapy for Children and Adolescents with Anxiety Disorders." *Journal of Clinical Psychology*, 58: 525–34. DOI: 10.1002/jclp.10030

Jungbluth, Nathaniel J., and Steven Shirk. 2012. "Promoting Homework Adherence in Cognitive Behavioral Therapy for Adolescent Depression." *Journal of Clinical Child & Adolescent Psychology* (published online December 13): 545–53. DOI: 10.1080/15374416.2012.743105

Kazantzis, Nikolaos, Georgios K. Lampropoulos, and Frank P. Deane. 2005. "A National Survey of Practicing Psychologists' Use and Attitudes Toward Homework in Psychotherapy." *Journal of Consulting and Clinical Psychology*, 73: 742–8. DOI: 10.1037/0022-006X.73.4.742

Kazantzis, Nikolaos, Craig Whittington, and Frank Datilio. 2010. "Meta-Analysis of Homework Effects in Cognitive and Behavioral Therapy: A Replication and Extension."

Clinical Psychology: Science and Practice, 17: 144–56. DOI: 10.1111/j.1468-2850.2010.01204.x

Kazantzis, Nikolaos, Frank Datilio, A. Cummins, and X. Clayton. 2013. "Homework Assignments and Self-Monitoring." In Stefan G. Hofmann (Ed.), *The Wiley Handbook of Cognitive Behavioral Therapy* (pp. 311–30). New York: Wiley.

Kazantzis, Nikolaos, Frank P. Deane, Kevin R. Ronan, and Luciano L'Abate. 2005. "*Using Homework Assignments in Cognitive Behavior Therapy.*" New York: Routledge/Taylor and Francis Group.

Kearney, Christopher A. 2008. "School Absenteeism and School Refusal Behavior in Youth: A Contemporary Review." *Clinical Psychology Review*, 28: 451–71. DOI: 10.1016/j.cpr.2007.07.012

Kearney, Christopher A., and Anne Marie Albano. 2007. *When Children Refuse School: A Cognitive–Behavioral Therapy Approach Therapist Guide.* New York: Oxford University Press.

Kendall, Philip C., and Andrea J. Barmish. 2007. "Show-That-I-Can (Homework) in Cognitive–Behavioral Therapy for Anxious Youth: Individualizing Homework for Robert." *Cognitive and Behavioral Practice*, 14: 289–96. DOI: 10.1016/j.cbpra.2006.04.022

Kendall, Philip C., and Kristina A. Hedtke. 2006a. *Cognitive–Behavioral Therapy for Anxious Children: Therapist Manual* (3rd ed.). Ardmore, PA: Workbook Publishing.

Kendall, Philip C., and Kristina A. Hedtke. 2006b. *The Coping Cat Workbook* (2nd ed.). Ardmore, PA: Workbook Publishing.

Kendall, Philip C., Muniya Choudhury, Jennifer Hudson, and Alicia Webb. 2002. *The CAT Project Manual for the Cognitive Behavioral Treatment of Anxious Adolescents.* Ardmore, PA: Workbook Publishing.

Kendall, Philip C., Elizabeth Gosch, Jamie M. Furr, and Erica Sood. 2008. "Flexibility within Fidelity." *Journal of the American Academy of Child Psychiatry*, 47: 987–93. DOI: 10.1097/CHI.0b013e31817eed2f

Lambert, Michael J., and Kara Cattani. 2012. "Practice-Friendly Research Review: Collaboration in Routine Care." *Journal of Clinical Psychology*, 68: 209–20. DOI: 10.1002/jclp.21835

Lewin, Adam B., Tara S. Peris, R. Lindsey Bergman, James T. McCracken, and John Piacentini. 2011. "The Role of Treatment Expectancy in Youth Receiving Exposure-Based CBT for Obsessive Compulsive Disorder." *Behaviour Research and Therapy*, 49: 536–43. DOI: 10.1016/j.brat.2011.06.001

March, John S., and Karen Mulle. 1998. *OCD in Children and Adolescents: A Cognitive–Behavioral Treatment Manual.* New York: Guilford Press.

Mausbach, Brent T., Raeanne Moore, Scott Roesch, Veronica Cardenas, and Thomas L. Patterson. 2010. "The Relationship between Homework Compliance and Therapy Outcomes: An Updated Meta-Analysis." *Cognitive Therapy and Research*, 34: 429–38. DOI: 10.1007/s10608-010-9297-z

Medical University of South Carolina. 2005. "TF-CBT Web: A Web-Based Learning Course for Trauma-Focused Cognitive Behavioral Therapy," http://tfcbt.musc.edu (accessed September 12, 2012).

Puleo, Connor Morrow, and Philip C. Kendall. 2011. "Anxiety Disorders in Typically Developing Youth: Autism Spectrum Disorders as a Predictor of Cognitive–Behavioral Treatment." *Journal of Autism and Developmental Disorders*, 41: 275–86. DOI: 10.1007/s10803-010-1047-2

Puleo, Connor Morrow, Bradley T. Conner, Courtney L. Benjamin, and Philip C. Kendall. 2011. "CBT for Childhood Anxiety and Substance Use at 7.4-Year Follow-Up: A Reassessment Controlling for Known Predictors." *Journal of Anxiety Disorders*, 25: 690–6. DOI: 10.1016/j.janxdis.2011.03.005

Sburlati, Elizabeth S., Carolyn A. Schniering, Heidi J. Lyneham, and Ronald M. Rapee. 2011. "A Model of Therapist Competencies for the Empirically Supported Cognitive Behavioral

Treatment of Child and Adolescent Anxiety and Depressive Disorders." *Clinical Child and Family Psychology Review*, 14: 89–109. DOI: 10.1007/s10567-011-0083-6

Simons, Anne D., C. Nathan Marti, Paul Rohde, Cara C. Lewis, John Curry, and John March. 2012. "Does Homework 'Matter' in Cognitive Behavioral Therapy for Adolescent Depression?" *Journal of Cognitive Psychotherapy*, 26: 390–404. DOI: 0.1891/0889-8391. 26.4.390

Skinner, Burrhus F. 1969. *Contingencies of Reinforcement: A Theoretical Analysis*. New York: Appleton.

Stark, Kevin, Philip C. Kendall, Mary McCarthy, Mary Stafford, Rachel Barron, and Marcus Thomeer. 1996. *Taking Action: A Workbook for Overcoming Depression*. Ardmore, PA: Workbook Publishing.

Weck, Florian, Samantha Richtberg, Sebastian Esch, Volkmar Höfling, and Ulrich Stangier. 2013. "The Relationship between Therapist Competence and Homework Compliance in Maintenance Cognitive Therapy for Recurrent Depression: Secondary Analysis of a Randomized Trial." *Behavior Therapy*, 44: 162–72. DOI: 10.1016/j.beth.2012.09.004

Part III
Specific CBT Techniques

12

Managing Negative Thoughts, Part 1

Cognitive Restructuring and Behavioral Experiments

Sarah Clark, Gemma Bowers, and Shirley Reynolds

Introduction

Negative thoughts are characteristic features of depression and anxiety and within the CBT model are seen to play a role in maintaining these conditions. This means that they are a key target for change. This chapter outlines ways of working with children and adolescents that help them manage and reduce their negative thoughts. The use of thought diaries, thought challenging, and behavioral experiments is described in relation to working with both children and teenagers across the anxiety disorders and depression.

Key Features of Competencies

Cognitive restructuring

The core principle of cognitive behavioral therapy (CBT) is that one's emotions and behaviors are influenced by cognitions or the meaning that we attach to certain events. Helping individuals find alternative meanings or ways of thinking about events is central to changing the associated emotions and behaviors (see Chapter 8 for more detail on the theory behind CBT). However, young people often come to therapy expressing a desire to change how they feel rather than to change what they are thinking. The idea of changing their thoughts is usually not at all familiar. Therefore it is important to spend time explaining the basic CBT model and rationale. Time spent on this and on helping to develop, together with the young person, a basic formulation of his/her

Evidence-Based CBT for Anxiety and Depression in Children and Adolescents: A Competencies-Based Approach,
First Edition. Edited by Elizabeth S. Sburlati, Heidi J. Lyneham, Carolyn A. Schniering, and Ronald M. Rapee.
© 2014 John Wiley & Sons, Ltd. Published 2014 by John Wiley & Sons, Ltd.

problems is vital and must occur before any work to challenge cognitions can begin. A description of the steps required for cognitive restructuring will be given below.

Identifying cognitions

Children and adolescents, like adults, can benefit from having some help with identifying their thoughts and finding a way to talk about them.

Talking about a recent situation in which the child or young person experienced a distressing emotion or an unwanted behavioral reaction can be a very helpful way of identifying his/her negative automatic thoughts. It can also help to socialize him/her to the CBT model and make him/her start to develop a basic formulation of the maintenance cycle (see below). In many instances, especially with younger children, including parents in this process can also be valuable, as parents may be able to offer suggestions as to what the young person was reporting at the time, while developing their own understanding of how thoughts, feelings, and behaviors are linked and how their own behaviors may be acting to maintain the young person's difficulties.

Case example

Emily, a 14-year-old girl with social anxiety, attended weekly CBT appointments with her mother. She described feeling very uncomfortable at school, particularly in group activities or in lessons with people she described as acquaintances (rather than close friends or strangers). In order to develop a basic understanding of Emily's experiences at school and to socialize her to the CBT model, a basic maintenance cycle was collaboratively constructed with her (see Figure 12.1). Emily's mother also contributed to the development of the maintenance cycle by reminding her of things that she had told her about the situation being discussed.

Linking thoughts and feelings

As illustrated above, Emily, like many young people, identified a range of thoughts and feelings that she experienced. One of the challenges for us, as clinicians, is to identify which thoughts match with which emotions, and consequently with which behavioral responses. For example, if the young person is reporting feelings of anxiety, we would expect the associated cognitions to have themes of anticipation of harm, whereas feelings of sadness are more likely to be accompanied by thoughts of loss (actual or impending) or self-criticism. Trying to challenge a cognition that is not linked with the target emotion is likely to have little if any effect on reducing that emotion. Although Emily reported experiencing both worry and upset in the situation described in Figure 12.1, the content of her thoughts might best be categorized as related to potential social harm coming to her; her thoughts are therefore likely to be more strongly associated with anxiety than with sadness or feeling upset.

Learning to use emotion words

Young people often have their own words for certain emotions, and it is important not to assume that their interpretation of emotional words is the same as our own. Spending time talking through a list of common emotions can be very helpful, particularly when working with younger children. Asking where they feel certain emotions in their body, or asking them to draw on a picture of the human body and coloring in where they feel certain emotions can help the therapist and the child identify

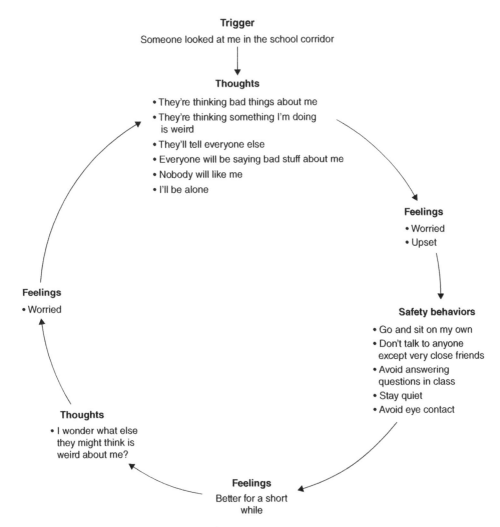

Trigger
Someone looked at me in the school corridor

Thoughts
- They're thinking bad things about me
- They're thinking something I'm doing is weird
- They'll tell everyone else
- Everyone will be saying bad stuff about me
- Nobody will like me
- I'll be alone

Feelings
- Worried
- Upset

Safety behaviors
- Go and sit on my own
- Don't talk to anyone except very close friends
- Avoid answering questions in class
- Stay quiet
- Avoid eye contact

Feelings
Better for a short while

Thoughts
- I wonder what else they might think is weird about me?

Feelings
- Worried

Figure 12.1 Emily's maintenance cycle.

together the different emotions that the child is experiencing – quite apart from the fact that it offers a fun and engaging task early in therapy. Asking young people to rate the intensity of their different emotions can also be helpful: it may contribute to identifying the most salient emotion. Then the therapist may consider which thoughts link with this particular emotion. Images such as a feelings' "thermometer" or building blocks that show higher and lower levels of emotion, can help children and young people understand that feelings and emotions can vary in intensity (hot versus cool, high versus low) and are useful ways of helping the young person start focusing on his/her own emotions and start monitoring how (s)he changes in different situations, with different people, and in the course of a day.

Identifying images
It is also important to remember that many young people will find it easier to describe images than to describe thoughts. Asking questions such as "What was going through

your mind?" or "What did you see in your mind's eye?" encourages young people to report images as well as verbally based thoughts. More specific questions, such as "Did you notice any pictures in your mind?" or "Can you draw what was going through your mind?" can be valuable. When Emily was asked if she had any images in her mind during the situation she described above, she evoked an image of everyone at school standing in a group, looking down on her. In her image, everyone else was much bigger than her, and they were all laughing at her. When she described this image, she became visibly upset, in a way that she had not when describing her thoughts. This image, therefore, seemed important to add to the maintenance cycle formulation.

Thought diaries

Sometimes, even when therapists are creative and draw on many different methods to elicit thoughts from their clients, children and teenagers – and adults, too – struggle to identify what was going through their mind during a given situation. Here it is often helpful to encourage them to keep a record of their experiences outside of therapy sessions. This is because it is generally easier to access thoughts and images when you are as close to the situation as possible. In CBT, diaries and worksheets are often used between sessions, to record thoughts and images. These help the young person keep track of what was happening at the time – that is, of what the situation was – and of how they felt, how strong that feeling was, and what they noticed was going through their mind. There are numerous thought diaries designed for use with young people (see, e.g., Stallard 2002). However, particularly when working with adolescents, it is important to discuss with them how they would like to record their thoughts. For many, recording their thoughts on a mobile phone or on a dictaphone may be preferable to completing a paper version of a thought diary and may feel less like a school homework task. An example of a thought diary completed by Emily is shown in Table 12.1.

Apart from what goes on outside of therapy sessions, there are also important emotional shifts that occur during therapy. These give much more immediate access to the child's ongoing thoughts and images, and therefore it is very important for therapists to be aware of changes of emotion and to be prepared to explore what the young person notices is going through his/her mind at such times. If the therapist is helping young people link thoughts and feelings within sessions, any thought-recording homework task is likely to be much more successful.

Table 12.1 Emily's thought diary: Part 1.

Situation	Feelings	Intensity of feeling	Thoughts	Distress caused by thought
Sitting in a French lesson	Worried	90%	People are looking at me	75%
	Upset	80%	They are talking about me	80%
			They will tell everybody else what they are saying about me	80%
			Nobody will like me	85%
			I won't have any friends	90%

Working with negative thoughts

When the thoughts and images that are associated with the target emotion have been identified, it is important to spend time with the child or young person to acknowledge and recognize the emotional impact of these negative cognitions. This helps to validate the young person's experience and makes him/her feel understood and "heard." Moving on to challenging thoughts too quickly can feel dismissive to young people and may imply – or be understood as – a form of indirect criticism. Time should be given to discussing the thoughts they are experiencing in the context of their experiences and to accepting that, given their specific experiences, it is understandable that they might think the way they do.

For Emily, it was important to consider the events that precipitated the onset of these worried thoughts and feelings. She described finding the move up to high school difficult because she was separated from her close friends and remembered experiencing high levels of anxiety. At about the same time, Emily's older brother, with whom she had previously had a close relationship, started going out more with his peers and spending less time with Emily. He also started teasing Emily about her taste in clothes and music and regularly referred to her as "weird." Within the therapy session where this was discussed, the clinician and Emily spent time exploring how difficult this had been for Emily and how natural it was that she should tend to believe her older brother's opinion of her. The clinician and Emily also acknowledged that, if Emily believed what her brother was saying about her, then it was understandable that she might think others were thinking similar things about her. This was even more understandable in the specific context, which was that she has started a new school and did not have the support of close friends.

Following this process of acceptance and validation, the next stage is to consider which one of the thoughts identified would be appropriate and effective to work on. A common mistake in CBT is for therapists to try to challenge thoughts that, for some reason, are difficult to shift. For example, it is not possible to challenge facts (e.g., "My mum is dead") or questions (e.g., "Why me?"). However, questions can be turned into statements that may be challengeable; this can be done by asking questions such as: "What does it mean that this has happened to you?" Similarly, with careful questioning about the impact of events (such as a parent dying, or being bullied at school) and the meaning these events have for the young person, thoughts that are challengeable can be identified (e.g., unrealistic thoughts that have developed as a result of the event). It is also difficult to challenge central beliefs, such as "I am worthless," early on in therapy, as these beliefs tend to be more global and rigid. Working on such beliefs too early in therapy can be overwhelming for the young person, and any shift is likely to be very small – if it occurs at all. Therefore selecting a thought that can be more easily challenged is likely to be helpful in the first instance and will instill a sense of hope in the young person that CBT might be a useful process for him/her.

Challenging thoughts

While it is important to understand and validate the reasons why a young person might be experiencing certain thoughts, it is also important to help that person develop a sense of distance from these thoughts and an understanding that thoughts are transient and fluid rather than being facts. This process was referred to by Beck, Rush, Shaw and Emery (1979) as "decentering." A useful technique here can be asking the young person if there was ever a time when (s)he didn't experience these thoughts in similar situations. Or "Before you felt anxious, what would have gone through your mind in this situation?" "What would your best friend/your brother/your mum think in this situation?"

Through a process of decentering, it is likely that the young person's belief in his/her thoughts will be diminished or shaken and his/her thinking about the target situations will become more flexible. Being able to stand back from negative automatic thoughts can be very powerful. Once a sense of distance from the thought has been created and the young person has developed an understanding that thoughts are just thoughts rather than being facts, that person is much more likely to engage with the process of thought challenging and with the development of alternative thoughts and perspectives. Given that thoughts have been previously considered to be powerful and to represent reality and "truth," the ability simply to accept that thoughts are not reality is an important shift.

Young people usually find it relatively easy to identify the evidence that supports their thoughts and to draw upon it. This process sometimes leads to their feeling even more anxious or depressed, since they focus on the evidence for the thoughts that are related to the target emotions. It is therefore important to provide young people (and their parents) with psycho-education about the fact that this is a common reaction prior to commencing this task. As a therapist, it is essential to offer a great deal of empathy during this process and to build a sense of validation – a sense that, given these experiences and this evidence, it is understandable that the young person developed such thoughts.

Finding evidence against the disturbing thought can be much more challenging. Often young people cannot think of any evidence that goes against a thought or idea they have believed in so strongly. Elaborating on, and developing, the questions that were used at the decentering stage can be useful at this point: it may help the young person gain a wider perspective.

Box 12.1   Examples of questions that can help the young person identify evidence against his/her thoughts

1   If your best friend had this thought, what might they say to themselves?
2   What advice would you give your best friend if they did have this thought?
3   What do you think your best friend/your mum/your sister would say if you told her about this thought?
4   Has there ever been a time when you've been in a similar situation and not been worried or upset?
5   What do you think you would think if you were less depressed?
6   Now that you are no longer in that situation what do you think?
7   If this were to happen tomorrow, what do you think you would say to yourself?
8   Are you blaming yourself for something that is not under your control?

Table 12.2 Emily's thought diary: Part 2.

Evidence that supports the thought	Evidence that does not support the thought	Alternative thoughts	Mood rating now
My own negative thoughts about what I look like	I have a group of good friends	Sometimes people could be thinking bad things about me or think something I'm doing is weird but I won't be left without any friends	Worried (10%) Upset (20%)
My brother's comments that I look weird	I've always had friends even though I've done things that people might have thought were weird	(Belief = 75%)	
Hearing people at school make nasty comments about how my friend looks	My friend, whom I heard bad comments about, still has friends and people that like her		

In addition to working directly with the young person, it can be helpful to invite the parents to make suggestions about evidence that does not support the target thought. A useful homework task might be for the young person to collect evidence during the week that does not support the thought, or to ask friends for their views and opinions.

Once the evidence for and against the thought has been collected, it is important to support the young person to develop a new, more balanced thought. Again, parents may be useful by suggesting alternative thoughts on the basis of the available evidence. Once an alternative thought has been constructed, the young person should be asked how much (s)he believes the new thought and how intense his/her target emotion gets when thinking this thought. The second section of Emily's thought diary, which reviewed the evidence for and against the thought "I won't have any friends," is shown in Table 12.2.

Although cognitive restructuring can be a very powerful and useful process, young people often report that they understand logically that their old thoughts are not 100 percent true and that there is evidence that does not support them, but they explain that this exercise has not caused a significant shift in their emotions. It is therefore essential that this process is followed up by a process of testing out the new thought or of continuing to gather evidence to support it (this can be used in future cognitive restructuring tasks, if appropriate). Encouraging young people to think of ways in which they could test out the thoughts through behavioral experiments is likely to lead to a much larger emotional shift than a pen-and-paper exercise would.

Behavioral experiments

Giving the rationale for behavioral experiments
Once the child (and the parent) is (are) familiar with a coherent formulation, the foundations are laid for designing a behavioral experiment. The formulation is vital for establishing the reasons to carry out the behavioral experiment, which are (i) to increase

the motivation for testing out an alternative behavior; and (ii) to set up a context for the meaningful interpretation of the experiment's outcomes, once it has been carried out. This process is most effectively (and efficiently) conducted by focusing on the maintenance cycle (as already described). By drawing out the maintenance cycle in a circular format, the child – and, where appropriate, the parent(s) – can reflect on the circularity of the safety behavior(s). The child can then be encouraged to use his/her own problem-solving abilities to break the cycle. This transfer, to the child, of the responsibility for change at such an early stage can help reduce apathy or lack of confidence, which can be common reactions at the beginning of therapy, when the child and the parent are desperate for a "quick fix" from the therapist. It also encourages confidence and self-belief – that is, young people's belief that they themselves can improve things, and therefore can continue to do so after therapy has ended:

THERAPIST: Where do you think the weakest part of this trap is? Where would it be best to try to break the cycle?

The child has three options: thoughts, feelings, or safety behaviors, to which the therapist can respond accordingly:

CHILD: Stop the thoughts?
THERAPIST: That would seem logical, wouldn't it? Why don't we try to test that out, to see if it would work?

This response may be more common in younger children, who are more likely to believe they can have control over their thoughts. It is now the therapist's role, while validating their suggestion, to introduce an alternative option. In doing so, the therapist is already modeling the CBT approach of open-mindedness and the consideration of other possible answers to a seemingly obvious question. At this point the Pink Elephant experiment can helpfully show that, when we try to stop thinking about something, our minds paradoxically think even more about the unwanted thought. The Pink Elephant experiment involves the therapist inviting the child (and the parent) to close his/her eyes and try to clear his/her mind. The therapist then asks him/her to spend the next minute (or less, depending on the child's age and attention span) thinking of anything (s)he would like to, *apart from* pink elephants. In most cases, the child will laugh after the first few seconds, quickly realizing that the more (s)he tries to avoid a thought, the more fierce and intrusive it becomes. Indeed, children with a more vivid imagination may even make comments such as "the elephants are multiplying ... and they're all flying around in circles."

These reflections can serve as a good introduction to behavioral experiments: the Pink Elephant experiment provides an experiential opportunity of putting a belief to the test – in this case, the belief that we can stop our thoughts – and of noting the similarities between pink elephants and unwanted thoughts. In the rare case where a child denies any "pink elephant" thoughts, it may be useful to ask the parent to reflect on their own experience, or to overtly drop in the words "pink elephant" into the middle of sentences throughout the remainder of the session, to highlight the difficulty and annoyance of trying to "get rid" of the thoughts. Additionally, the findings recorded in a useful piece of research carried out by Crye, Laskey, and Cartwright-Hatton (2010) can be shared with older children and teenagers. Crye and colleagues found that, among young people aged 12 to 14, 77 percent reported that they had intrusive and unwanted thoughts, thus highlighting how "normal" it is to have unwanted thoughts.

Realizing now that thoughts may not be the easiest place to start breaking the maintenance cycle, the child may suggest:

CHILD: Stop the feelings?
THERAPIST: That would make sense too, wouldn't it?

At this point, it is again helpful to ask the child to think of a recent example of their anxiety or depression showing up, and to reflect on how hard it would have been to stop the feeling. Directing the child to a recent example can help to elucidate the point that, just as with our thoughts, it is very hard to stop or change our feelings on demand:

THERAPIST: Maybe you could think of a recent example of a strong feeling that you've had, and think about whether you would have been able to stop it.

If the child struggles to come up with an example, a useful analogy to use here is that of our feelings on a rollercoaster. That is, while you may be able to suppress the overt expression of a feeling, the feeling itself cannot be prevented, as it is a near-automatic response to the environmental trigger.

By this stage the child will gradually be realizing that there is only one other place where the cycle can be broken:

CHILD: Stop the safety behaviors?
THERAPIST: Have you ever tried that before?

At this point it can be shared with the child that this is indeed the weakest part of the cycle, and an arrow can be drawn on the maintenance cycle to show how "doing something different" can help to determine whether the thoughts and beliefs are indeed as accurate as currently believed (Figure 12.2). The aim is to begin to invite curiosity in the child about the trustworthiness of his/her thoughts. This sets up the reason for devising the first behavioral experiment.

Depending on the duration and severity of his/her anxious or depressive thoughts and feelings, the child may find it difficult to think of a time when (s)he did not use his/her safety behaviors. (S)he may not remember a time when (s)he did not have a problem with anxiety or low mood; (s)he may not be able to imagine dealing with things differently. However, there may be exceptions – times when safety behaviors have not been used; and the therapist can help find information about these "exceptions" by discussing situations where environmental factors have prevented the child from using his/her safety behaviors – for instance being on holiday or at school, being distracted, being with certain people, and so on.

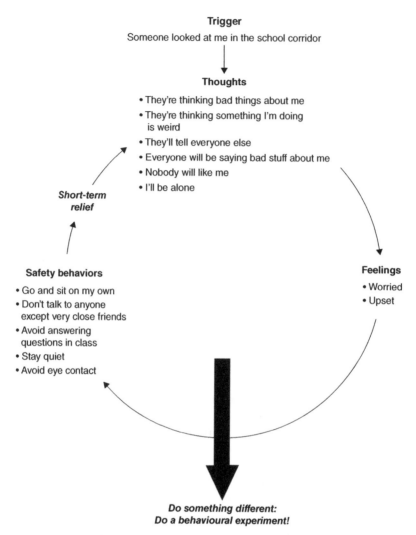

Figure 12.2 Emily's formulation, showing a possible exit route.

   Typically the child or young person will feel daunted and alarmed at the prospect of removing his/her safety behaviors. Safety behaviors do provide short-term relief from distressing symptoms and have become habitual and comforting. Therefore the idea that they would not be available to use is frightening and may be resisted by both children and parents. It is important to remind the child and the parent(s) that the therapy will continue to be guided by *them*, will be going at *their* pace, and that, while it is necessary to challenge their thoughts, this will not be done by "jumping in at the deep end." An honest explanation of what a behavioral experiment is must be shared, both in order to socialize the child and the parent(s) to this part of the model and to enable informed consent (which, again, will increase the child's feelings of mastery over the therapeutic interventions thereafter).

   It can be helpful to draw out a basic graph to show how safety behaviors are successful and effective at reducing distress in the short term, but that behavioral

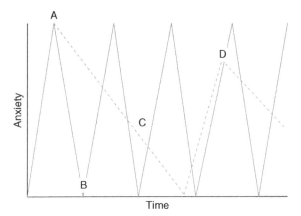

Figure 12.3   The effect of safety behaviors and behavioral experiments on anxiety.

experiments are much more effective at reducing distress from unwanted thoughts in the long term (Figure 12.3). The graph shows how, at the peak of anxiety (A), the use of a safety behavior will often reduce the anxiety quickly to a near-normal level (B), but, because it does not "fix" (get rid of) the anxious thought, the levels of anxiety will soon reach their peak again whenever the thought reappears. Alternatively, the dashed line shows how refraining from using the safety behavior (i.e. "doing something different" via a behavioral experiment) will result in a more gradual decrease in anxiety (C), but one that is much more likely to last; each time the thought reappears, the initial level of anxiety decreases (D).

Once the child is in agreement to start using behavioral experiments, it is useful to set a long-term agenda to plan his/her experiments in a way that feels challenging, yet not out of his/her "comfort zone." Loosely speaking, this may be referred to as graded exposure: beginning with the least challenging tasks and working up to the most challenging (see Chapter 14 for more details on exposure). It is useful to place this long-term plan in a context of specific short-, medium-, and long-term goals – again, in order to help the child create motivation for change and provide tangible reasons for carrying out the behavioral experiments.

A useful task to set as an initial piece of homework is for the child to pin up their main-tenance cycle somewhere at home. The aim is for him/her to start trying to "observe" his/her thoughts, feelings, and behaviors just as they happen, using this cycle as a reference point. This helps the child to gain a "bird's eye view" of his/her maintenance cycle when it is in action. Consequently the child will become able to notice when they are 'at risk' of using a safety behavior, slow down this 'usual' response to their anxious/ depressive thoughts and feelings, and disengage from the process of using safety behaviors (which are likely to have become more and more automatic over time). This means that, even before (s)he begins to carry out behavioral experiments, the child is able to increase the period between the onset of an anxious or negative thought and the start of the safety behavior. This gives him/her more time to make a choice to "do something different."

Devising behavioral experiments
If the therapist refers to the formulation together with the child and revisits the child's goals in therapy, this will enable an informed decision about the most effective type

of experiment to carry out. For example, a child with depression who has a number of negative beliefs about him-/herself may find it useful to gather information (e.g., from school reports) before moving on to more challenging, proactive experiments.

Depending on the child's level of willingness and enthusiasm to carry out a behavioral experiment, the therapist may wish to model the process by devising, with the child, an experiment designed to test out one of the therapist's own thoughts. The child may well enjoy designing an experiment that really challenges the therapist, giving the therapist permission to return the challenge in good humour at a later date. This can be a good way of introducing different types of experiments, which, in themselves, will require varying levels of bravery.

Careful and thorough planning is key to an effective behavioral experiment. That is, the details of the experiment must be discussed in depth and recorded in order that the experiment can be carried out accurately and effectively. The analogy with a "curious scientist" can be used here to explain to older children and teenagers the aim of "testing out" a theory: the therapist explains that, when a scientist does not know the answer to a question, his/her task is to devise ways of gathering information that would help him/her work it out. This analogy can make the child improve the quality of his/her experiment; it may also make the task feel less threatening and unfamiliar. Most children of middle school age and older have had the experience of carrying out experiments at school. This can then be used to facilitate the planning of future experiments and more *ad hoc* thought challenging in the future: "What would the curious scientist in you say?"

It is useful to carry out the first behavioral experiment with the child in a session, to make sure that the experience is positive and that the child understands the procedure and its rationale. Later on in therapy, behavioral experiments can be used as homework tasks. Some children may be more willing to complete homework than others. It is therefore useful to discuss with the child the best way to incorporate the homework into their day, and how on school days this process might be different from incorporating it at weekends. To encourage maximum feedback, the worksheet below (Figure 12.4) can help the child to briefly summarize predictions about the experiment, increase the likelihood of his/her carrying out the experiment (by minimizing potential barriers), and provide a space for the child to note his/her findings along the way. It also encourages him/her to carry out the experiment more than once between therapy sessions, on the premise that "practice makes perfect." All this provides useful information about the effect, on the child's troubling thoughts and feelings, of not using the safety behavior. This effect can be plotted on a graph over the course of therapy (if this is appropriate for the child's age and ability); and any patterns can be noted along the way (e.g., behavioral experiments may be easier to carry out at certain times of day or in certain places).

Involving parents can both assist the process and hinder it. Again, the formulation is key in determining the extent of parental involvement in the experiments. Parents may opt for having minimal input by acting in a "support from the sidelines" role; by offering encouragement while not getting involved in the actual experiment; or by offering their own alternative responses to similar situations. A more involved input may take the form of a "dual experiment," where the parent simultaneously carries out his/her own behavioral experiment in order to test out his/her own beliefs

Thought to be tested:	
Rate your belief in the thought (0–100%)	
How can you test out your thought?	
What might get in the way of you doing this?	
How can you get over this barrier to continue with the behavioral experiment?	

Days and times that you will do your experiment:	What was the outcome of your experiment? / What happened when you didn't use your safety behavior(s)?	Re-rate your belief in the thought that you were testing (0–100%)

Figure 12.4   Behavioral Experiment Worksheet. Adapted from Greenberger and Padesky (1995).

Box 12.2   Evaluation of behavioral experiments

Ask yourself these questions each time you have completed a behavioral experiment:

1 What was your experiment? What did you do?
2 What went well?
3 What did not go so well?
4 What did you think would happen?
5 What actually happened?

in relation to the child's behavior. The former kind of input may be more useful in situations where developing confidence and independence is important (e.g., with children experiencing low self-esteem or separation anxiety), whereas the latter may be particularly useful in situations where the parents themselves may be involved in maintaining the behaviors (e.g., by offering reassurance in obsessive compulsive disorder). It may also be useful, particularly with younger children, to devise a reward system upon completion of the experiment: a system that rewards new, non-avoidant behaviors, and therefore increases the motivation for further behavior change.

Reflection on the experiments

To maximize the impact of experiential learning, it is vital to "make sense" of the behavioral experiment after it is completed. Ideally this should be done immediately after, when the most accurate reflections can be recovered. A simple prompt sheet can be given as part of the behavioral experiment homework (Box 12.2), or the notes made on the behavioral experiment worksheet can act as prompts at the next session. The child can then be encouraged to compare previous safety behaviors and thoughts to updated behaviors and thoughts, again referring back to the maintenance cycle and to the goals originally set by the child. This then invites the child to move on to the next behavioral experiment.

Competence in Treating Anxiety Disorders and Depression

Most evidence-based treatments for children and adolescents have focused on anxiety disorders; the treatment of depression in children and adolescents is relatively under-researched. Depression is rarely seen before adolescence, and around three quarters of those diagnosed with it are girls. Young people who are depressed often have comorbid mental health problems such as anxiety disorders, eating disorders, self-harm, and conduct problems (National Institute for Health and Care Excellence 2005). Therefore the presentation of depression in young people can be extremely varied and complex. Young people with depression show low mood, low levels of energy and motivation, pessimism, and disengagement from social and educational activities. All CBT is based on the development of the therapeutic alliance (see Chapter 6), and this is the first priority in CBT for depression.

Cognitive restructuring with young people who have anxiety disorders typically focuses on perceptions of threat or harm coming to the self or to loved ones. Threats can be social ("they will ignore me, everyone will think I'm weird") as well as physical ("I'll be so frightened I'll stop breathing"). Behavioral experiments to test these thoughts can include trying out new behaviors and seeing how other people react (e.g., do they ignore me?), carrying out informal surveys to ask people their opinions about the perceived threat, researching the medical literature to find out if it is possible to stop breathing through fear, or checking out beliefs with "experts."

In depressive disorders, negative automatic thoughts are often associated with failure ("I'll never pass my exams, I'm stupid/useless") or loss ("no one will like me; I'll be alone"). The key characteristics of depression coalesce around the cognitive triad: negative thoughts about the self, the world, and the future (Beck et al. 1979). Young people who are depressed are more likely to attribute any success or positive outcomes to luck or to other people, or to assume that such results are "random." For example, a compliment about a young person's behavior or performance ("You did that really well") may be minimized by attributing it to kindness in the other person ("They're just saying it to be nice"), or to a fluke or luck, rather than to a real skill or ability in the young person. In contrast, such a person is likely to attribute negative life events, for instance failures, to his/her own faults ("That just shows how rubbish I really am"). Cognitive restructuring should therefore examine alternative causal pathways for both positive and negative events, which balance internal global and stable attributions for negative events with external, specific, and unstable attributions for positive events.

Competence in Treating both Children and Adolescents

Cognitive behavior therapy relies upon the ability of the client and his/her therapist to be able to stand back from ongoing experiences and to notice and attend to the thoughts and the feelings that are being experienced. In other words, it is necessary to be able to think about your thinking. This ability of *metacognition* develops during childhood and adolescence and into adulthood (Cartwright-Hatton et al. 2004). It is influenced by our environment as well as by the increasing complexity and sophistication of our cognitive structures, and therefore therapists need to be able to work in a flexible way to meet the skills and developmental stage of their young clients.

CBT with children often relies more heavily on the behavioral than on the cognitive components. However, there is evidence that young children are able to identify thoughts and feelings and to discriminate among thoughts, feelings, and behaviors if they are given appropriate and child-friendly tasks. Ways of making the task more accessible to children include using puppets or toys, using drawings, cartoons, and especially thought bubbles. This ability has been observed in children of 6 and 7 years, who have high levels of behavioral or emotional problems and, therefore, are at risk of mental health difficulties (Reynolds, Girling, Coker, and Eastwood 2006). This suggests that many young children do have the fundamental metacognitive abilities to engage in CBT work. However, despite this basic understanding, children tend to find it easier to identify what they did in response to a certain situation, and even how they felt at the time; it is often more difficult for them to identify what they were thinking at that time. Therapists therefore need to be able to relate things to concrete incidents and to use simple and direct language when working with children and adolescents.

Children are also influenced by their social networks: their family, school, and peer group. Younger children tend to be more influenced by their parents, whereas older children and adolescents become more concerned about their peers and the external world. The involvement of parents in CBT can be helpful and will be discussed later (see Chapter 19). However, for adolescents, the involvement of parents may require careful negotiation. Adolescents often wish (and need) to develop autonomy from their parents and may be in conflict with them. Parents, on the other hand, may resent being excluded from therapy, may inadvertently contribute to the maintenance of difficulties, and frequently have their own mental health needs, which impact on the child. Where possible, the role of the family in maintaining difficulties should be explicitly considered in the formulation, and this information should highlight if, how, and when parents and other family members are involved in treatment sessions. Where the parents are not directly involved in treatment, it is often helpful to arrange occasional "catch-up" sessions in which the young person and the therapist jointly provide feedback to the parents.

Common Obstacles to Competent Practice and Methods to Overcome Them

There are likely to be a number of setbacks in therapy, which must be problem-solved if improvement is to be made. Just as we would guide the child back to his/her formulation if they faced a difficulty, a return to the formulation is likely to be helpful for the therapist in resolving barriers to progress in therapy.

Perhaps the most common difficulty is a lack of motivation – manifest for instance in not completing homework tasks, refusing to complete behavioral experiments, or missing appointments. This is an alternative example of avoidance, which can quickly be elucidated as a form of safety behavior in the maintenance cycle. The child must acknowledge that it is his/her choice to decide whether the anxiety or depression (s)he is experiencing is disabling enough to warrant change. This decision can be made by establishing the pros and cons of change by comparison to the pros and cons of continuing with current coping mechanisms. Additionally, modeling proactive behavior in sessions, either via role-play where the therapist and child swap positions or via an *in vivo* behavioral experiment, can serve to increase motivation by showing that change is often not as difficult as it was predicted to be.

Another difficulty that may arise is a difference of opinion between parent and child as to how much the parent should be involved in these therapeutic tasks. Again, a revision of the formulation will help to determine just how effective parental involvement will be. Ultimately the therapist must help the child and his/her parent to come to a compromise that enables the child to feel in control of the therapeutic interventions while the parent does not feel abandoned or replaced by the therapist. Some children may wish for parents to come to the first session, in order that they understand the rationale and procedure of the therapy, while others may like their parents to come to the first or last five minutes of the sessions, to remain "in the loop." Maintaining parental involvement to some extent may also help the family to adapt to the changes that may come about during the course of therapy. In successful cases, for example, children may quickly find that they have more time on their hands, and parents may feel less "needed" by their children; and there is also the potentially accelerated transition to autonomy and independence that may accompany a reduction in anxious or depressed symptoms.

One of the harder problems in therapy may arise when a behavioral experiment does not go to plan. This is usually the result of poor planning or of the child's not carrying out the experiment as planned. Using the prompt sheet (Box 12.2), the difficulties can be discussed and understood. Thereafter the behavioral experiment can be replanned and carried out, perhaps *in vivo* or with additional help from a parent, if necessary.

Conclusion

Negative and anxious thoughts are normal in children, as well as in adults. It is the interpretation of such thoughts that can lead to psychological distress. Problematic interpretations can be challenged by using techniques designed to broaden the perspective and to invite in new information. This can be done via conversation, via paper-and-pen cognitive restructuring exercises, or, more proactively, via behavioral experiments. The role of the family in such interventions can be useful, although the extent of involvement of family members must be agreed by all involved and in line with the information gained from the formulation – and particularly from the maintenance cycle. Children can then be guided in building a repertoire of skills that help them cope with negative and/or anxious thoughts as these crop up, thereby enabling a long-term strategy for managing difficult thoughts and feelings throughout their life.

References

Beck, Aaron T., A. John Rush, Brian F. Shaw, and Gary Emery. 1979. *Cognitive Therapy of Depression*. New York: Guilford Press.

Cartwright-Hatton, Sam, Alison Mather, Vicky Illingworth, Jo Brocki, Richard Harrington, and Wells Adrian. 2004. "Development and Preliminary Validation of the Meta-Cognitions Questionnaire – Adolescent Version." *Journal of Anxiety Disorders*, 18: 411–22.

Crye, Jenny, Ben Laskey, and Samantha Cartwright-Hatton. 2010. "Non-Clinical Obsessions in a Young Adolescent Population: Frequency and Association with Meta-cognitive Variables." *Psychology and Psychotherapy: Theory, Research and Practice*, 83: 15–26. DOI: 10.1348/147608309X468176

Greenberger, Dennis, and Christine Padesky. 1995. *Mind over Mood: Change How You Feel by Changing the Way You Think*. New York: Guilford Press.

National Institute for Health and Care Excellence. 2005. *Depression in Children And Young People: Identification and Management in Primary Community and Secondary Care*.

Reynolds, Shirley, Emma Girling, Sian Coker, and Lynne Eastwood. 2006. "The Effect of Mental Health Problems on Children's Ability to Discriminate amongst Thoughts, Feelings and Behaviours." *Cognitive Therapy and Research*, 30: 599–607. DOI: 10.1007/s10608-006-9037-6

Stallard, Paul. 2002. *Think Good – Feel Good: A Cognitive Behaviour Therapy Workbook for Children and Young People*. Sussex, England: Wiley-Blackwell.

13

Managing Negative Thoughts, Part 2

Positive Imagery, Self-Talk, Thought Stopping, and Thought Acceptance

Maria Loades, Sarah Clark, and Shirley Reynolds

Introduction

Intrusive negative thoughts play a core part in maintaining and exacerbating children's fears and their difficulties with low mood. A range of strategies have been developed that can be used with children and young people to help them identify, manage, or reduce their negative thoughts. Children's cognitive development is highly variable and individual; therefore therapists may need to try a range of strategies with each child before finding the one that works best for the individual child or young person (see Chapter 5 for more details on development). In addition, these strategies are likely to be much more useful and engaging if they are adapted to suit the individual needs and interests of each child. In this chapter we describe four different specific CBT techniques, drawn from Sburlati, Schniering Lyneham and Rapee (2011), that are designed to help children overcome or tackle their negative thoughts. We also provide examples of each strategy being used. These examples are offered in order to illustrate the techniques, help clinicians relate them to clinical work, and establish a basis for the creative adaptation of these techniques to each client's specific circumstances and needs.

In order to illustrate the use of the techniques described, we will present the following two cases:

1. Katie is a 9-year-old girl with separation anxiety. She is unable to sleep in her own room at night because she is afraid that that a burglar will break in and attack her and her parents. Therefore she insists on sleeping in her parents' room and cannot go for sleepovers at friends' houses.

Evidence-Based CBT for Anxiety and Depression in Children and Adolescents: A Competencies-Based Approach, First Edition. Edited by Elizabeth S. Sburlati, Heidi J. Lyneham, Carolyn A. Schniering, and Ronald M. Rapee. © 2014 John Wiley & Sons, Ltd. Published 2014 by John Wiley & Sons, Ltd.

2. Francis is a 16-year-old boy with depression and low self-esteem. He has little motivation for social events and friendships and sees himself as worthless and useless. Francis lives with his mother, who is a hotel manager, and with his 18-year-old brother, who is just about to leave home to study medicine.

Positive Imagery

Key features of the competency

The images that go through our minds are a key part of our cognitive architecture. They can be brought to mind deliberately, for example when we try to remember a happy event (such as a birthday party or a holiday), or they can come to mind unintentionally. Although we are sometimes unaware of their occurring, images can capture key emotions, memories, and beliefs and have a powerful impact on our mood and well-being. Images are often visual but can consist of (or include) sounds, smells, and movements. Fear is often linked to strong and powerful images that, for many people, evoke more emotional content than verbal descriptions of their fears. Therefore, if therapists do not access their client's images, they may miss their most significant thoughts. To illustrate, compare the image of a dog that a child who fears dogs might entertain with the image of a dog that is likely to be generated by a child who does not have a fear of dogs. These contrasting images are likely to include movement (say, tail wagging or biting) and sound (growling or barking) in addition to visual elements related to the dog's size, color, and shape. Similarly, a child frightened of needles and injections may associate these objects with visual images of frightening places (hospitals) and people (doctors and nurses), of themselves or their parents in pain or distress, or of the needle or injection itself.

Because our mental images have a powerful impact on emotions, they can be a useful tool for attenuating emotional distress. In therapy, positive images can be used in two ways. First, the therapist can work with his/her client to transform negative, unhelpful images – for example, an image of a scary monster under the bed – into positive or benign images – for example, a friendly cartoon character (Deblinger and Heflin 1996). Second, the therapist can work with his/her client to create new positive images – for instance, an image of the self as successful and competent – in order to help that client counteract his/her key psychological difficulties – for example, to replace negative images and beliefs about the self as useless. Therefore, rather than trying to eliminate negative images directly, therapy tends to build and develop new positive images that may replace them.

Clients do not always describe their images spontaneously, but therapists can elicit them. Standard cognitive techniques (see Chapter 12) can be adapted so as to include questions targeted specifically at eliciting imagery (Hackmann, Bennett-Levy, and Holmes 2011). The following excerpt from a session with Katie illustrates this procedure:

> THERAPIST: So when you heard a noise that evening, what went through your mind in that moment?
>
> KATIE: Ummm, I thought it was a burglar.

THERAPIST: Ok, so you thought it was a burglar making the noise. Was there a picture of that in your mind?

KATIE: Ummm, I'm not sure. Like what do you mean?

THERAPIST: Like could you paint me a picture, using words, of what you thought was happening when you heard that noise.

KATIE: Well, I thought ... that the burglar was outside, trying to open the front door.

Such questions can be followed by further questioning designed to explore the imagery more closely. This questioning can focus on physical features of a visual image ("What/whom else can you see there?" or "What color are her shoes?").

THERAPIST: Mmmhmm ... can you tell me what the burglar looked like in your mind?

KATIE: Yeah, he was like a really big man, wearing all black clothes, with a big axe in his hand.

Depending on the child's age and developmental level, it may be appropriate for the image to be drawn by the young person (see Figure 13.1 for an example).

The focusing questions can then be developed further, so that more of the emotional content emerges:

THERAPIST: What did you think was going to happen next?

KATIE: Ummm, I thought that he was going to break through the window.

THERAPIST: Ok, so you thought he would break through the window, and then?

KATIE: Then he would come running into the house ...

THERAPIST: Gosh! How did that picture in your mind make you feel?

KATIE: Well ... scared and worried.

THERAPIST: It does sound like a really scary picture to have in your mind. What did it make you do?

KATIE: I had to check if mum and dad were ok, and wanted to be close by them. I asked dad to check if the door was locked.

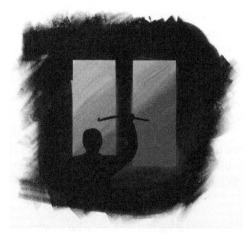

Figure 13.1 Image of the imagined intruder. © Christopher Jacobs. Reproduced with permission.

When the image has been described, the therapist can then help the young person explore what it means.

> THERAPIST: Ok, Katie, so when you have that scary picture in your mind of that big man with the axe, what does it make you think about: yourself or other people?
>
> KATIE: Ummm … I'm not really sure …
>
> THERAPIST: Well, if I had a scary picture in my head, I might start to worry about myself, or I might start to worry about other people, or both. Does that happen for you?
>
> KATIE: Oh, I worry about mum and dad, and me, and that we'll get hurt. That's why I always stay near to them.
>
> THERAPIST: Ok, so that picture in your mind makes you worry about yourself and mum and dad getting hurt.

Once the image has been elicited and its impact understood, rather than proceeding to challenge it, the next step is to collaboratively develop a transformation of the image, on the basis of what would have to change within the image for it to be less distressing.

> THERAPIST: So this really scary picture in your mind, Katie, what do you think would have to change to make it less scary for you?
>
> KATIE: Ummm, I don't know.
>
> THERAPIST: If we could change the story that comes up in your mind when you hear those scary noises at night, what would be a story that wouldn't be scary for you?
>
> KATIE: Well, mum once told me that there are lots of animals around in the night and that they make lots of noises, so maybe a story about the animals?
>
> THERAPIST: What kind of animals do you think move around in your garden at night?
>
> KATIE: I think that there was a hedgehog once …
>
> THERAPIST: Ok, so we could make a story about a hedgehog…what do you think this hedgehog would be up to in the night?

The final step is to introduce this transformation into the image (which could be done creatively, through role-play or drawing; see, e.g., Figure 13.2) and then rehearse the re-scripted image.

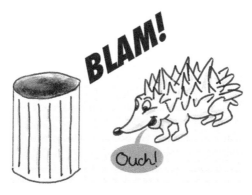

Figure 13.2 Transformed image of the night-time "intruder." © Christopher Jacobs. Reproduced with permission.

Transforming the frightening image is a process similar to cognitive restructuring (Chapter 12), although it focuses on nonverbal content and, rather than identifying evidence for and against the image content, the process concentrates on developing and elaborating a new image that is less distressing. The new image need not be realistic, provided that it feels helpful, gives a sense of control over the negative imagery, promotes image acceptance, and enables the client, rather than dismissing it, to "play" it through, mentally, past the worst point, facilitating a sense of resolution.

Positive images can also be developed in the absence of negative imagery. This can be useful for managing negative affective states, for reducing negative affect (for instance by inducing relaxation, which is a low negative state), and for promoting self-compassion and/or a sense of self-efficacy. For example, Gilbert (2009) has introduced the concept of self-compassion as a helpful way of countering self-criticism and feelings of isolation. In the session, the young person is encouraged to bring to mind a real or an imaginary character who personifies compassion and nurturing. This task involves brainstorming the qualities of an "ideal" nurturer, focusing on fostering feelings of warmth, acceptance, and compassion, then generating an image of what this figure would look like – its physical features and facial expression, its sensory characteristics (e.g., tone of voice, smell), its knowledge or wisdom – and finally exploring what being close to that figure would feel like. The compassionate character may be given a name or identity. In subsequent sessions the young person is encouraged to bring the compassionate image to mind and to focus on positive emotions that are associated with the image – such as warmth, safeness, and soothing (Lee 2005). When the image has been developed in therapy sessions, the young person is encouraged to bring it to mind outside sessions, when (s)he has a negative automatic thought or experiences distress.

Imagery can also be used to develop positive feelings about the self and the future. An example would be helping the young person develop a positive image of the self that the young person has not yet become. In such cases the image represents a positive self-image, which can be brought to mind and used in interpersonal problem-solving situations. The following extract illustrates how this technique was used successfully with Francis:

THERAPIST: Ok, Francis, we are going to do an imagery exercise now. Ideally, it would be good if you could keep your eyes closed throughout the exercise. But, if you don't want to close your eyes, then maybe you could pick a spot on the wall opposite you to stare at.

FRANCIS: Ok. [*closes his eyes*]

THERAPIST: Are you ready to begin?

FRANCIS: Yep. [*nods*]

THERAPIST: Ok Francis, while you are sitting there with your eyes closed, I would like you to imagine a TV screen in front of you. On this screen, I would like you to place an image – a picture of your future most developed self. Let me explain. This is a picture of yourself that you have not yet become. This is you. This future self has all the knowledge, coping, and experience necessary in life, to be fully in charge of himself in his life, and able to choose what he wants and how he wants to live his life.

FRANCIS: Mmmm, ok ... I'm not sure I know what you mean ...

THERAPIST: Like yourself as you most want to be in the future, yourself at your peak.

FRANCIS: Oh, I think I get it now.

THERAPIST: Ok, Francis, I'll give you a few minutes to think, so let me know when you have a picture on your screen of your future most developed self, yourself at your peak.

[*pause*]

FRANCIS: Mmm, I think I have it.

THERAPIST: Great, excellent. Now, let's spend a little time building this up into a clearer picture of your future most developed self.

THERAPIST: Tell me, what do you notice about your future, most developed self that is possibly different from how you are today? Is he doing anything? Standing? Sitting?

FRANCIS: I can see me but older, maybe 25. Sitting down.

THERAPIST: Ok, great, let's see if we can add in some more details. What is his hair like?

FRANCIS: Kind of short and neat, shorter than now.

THERAPIST: And his face?

FRANCIS: Well, like now but his skin is way better, no spots!

THERAPIST: What is your future most developed self wearing on his top half?

FRANCIS: Like a button up shirt.

THERAPIST: What color?

FRANCIS: It's like a blue color, pale blue.

THERAPIST: Buttoned up to the top?

FRANCIS: Mmmm ... top button open, like casual. Sleeves rolled up too.

THERAPIST: Ok, great, what is your future most developed self wearing on his bottom half?

FRANCIS: Ummmm ... like jeans I think.

Now that the therapist has developed the physical image, she starts to move onto questions to explore the emotional state of the future most developed self (FMDS) image.

THERAPIST: Now Francis, take a look at his face. What expression can you see?

FRANCIS: Yeah ... He looks happy, and quite chilled, I think ...

THERAPIST: So he looks happy, chilled. How does your future most developed self feel?

FRANCIS: Ummm ... this is tricky ...

THERAPIST: You're doing a great job so far. How do you think he feels?

FRANCIS: I think he feels happy and in control.

THERAPIST: Ok, so happy and in control. What tells you this? How can you see it?

FRANCIS: Well, he's like sitting back in the chair, his body looks relaxed, and he looks healthy, tanned and toned.

Having explored the emotional state of the FMDS image, the therapist continues to develop the image by exploring the relationships of the FMDS to self and others.

THERAPIST: Great, Francis. And how does your future most developed self feel toward others?

FRANCIS: Ummm, he gets on well with everyone. Is that what you mean?

THERAPIST: You got it. And how do others feel toward your future most developed self?

FRANCIS: Yeah, I think most people get on well with him and feel positive toward him.

THERAPIST: I wonder how your future most developed self feels toward himself?

FRANCIS: Mmmm, I think he is happy with himself, I think he likes himself, but not too much. [*little laugh*]

THERAPIST: What tells you that from what you can see?

FRANCIS: Just that he seems to be happy being himself.

The therapist now moves on to summarizing the FMDS image that has been created.

> THERAPIST: Now, using the information that you have given me, I'm going to try to pull together what you've described. Let me know if I have missed anything out or if there is anything else that needs adding, okay?
>
> FRANCIS: Mmmmhmmm. [*nods*]
>
> THERAPIST: So your future most developed self is yourself, in your mid-20s, wearing a pale blue button-up shirt, slightly open at the neck, and jeans. With good skin, tanned and a toned body, short and neat hair. Your future most developed self feels happy and relaxed, contented. He likes himself, but not too much, and gets on well with other people.

After checking out with Francis whether this is an accurate summary and whether he wants to add anything more to the image, the stage of image creation is completed, and the therapist moves on to use the image for problem-solving.

> THERAPIST: Ok, Francis, what I'm going to ask you next is to just step inside your future most developed self. I can't tell you how to do that, as each person will have his or her own way of doing it. But, once you are there, simply be in his body, looking out of his eyes and seeing what it feels like to be there. Let me know when you are there.
>
> [*pause*]
>
> FRANCIS: I'm there.
>
> THERAPIST: Excellent! Now, Francis, it's your job to be inside your future most developed self, looking out of his eyes and seeing what it feels like to be there.
>
> FRANCIS: Ok.
>
> THERAPIST: In a moment, we will revisit and re-run the problem situation that you chose to focus on today. This time, we will be watching and seeing how your future most developed self handles it and what it feels like for him. You are simply along for the ride, like an observer.
>
> FRANCIS: Ok.
>
> THERAPIST: So Francis, in your own time, simply re-run the scene right from its beginning through to its natural completion and then let me know when it is complete.

Finally, the therapist asks Francis to open his eyes, and he explores how the FMDS coped with the problem scenario, what the FMDS did that was different from what Francis himself did, and how this made the FMDS feel. Thus this image can be used to help the young person to take another perspective on the situation and, using his/her life values and what (s)he aspires to be, to develop his/her problem-solving ability.

Competence in treating anxiety disorders and depression

In treating anxiety disorders in children and young people, the focus of positive imagery is most likely to be on:

1.   transforming (de-catastrophizing) images linked to catastrophic thoughts about perceived danger (e.g., as we described above, an image of a burglar trying to break in, triggered by hearing a noise at night, could be transformed into an image of lots of nocturnal creatures going about their business);

2. developing a sense of ability to cope (e.g., teaching children to use their imagination to pretend that they have special powers that will help them to face the danger or perceived danger); this reduces anxiety by increasing the client's sense of self-efficacy;

3. inducing physiological relaxation via bringing to mind an image that is relaxing or enjoyable and thus lowers arousal levels (e.g., creating the image of playing in a place that the child finds relaxing: playing on the beach, with one's family, hearing the waves breaking on the sand, feeling the sun shining on one's back and the sand between one's toes…).

In treating depression, the focus of positive imagery is more likely to be on:

1. developing self-compassion as a means to counter self-critical thinking (e.g., creating a compassionate, nurturing figure, based on reality or entirely imagined, which can be brought to mind when the client recognizes that (s)he is being self-critical or is in distress, to help soothe and comfort the client, in his/her mind, in a compassionate way);

2. developing images of successful future performance, to counter hopelessness and apathy and to build self-confidence and motivation (e.g., generating images of interacting successfully in a social situation, such as a party).

Competence in treating both children and adolescents

Most young children are familiar with imaginary play, which develops naturally in early childhood. Younger children tend to approach imaginary tasks very directly (as compared to adults, who need to be more explicitly taught to use imagination), perhaps because they use imagination naturally in their daily lives (Ronen 1997). For example, a child who is afraid that a monster or a wild animal will enter their bed at night can be taught to draw a sword for protection; and this is likely to be much more effective than explaining that monsters or wild animals are very unlikely to be found in one's bedroom. What is critical to engaging children in harnessing their imagination successfully within therapeutic work is the language used and the explanations given, which should be at a developmentally appropriate level. The rationale behind introducing new imagined material is a fairly complex cognitive concept, which younger children may struggle to follow, and some imagery exercises (e.g., developing an FMDS) require sophisticated metacognitive skills. However, younger children tend to respond well to the idea of pictures or "movies" in the mind and, provided that appropriate adaptations are made in terms of the ways in which positive imagery techniques are introduced, such pictures can be used to good effect with children and young people.

Particularly important is the way in which imagery is labeled and framed for the young person. This can help maximize the chance of their developing and using new images in a deliberate way in order to deal with difficulties. For example, a "compassionate creature" may be a more appropriate and accessible way to describe the compassionate nurturer concept outlined above when working with younger children (like Katie), while an older adolescent (like Francis) might prefer the more adult terms "compassionate figure" or "compassionate nurturer."

With children and young people, eliciting negative imagery potentially raises concerns or questions about the client's safety or exposure to possible risks. The therapist needs to judge if the imagery is grounded in any real risk to the child or young person. To do so, (s)he will need to use other information about the child's wider context and to make an assessment on the basis of his/her own clinical judgment, therapy supervision, and relevant service guidelines.

Common obstacles to competent practice and ways to overcome them

Possibly the most common obstacle to using imagery effectively is not giving it enough time and attention. It is important to explore negative images with the child or young person and to help him/her develop and transform them, as well as develop and practice positive imagery. Imagery can encompass night-time imagery such as nightmares, which can be effectively addressed by using the approach outlined above for dealing with and re-scripting negative imagery (Hackmann et al. 2011).

With imagery, it is important to engage a number of sensory modalities – not just what the person can see, but also what (s)he can hear, feel, and smell and what feelings this evokes in him/her. Imagery is most successful when a vivid image is created and rehearsed, so that it becomes accessible to the client even when his/her arousal or distress levels are high.

Self-Talk

Key features of the competency

Vygotsky's (1962) seminal work highlighted the critical role of internalizing verbal commands in establishing voluntary control over one's own actions. In CBT, the specific CBT technique of self-talk – also known as "thought substitution" – focuses on changing what people say to themselves and is premised on the belief that behavior follows directly from this self-talk. Self-talk involves the use of short enabling statements that the client repeats to him-/herself during periods of distress. The statement counters his/her negative automatic thoughts and, through repetition, focuses his/her attention away from the negative thoughts and undermines them, without the client's using the explicit methods of evaluating and challenging negative thoughts that are characteristic of cognitive restructuring (Stallard 2009).

The use of self-talk with children and young people can be quite directive – that is, the therapist tells the client what to do or say – or it can be collaborative – in other words self-talk can be taught as a skill (Ronen 1997). The collaborative approach is more consistent with the collaborative stance of CBT. However, no matter how it is carried out, self-talk needs to be realistic and believable rather than simply a positive statement (Kendall and Hedke 2006; Rapee et al. 2006). For example, for an anxious child such as Katie, the self-statement "I'm afraid, but I can cope" is much more realistic and believable than "it's OK, I'm fine."

Competence in treating the anxiety disorders and depression

With children who are anxious, focused self-talk is most useful in preparation for, rather than during, anxiety-provoking situations. Anxious children tend to experience high rates of negative thoughts when they anticipate the situations they fear. The treatment of anxiety using CBT frequently involves the child or young person deliberately exposing him-/herself to things that (s)he is frightened of and this, not surprisingly, leads to high levels of anticipatory fear. Self-talk can be used to tackle distressing anticipatory anxiety in the lead-up to exposure exercises. For example, in treatment, Katie might be encouraged to replace anticipatory negative anxiety-increasing thoughts (say, the thought "I can't cope with being frightened when I'm on my own in bed") with more positive, anxiety-reducing self-talk (such as "I might be a bit frightened but I can manage it and stay in my own bed"). Such cognitions emphasize how the child will cope with feeling anxious, rather than getting rid of, or avoiding, anxiety and worry. This can help the child to feel more self-confident and encourage him/her to face his/her worries or fears rather than to escape or avoid them (Stallard 2002).

Self-talk for children with anxiety can be a useful part of the overall anxiety management strategy; for example, Kendall and Hedtke's Coping Cat 16-session treatment program for anxious children (2006b, p. 37) uses the FEAR acronym to prompt the child to a four-step coping process. In this acronym,

- F stands for "feeling frightened" (i.e., developing awareness of physiological cues to identify anxiety and learning to relax);
- E represents "expecting bad things to happen?" (i.e., identifying unhelpful thoughts and self-talk);
- A is for "attitudes and actions that can help" (i.e., positive self-talk and problem-solving); and
- R stands for "results and rewards" (i.e., facing fears, self-evaluation, managing failure).

Similarly, children who are depressed can be supported to replace anticipatory cognitions that predict failure (such as "I will fail this test") with more helpful self-talk such as ("I will do my best"). Furthermore, positive self-talk (as compared to coping self-talk) can also help children who are depressed to notice and celebrate their achievements. For example, in response to Francis's negative automatic thought "I'm no good at anything and will fail this test," positive self-talk could be developed – for instance "all I can do is to try my best." This is useful in eroding all-or-nothing thinking patterns by helping children to develop more flexible and less negative predictions (Stallard 2002).

Competence in treating both children and adolescents

Self-talk does not require complex or advanced thinking skills; for this reason it may be particularly helpful for younger children or children with a cognitive delay. The use of self-talk can help reduce avoidance and anticipatory anxiety as well as to develop confidence and self-esteem. Children's use of self-talk is more likely to be successful if parents, teachers, and therapists encourage children to use self-talk in real situations, recognize when they have used it, and reinforce their positive self-talk and associated behaviors through comments such as: "It's great that you had a go at sleeping on your own"; "Well done for having a go at that."

Self-talk can be developed creatively; Friedberg and McClure (2002) suggested a treasure-chest metaphor to promote the use of self-talk in children. They made an analogy between forgotten or misplaced coping thoughts and lost treasure. The child is supported to draw or construct a treasure chest during therapy sessions and to develop new positive self-coping statements (which are his/her "loot") to go in the chest. The child is then taught to go to the chest and pull out his/her positive "loot" whenever (s)he feels low.

Common obstacles to competent practice and ways to overcome them

When developing self-talk with a child or young person, it is important to engage the parents. Some children prefer to use self-talk out loud, and this can worry parents if they are not forewarned. Parents can also help their child develop self-talk strategies in new situations and encourage them when they use self-talk in real situations outside the therapy room. It is important that they praise the child for his/her attempts to face his/her fears – that is, for his/her *efforts* – rather than for *success* in facing these fears. Parents can also engage the child's teachers to explain the use of self-talk in the classroom.

The development of a child's skills of positive self-talk will take time. It is common that the child would not believe the self-talk statements at first. However, (s)he should be encouraged to continue to practice and develop his/her self-talk. The child's natural tendency toward negative beliefs ("I can't do it!") will be strong, particularly when the child is in a feared situation. Overcoming this tendency will therefore require regular practice and support, initially outside of, as well as within, trigger situations, and it is important that any attempts to use self-talk are reinforced.

For children and young people who find it difficult to think of helpful self-talk to develop, Vivyan (2009) has produced a helpful list of "positive affirmations," which may give the young person (or at least the therapist) some ideas of possible starting points in the development of one's own idiosyncratic self-talk.

Thought Stopping

Key features of the competency

Thought stopping, a specific CBT technique also known as "thought suppression" or "thought interruption," is a process of intentionally trying to stop thinking certain thoughts. Thought stopping is premised on recognizing the occurrence of negative or unhelpful thoughts, and then breaking the cycle of negative thinking. It can be used as a distraction technique, in which it is first necessary to identify a positive thought or image (like a holiday experience). The client is then instructed to notice negative thoughts as they arise and, each time (s)he notices a negative thought, (s)he is asked to instruct him-/herself to "stop" and switch his/her thinking to the positive thought or image (Verduyn, Rogers, and Wood 2009). Stallard (2002, p. 115) suggests that thought stopping is like changing the tape inside your head and learning "how to turn the tape off." He suggests the following steps:

- Notice the negative thought.
- Immediately say "stop."
- This can be emphasized by "banging the table, or holding a chair or table tightly" (Stallard 2002, p. 105).
- Remind yourself of a more positive or balanced thought in response to this negative thought (this could be developed and agreed upon in collaboration with the therapist in the form of self-talk) and say it loudly.

An alternative method, also suggested by Stallard (2002), is to pair negative thoughts with a mildly aversive experience (e.g., snapping an elastic band against one's wrist) while saying "stop."

Competence in treating anxiety disorders and depression

In anxiety disorders the patterns of negative automatic thoughts tend to be about events in the future. Further, by definition, our anxiety system promotes survival. It is therefore very difficult to override anxiety by simply instructing your brain to "stop." What may be more effective is catching the anxious thoughts (worries) and putting them to one side, for consideration within a problem-solving framework, during dedicated worry time (Clarke, Lewinsohn, and Hops 1990). Thus, rather than trying to dismiss or ignore the intrusive negative thoughts, one should treat them as important and validated; but one should set them aside so as not to allow them to interrupt daily living constantly.

In depression, the patterns of negative automatic thoughts tend to be ruminative, going over past events. Conceptually this mechanism has less survival value; in consequence it may be easier to override the pattern through thought stopping.

Competence in treating both children and adolescents

Thought stopping may be useful with younger or less cognitively able clients – such as Katie, who could be instructed to imagine pressing "stop" on the tape in her head that begins to play a story about danger at night-time. Alternatively, with younger children, it may be helpful to introduce a worry box into which they can post their worries, for discussion with an adult at a pre-arranged time.

Common obstacles to competent practice and ways to overcome them

Despite the inclusion of the thought-stopping technique in empirically supported treatment manuals, significant concerns have been raised about the use of thought stopping as a cognitive technique. Wegner, Schneider, Carter, and White (1987) observed that research participants who were instructed not to think about a "White Bear" reported significantly higher White Bear intrusions than participants who were not given the thought-stopping instruction. Thus intentional thought stopping may have paradoxical impacts and increase the frequency of negative thoughts. In a review of the literature with clinical participants, Aldao, Nolen-Hoeksema, and Schweizer (2010) reported that attempts to avoid, suppress, or neutralize thoughts resulted in their returning more strongly than before. Thought suppression strategies were also associated with greater anxiety and depression. The paradoxical effect of thought stopping or suppression is imperfectly understood. However, because of the potential negative effects of thought stopping, many clinicians advise that it is better to *ignore* negative and unhelpful thoughts or to *accept* them and move on, rather than to try to simply stop or suppress them (see, e.g., Marcks and Woods 2005).

Thought Acceptance

Key features of the competency

Thought acceptance contrasts with thought-stopping strategies in the way described above. Thought acceptance can be defined as the ability to see thoughts as thoughts or opinions, not as facts. Thought acceptance as a therapeutic strategy involves allowing intrusive thoughts simply to "be" in the mind. Thus, rather than engaging and interacting with his/her negative and unhelpful thoughts, the individual develops a strategy of non-attachment to the thoughts and in this way alters his/her relationship with those thoughts.

Thought acceptance can be achieved by developing the skill of mindfulness. Mindfulness has three interdependent elements (Germer 2005, pp. 6–7):

1. awareness (i.e., stopping and observing sensations, thoughts, and feelings and re-orienting attention)
2. of the present moment,
3. with acceptance (i.e., so as "to receive our experience without judgment or preference, with curiosity and kindness").

In other words, mindfulness involves paying attention in a specific way. Mindfulness can be developed by using focused exercises that are based on principles of meditation. This can be a lengthy process, but young people can be helped to develop mindfulness skills without full training in mindfulness meditation (Bögels, de Bruin, and van der Oord 2013). Developing mindfulness can help the young person to recognize his/her habitual or automatic responses to events, and thus it gives him/her the opportunity to choose to respond differently. For example, a young person might recognize a negative automatic thought such as "I'm going to mess this up." The use of mindfulness would allow this person to notice that intrusive thought as a thought, not a fact, and to observe it dispassionately. This mindful response would replace the person's habitual response, which is to tend to elaborate on the negative thought and to catastrophize about it. The use of mindfulness techniques to deal with intrusive thoughts can help young people recognize that their thoughts need not be accorded importance, significance, or power (Verduyn et al. 2009).

Competence in treating anxiety disorders and depression

Thought acceptance and the awareness that thoughts are not facts can help make individuals distance from their intrusive and repetitive negative schemata (Mason and Hargreaves 2001). Mindfulness-based cognitive therapy (MBCT) has been used to reduce relapse in adults with recurrent depression (Kuyken et al. 2008).

Thought acceptance has also been advocated for use in anxiety disorders such as obsessive–compulsive disorder (OCD) (March and Mulle 1998). Intrusive negative thoughts are common in this population (Berry and Laskey 2012). However, people who have OCD attribute particular significance to normal intrusive thoughts and interpret them as indicating danger or risk, either to themselves or to their loved ones. This belief then leads to distress and anxiety, and people with OCD typically develop rituals and repetitive behaviors that are designed to prevent danger and harm. By cultivating thought acceptance, the young person can learn to allow his/her intrusive thoughts to pass through his/her mind without interacting with them or attributing meaning to them; thus the young person can break the cycle of OCD.

Competence in treating both children and adolescents

Within the safety of therapy and of the therapeutic alliance, young people may be encouraged to take risks and to experiment with their negative intrusive thoughts by dealing with them differently. The therapist needs to validate the power of his/her client's negative intrusive thoughts to create distress. In addition, therapy provides a safe place for young people to explore the potential effect of leaving their trouble-some, intrusive thoughts alone while they carry on with their lives – instead of responding to these thoughts or trying to push them away. Behavioral experiments (see Chapter 12) can be useful in this respect: they help young people explore the effect of engaging with the troublesome thoughts versus accepting them, noticing that they are there, and carrying on with life. A number of useful metaphors can be used to convey this idea:

1. The "rude guest": here an analogy is drawn between intrusive thoughts and a rude guest who visits the family home without being asked and says lots of annoying and rude things. The child is asked to think about how they would handle this guest. They may suggest arguing (to which the rude guest responds by arguing back more loudly); throwing the guest out (which the guest resists and tries to come back in); or ignoring the guest until the guest gets bored and leaves. The child is then asked how this guest is similar to his/her intrusive thoughts, and what the best way to deal with intrusive thoughts that come into his/her mind uninvited might be; and the take-home message is "leave thoughts alone and let them come into your mind when they want to" (Atkinson 2009, p. 87).
2. The "nasty parrot," which repeats phrases it has learned without any understanding of their meaning. The nasty parrot has only learned the unhelpful, negative, and critical phrases that the child experiences as intrusive thoughts (e.g. "You're rubbish," "They won't like you," "You're a failure") and repeats them over and over. The child is asked to imagine the parrot coming to live with him/her, how

long (s)he would tolerate this abuse before ignoring the parrot, and what would happen if (s)he did ignore the parrot (it would get louder, to try to get attention, but if it was ignored for long enough, it would give up). The child is then asked how this is similar to his/her negative thoughts; and the concept of thought acceptance is conveyed through the metaphor of ignoring (e.g., by throwing a towel over its cage) rather than listening to the parrot (Vivyan 2010).

3. Turning down the volume: rather than listening to the constant negative tracks, the album selection can be replaced with something more balanced. In practice, this could involve establishing the means by which the child or young person listens to music (e.g. iPod, MP3 player, CD player) and asking him/her to describe this device in as much detail as possible: what it looks like, where the controls are, how to switch it on and off, how to change tracks and albums, and how to adjust the volume. The negative-thought tracks or albums can then be manipulated by the young person as (s)he imagines him-/herself turning the volume up and down, switching off the device, turning it back on again, changing the album or track selection, and so on.

Common obstacles to competent practice and ways to overcome them

The idea of thought acceptance requires the young person to be able to stand back from his/her own thoughts and to gain some distance from them. This skill demands quite developed metacognitive abilities and therefore is likely to be more useful with teenagers than with younger children. Thought acceptance is most likely to be useful with intrusive thoughts that are destructive, ruminative, self-referential, and undermining. These thoughts are likely to be self-generated and self-defeating and to get in the way of the young person's development and life goals.

It is important to help the young person understand that not engaging with, or paying attention to, negative thoughts about the self does not mean that one should accept negative events and circumstances in one's life. Rather the emphasis of accepting and letting go of negative intrusive thoughts is to make room for engagement in more active, goal-oriented behaviors and plans. Thus it is important that thought acceptance is promoted in a way that explicitly balances acceptance with action and positive future goals, for example through the development of the image of the positive and most developed self (see above).

Conclusion

Successfully engaging children and young people with the cognitive elements of CBT draws on a wide range of therapeutic skills and knowledge. We have outlined a range of strategies that can be used to help children and young people recognize, challenge, and manage their negative thoughts. Therapists will typically find some strategies more appealing than others, and individual children and young people are also likely to engage with some strategies in preference to others. We would tend to favor behavioral experiments (see Chapter 12) as a core strategy to bring about cognitive change, and to use the other strategies to support and expand on behavioral experiments. Behavioral experiments provide immediate and powerful learning experiences, which can feel more "real" than pure cognitive work: such work may appear to take a more abstract or theoretical approach to change.

Blending behavioral experiments and other cognitive strategies to help children overcome anxiety and low mood builds on a core therapeutic relationship. A strong therapeutic alliance with the child and his/her family provides a safe environment to introduce behavioral experiments and other interventions (see Chapter 6 for details on building a therapeutic alliance). Thus CBT relies on the basic therapy skills of warmth and empathy, which in turn provide the foundation for a positive therapeutic alliance with the child and his/her family. Therapists must be able to adapt their style and method of work to the needs and characteristics of each child and family. These include age and developmental level of the child, parental beliefs and mental health, the family's immediate social and cultural environment (e.g. class, religious beliefs, and language) and the wider environmental norms and expectations on children and their families. Ideally the child's wider environment at home and at school will support and encourage therapeutic work outside and beyond sessions; hence involving the parents and sometimes the teachers is generally recommended.

These various complexities of using CBT with children and young people mean that therapists require high levels of therapist skills, knowledge, and personal qualities. Like any form of psychotherapy, the delivery of CBT makes significant emotional and cognitive demands on therapists. Therefore in our view all CBT therapists, whether experienced or not, should receive regular and focused CBT supervision. In our view, supervision for CBT therapists working with children, young people, and their families should include direct or indirect observation of treatment sessions. In addition, supervision should focus on the development and maintenance of the therapeutic alliance as well as on the use of specific CBT techniques.

Acknowledgments

The authors would like to thank Christopher Jacobs for Figures 13.1 and 13.2.

References

Aldao, Amelia, Susan Nolen-Hoeksema, and Susanne Schweizer. 2010. "Emotion-Regulation Strategies across Psychopathology: A Meta-Analytic Review." *Clinical Psychology Review*, 30: 217–37. DOI: 10.1016/j.cpr.2009.11.004

Atkinson, Linda J. 2009. "CBT with younger children." In Polly Waite and Tim Williams (Eds.). *Obsessive Compulsive Disorder: Cognitive Behaviour Therapy with children and young people* (pp. 77–96). London: Routledge.

Berry, Lisa-Marie, and Benjamin Laskey. 2012. "A Review of Obsessive Intrusive Thoughts in the General Population." *Journal of Obsessive–Compulsive and Related Disorders*, 1: 125–32. DOI: 10.1016/j.jocrd.2012.02.002

Bögels, Susan M., Esther I. de Bruin, and Saskia van der Oord. 2013. "Mindfulness Interventions in Child and Adolescent Psychopathology." In Philip Graham and Shirley

Reynolds (Eds.), *Cognitive Behaviour Therapy for Children and Families: Current Trends* (pp. 371–84). Cambridge: Cambridge University Press.

Clarke, Gregory, Peter M. Lewinsohn, and Hyman Hops. 1990. *Leader's Manual for Adolescent Groups: Coping with Depression Course.* Portland, OR: Kaiser Permanente Center for Health Research.

Deblinger, Esther, and Ann Heflin. 1996. *Treating Sexually Abused Children and their Non-offending Parents.* Thousand Oaks, CA: Sage.

Friedberg, Robert D., and Jessica M. McClure. 2002. *Clinical Practice of Cognitive Therapy with Children and Adolescents: The Nuts and Bolts.* London: Guildford Press.

Germer, Christopher K. 2005. "Mindfulness: What Is It? What Does It Matter?" In Christopher K. Germer, Ronald D. Siegel and Paul R. Fulton (Eds.), *Mindfulness and Psychotherapy* (pp. 3–27). New York: Guildford Press.

Gilbert, Paul. 2009. "Introducing Compassion-Focused Therapy." *Advances in Psychiatric Treatment,* 15: 199–208. DOI: 10.1192/apt.bp.107.005264

Hackmann, Ann, James Bennett-Levy, and Emily Holmes. 2011. *Oxford Guide to Imagery in Cognitive Therapy.* Oxford: Oxford University Press.

Kendall, Philip C., and Kristin A. Hedke. 2006a. *Cognitive Behaviour Therapy for Anxious Children: Therapist Manual* (3rd ed.). Ardmore, PA: Workbook Publishing.

Kendall, Philip C., and Kristin A. Hedtke, 2006b. *The Coping Cat Workbook.* Ardmore, PA: Workbook Publishing.

Kuyken, Willem, Sarah Byford, Rod S. Taylor, Ed Watkins, Emily Holden, Kat White, ... John D. Teasdale. 2008. "Mindfulness-Based Cognitive Therapy to Prevent Relapse in Recurrent Depression." *Journal of Consulting and Clinical Psychology,* 76: 966–78. DOI: 10.1037/a0013786

Lee, Deborah A. 2005. "The Perfect Nurturer: A Model to Develop a Compassionate Mind within the Context of Cognitive Therapy." In Paul Gilbert (Ed.), *Compassion: Conceptualisations, Research and Use in Psychotherapy* (pp. 326–51). London: Routledge.

March, John, and Karen Mulle. 1998. *OCD in Children and Adolescents: A Cognitive-Behavioural Treatment Manual.* New York: Guildford Press.

Marcks, Brooke A., and Douglas W. Woods. 2005. "A Comparison of Thought Suppression to an Acceptance-Based Technique in the Management of Personal Intrusive Thoughts: A Controlled Evaluation." *Behaviour Research and Therapy,* 43: 433–45. DOI: 10.1016/j.brat.2004.03.005

Mason, Olivia, and Isobel Hargreaves. 2001. "A Qualitative Study of Mindfulness-Based Cognitive Therapy for Depression." *British Journal of Medical Psychology,* 74: 197–212.

Rapee, Ronald M., Heidi J. Lyneham, Carolyn A. Schniering, Viviana Wuthrich, Maree A. Abbot, Jennifer L. Hudson, and Ann Wignall. 2006. *Cool Kids "Chilled" Adolescent Anxiety Program.* Sydney: Centre for Emotional Health, Macquaire University.

Ronen, Tammie (1997). *Cognitive Developmental Therapy with Children.* Chichester, England: Wiley.

Sburlati, Elizabeth S., Carolyn A. Schniering, Heidi J. Lyneham, and Ronald M. Rapee. 2011. "A Model of Therapist Competencies for the Empirically Supported Cognitive Behavioural Treatment of Child and Adolescent Anxiety and Depressive Disorders." *Clinical Child and Family Psychology Review,* 14: 89–109. DOI: 10.1007/s10567-011-0083-6

Stallard, Paul. (2002). *Think Good – Feel Good: A Cognitive Behaviour Therapy Workbook for Children and Young People.* Chichester, England: John Wiley & Sons.

Stallard, Paul. 2009. *Anxiety: Cognitive Behaviour Therapy with Children and Young People.* London, England: Routledge.

Verduyn, Chrissie, Julia Rogers, and Alison Wood. 2009. *Depression: Cognitive Behaviour Therapy with Children and Young People.* London and New York: Routledge.

Vivyan, Carol. 2009. "Affirmations," www.getselfhelp.co.uk/affirmations.htm (accessed December 2, 2013).

Vivyan, Carol. 2010. "The Poisoned Parrot," http://www.get.gg/parrot.htm (accessed December 2, 2013).

Vygotsky, Lev S. 1962. *Thought and Language*. Cambridge, MA: MIT Press.

Wegner, Daniel M., David J. Schneider, Samuel R. Carter, and Terry L. White. 1987. "Paradoxical Effects of Thought Suppression." *Journal of Personality and Social Psychology*, 53: 5–13.

14

Changing Maladaptive Behaviors, Part 1

Exposure and Response Prevention

Brennan J. Young, Thomas H. Ollendick, and Stephen P. Whiteside

Introduction

Working with anxious children through exposure therapy is at once inherently challenging and rewarding. Children by nature desire to learn, grow, and gain mastery over their world; but children with anxiety must work harder to approach and effectively interact with their world. For those of us who are called upon to help anxious children, our reward is to see them push through the fear to grow in both confidence and competence; our challenge is to enable them to do so.

Just as it is inherently difficult for a child to face his fears, it can be difficult for clinicians to effectively implement exposure therapy with children, and many clinicians choose not to adopt this approach (Addis and Krasnow 2000; Valderhaug, Gotestam, and Larsson 2004). For some, exposure does not fit their theoretical orientation or therapeutic style. Others may be reluctant to deliberately induce additional distress in children who are already fearful. Nevertheless, exposure therapy in anxiety has garnered both theoretical and empirical support. Avoidance of fearful stimuli is regarded as a core feature in the etiology and maintenance of anxiety disorders. According to Lang's (1967) tripartite model, behavioral avoidance serves to negatively reinforce the anxiety response. Exposure, on the other hand, is incompatible with avoidance and, when performed competently and effectively, results in the extinction of the anxiety response through habituation. Indeed, empirical data support the efficacy of exposure in reducing fear and anxiety (see In-Albon and Schneider 2007; Kendall et al. 2005; Seligman and Ollendick 2011). For these reasons, exposure is considered the treatment of choice for childhood anxiety.

Our goal in the current chapter is to lay a clear road map for clinicians training to acquire competence in exposure therapy with children and adolescents. We begin by

Evidence-Based CBT for Anxiety and Depression in Children and Adolescents: A Competencies-Based Approach, First Edition. Edited by Elizabeth S. Sburlati, Heidi J. Lyneham, Carolyn A. Schniering, and Ronald M. Rapee. © 2014 John Wiley & Sons, Ltd. Published 2014 by John Wiley & Sons, Ltd.

describing an evidence-based approach to conducting exposure therapy, highlighting key factors for successful implementation as well as key areas of competence for the successful clinician. We then discuss variations on this theme, describing the application of these central principles to treating specific types of anxiety. Next, we examine some developmental considerations that arise in work with children and adolescents and can further complicate the design and delivery of exposure therapy. Finally, we identify and suggest ways to overcome obstacles commonly encountered while delivering exposure therapy to children and adolescents.

Key Features of the Competencies: Behavioral Markers of Competently Delivering Exposure Therapy

Successfully delivering exposure therapy requires competence in several specific areas. Each area of competence will be discussed, but we begin with a general overview of the principal elements of exposure therapy. First, providing a strong rationale for engaging in exposure builds motivation for therapy, orients the child and her parent to their active role in therapy, and promotes tolerance for the distress that inevitably accompanies exposure. Next, the clinician conducts a functional analysis of the child's anxiety, paying careful attention to the ways in which the child actively avoids facing her fears. The goal of this analysis is to build a graded fear hierarchy that specifies the steps by which the child will begin facing her fears. The clinician then guides the child through the appropriate form of exposure (e.g., *in vivo*, imaginal, narrative – see below), targeting her specific fears. In doing so, the clinician ensures that the child perseveres with each exposure until her subjective distress has decreased. During each exposure, the clinician is watchful for any safety behaviors the child engages in to avoid the situation or otherwise reduce her fear without directly facing it. The successful exposure session is then rewarded so as to reinforce the child's new behavior, and the clinician ensures that the child learns the necessary lessons (e.g., the feared consequences do not occur; the distress can be tolerated). Finally, exposures within a particular step are repeated until the task no longer elicits significant fear or avoidance; when this is achieved, the child is ready to progress to the next step on her fear hierarchy. Ultimately, exposure therapy can be considered successful when an unplanned confrontation with the feared stimulus no longer produces a heightened anxiety response or significant behavioral avoidance.

Functional analysis

Each child will display a unique set of fears as well as unique behavioral reactions when confronted with his fears. Thus an idiographic (versus a nomothetic) approach should be taken to designing the exposure plan, and the careful diagnosis and detailed conceptualization of the child's fear and behavioral avoidance should be considered an important area of clinical competence. A thorough functional analysis of the child's fear will include a description of the context in which fear and anxiety are triggered. It is also important to build as good an understanding as possible of what the child anticipates will happen in these situations. Finally, it is important to identify current strategies the child employs to reduce his fear. These strategies may be ways in which he is able to avoid the situation altogether, to escape from the situation when it occurs, or to seek reassurance. It may also be necessary to elicit from parents their own reactions to the situation and to the child's fears, looking for ways in which parents themselves reinforce the child's anxious responses and avoidance.

It is important that the functional analysis of the child's fear be as detailed and specific as possible. In fact a clinician may think of this assessment as "drilling down" or "peeling the layers of an onion" to find a core, underlying fear that lays at the heart of many of the child's fears and avoidant behaviors (Beidel and Turner 2007). For example, consider the case of a 12-year-old boy who presented himself to an outpatient clinic with symptoms of social anxiety. This child became very anxious when interacting with strangers outside the home. Behaviorally, he withdrew from social interaction by hiding behind his parent, often had difficulty in making eye contact, and spoke in a whisper that was very difficult for others to hear. After the interview, the child and his parents were both in agreement about the range of situations that presented difficulties for the child, as well as about his behavioral reactions to those situations. The clinician continued to seek more information, asking *why* these situations were difficult for the child, what reactions the child feared he would receive from others, or what may happen as a result of interacting with others. The clinician also followed the matter up with questions such as: "And if that were to happen, what would be difficult about it?" Thus it is important to identify not only the negative outcome initially expected, but also the expected consequences of that outcome.

Over the course of interviewing and working with this child and his parent, it became clear that the child feared that he would say something incorrect or would make a mistake in front of a stranger, who would then form the impression that the boy was "dumb." Understanding this core feature of the boy's anxiety led to exposures in which he deliberately began making incorrect statements and other mistakes while interacting with strangers. Once his anxiety about making mistakes began to dissipate, his anxiety and behavioral avoidance began to improve across a variety of social situations that were not specifically targeted through exposure. Thus, when a specific fear can be identified through functional analysis, exposures can more directly target the child's fear, and therapy can move more quickly and effectively. Often the process of getting to know a child's anxiety continues to unfold over the course of treatment and, as the child's trust in the clinician develops and rapport continues to be built, the child's own insight and ability to identify thoughts and fears start to improve.

Fear hierarchy

Functional analysis will lead naturally to the next step in the therapy, which is to create the fear hierarchy – another area in which clinicians new to exposure therapy will need to achieve competence. The fear hierarchy delineates a series of exposures that target a specific type of anxiety or fear and progressively move the child closer to confronting his core fear; in the previous example, a hierarchy would have been created targeting the child's fear of making mistakes in front of strangers. The clinician works with the child and his parent to identify a range of specific activities that center upon the identified fear and produce varying levels of anxiety or avoidance in the child. The child and his parent then provide a subjective rating of the level of the child's anxiety for each activity (typically such a rating ranges from 0 to 10 and is referred to as the Subjective Units of Distress Scale – SUDS). Once each activity has been assigned a SUDS rating, the situations are in effect ordered from the least to the most distressing or impairing. Each step along the hierarchy progressively activates greater anxiety or fear in the child, since, with each exposure, he confronts his core fear more directly. It is important to bear in mind that the child's level of distress for the later steps in the hierarchy may actually diminish as a result of his having progressed through the earlier steps. Thus a fear that originally was assigned a SUDS rating of "8" may actually be lower and more manageable by the time the child is ready to begin work on that step of the hierarchy.

A well-crafted hierarchy will include items that are easy enough for the child to engage with immediately; items that are more challenging than those encountered in a typical daily experience; and enough intermediate steps for the child to move from the former to the latter gradually. Taking good care to identify steps that produce lower levels of anxiety is very important for engaging the child and for starting to build confidence. By the same token, each step in the hierarchy should not be too far above the previous step in terms of the child's anxiety. Finally, the last steps may include very challenging exposures, which directly target the child's core fear and serve to dramatically disconfirm the consequences feared by the child. An example of this would be asking a child who is afraid of germs and contamination to put her hand in a toilet bowl – in the child's mind possibly the dirtiest and most germ-laden place imaginable. This overlearning may enhance symptom improvement and maintain treatment gains.

Having stated the importance of a well-developed hierarchy, it is also true that the process of getting to know a child's anxiety continues to unfold over the course of treatment, as rapport and trust continue to grow and the child's own insight and ability to identify thoughts and fears begin to improve. Thus the initial fear hierarchy is also a work in progress, and, in training new clinicians, it will be important to encourage flexibility when they plan and deliver exposures. In addition, many anxious children show multiple fears, which often encompass several domains and thereby necessitate several fear hierarchies (Kendall, Brady, and Verduin 2001). Beginning with exposures that are easily controlled by the clinician and that present a high likelihood of success for the child will help build confidence and motivation early on in therapy. The clinician should also consider beginning with fears that, once reduced, can liberate the greatest potential for regaining daily functioning. Clinicians are encouraged to focus on one set of fears at a time, so that the child can achieve success in an identified area. However, due to practical constraints on conducting exposures, a child might work on several hierarchies at the same time in therapy.

The need for flexibility is often encountered when beginning exposures or moving from one step of the hierarchy to another. Children often underestimate the degree of situational anxiety they experience until they are actually experiencing it. Take, for example, a child who is afraid of heights, has rated looking down from a tenth-floor window as 3 on a scale from 0 to 10 (a good starting point for exposures), but experiences significantly higher anxiety when the time comes to actually approach the window on the tenth floor and is unable to do it. To change the exposure activity altogether would reinforce the child's notion that he cannot cope with his anxiety and that avoidance is a solution. As a general rule, every step on the hierarchy can be further broken down into smaller, less anxiety-provoking steps. In the previous example, several intermediate steps are possible, such as allowing the child the first time round to hold onto a piece of office furniture or to the clinician's hand. Alternatively, a subhierarchy could be quickly established by rating the child's anxiety when he stands 5 feet from the window, then 4 feet, 3 feet, and so on; this method would allow the child to approach the window incrementally. Similarly each step of a hierarchy contains in itself a subhierarchy whose steps are small enough not to be overwhelming.

Psycho-education and building motivation

The anxiety experienced by both children and their parents may be a significant obstacle to promoting motivation and engagement in exposure therapy. Parents are asked to deliberately put their children in situations that cause distress, and children are asked to endure that distress. Thus both the children and the parents may need a strong motivation to engage in exposure therapy. A clinician's ability to effectively deliver an explanation (or rationale) of exposure therapy that gives both children and parents this kind of motivation is another important area of competence.

Clinicians should be well versed in the theory underlying exposure therapy and should be able to explain it coherently both to parents and to children. As discussed more fully elsewhere, exposure is generally thought to work by modifying associations between fearful emotions, cognitions, and behavior that maintain anxiety reactions. Repeated and prolonged exposure modifies these associations by presenting information and experiences that are incompatible with the fear response. It can be helpful to introduce the cognitive behavioral conceptualization of anxiety and of its maintenance through a concrete example that does not provoke anxiety, such as fear of dogs (assuming the child does not have this fear). Using an illustration, the clinician begins by explaining that some people are afraid of dogs because they believe that dogs are likely to bite people. When they see a dog and become fearful, they naturally run away or avoid the dog. This reaction is quite successful in reducing anxiety for the moment. However, as these people still believe that dogs are likely to bite people, they remain scared of dogs and stuck in this cycle of fear and avoidance. The clinician emphasizes that (i) it is the thought (not the dog) that causes anxiety; (ii) avoiding dogs prevents people from learning through their own experience that dogs are relatively safe; and (iii) because avoidance is so effective at reducing unpleasant anxiety, people rely on this strategy more and more frequently. The majority of families, even those with fairly young children, can readily understand the self-perpetuating nature of the anxiety cycle as it applies to a fear of dogs.

The clinician can then describe how the cycle is broken through exposure. Here it should be explained to the child and his parents that exposure will be a gradual process; for example, it will begin with looking at pictures of dogs, then progress to being near a small dog in a cage, then to petting a small dog, then to petting a larger dog. The importance of continuing to pet the dog until the child feels safe *without* running away and realizes that the dog does *not* bite should be underscored. It is often helpful to have the child explain the model in his own words, to demonstrate understanding. At this point the clinician can work with the family to map the child's anxiety triggers, maladaptive beliefs, and safety behaviors onto the cycle (see the section on exposure with response prevention, below) and to explain the persistence and exacerbation of symptoms in terms of a natural learning process involving negative reinforcement. This model for understanding anxiety is particularly valuable because it provides a clear rationale for treatment through exposure.

Becoming competent in exposure therapy will also require involving the parents as coaches in their child's treatment. By first observing the clinician in session and then gradually taking over more responsibility for exposure, the parent can become an active contributor to therapy. In addition, the clinician can coach the parent on effective techniques for responding to a child's anxiety – such as removing the child's attention from anxious behavior, breaking down the fear into manageable steps, and rewarding the child's approach behavior. Ultimately the clinician may not treat all of the child's anxiety symptoms or complete the treatment of all the steps in the child's hierarchy. As the parent takes over coaching and the child continues to make improvements, the family can make a plan to continue the treatment on its own, holding occasional check-ins with the clinician as necessary. As we will discuss below, the extent of a parent's involvement as a coach will depend upon the child's developmental level; parents will likely play less of a role with more autonomous adolescents.

Variations on a Theme: Competent Exposure in the Context of Different Anxiety Disorders

The principles discussed above are elements common to, and important in, all forms of exposure therapy; but variations on delivering exposure therapy do exist, depending upon the type of anxiety to be treated. As many patients require exposure in multiple formats, clinicians should be competent in each area. In the following paragraphs we provide an overview of available techniques. For a more detailed discussion of these techniques, we refer the reader to Abramowitz, Deacon, and Whiteside (2011).

In vivo or situational exposure

Treatment of the majority of anxiety disorders includes having the child directly confront places, situations, animals, or objects that produce anxiety – that is, *in vivo* exposure. Conducting this type of exposure generally requires pre-planning from the clinician in order to arrange a situation that corresponds to a step from the child's fear hierarchy and to have available the object that causes the child to be anxious. Many of these items may not exist in the office and the clinician should be prepared to make "field trips" into the community.

We generally recommend a gradual approach that begins with moderately distressing stimuli and progresses to more and more difficult exposures as soon as the child is ready (the child's ability to successfully confront previously feared and avoided stimuli generally indicates that he is ready to move on). There are, however, instances when a more rapid approach is appropriate, and even recommended. Many specific phobias – fears of balloons or dogs, for example – can be treated effectively and efficiently in a single prolonged session of rapid exposure (e.g., Ollendick et al. 2009). Other instances may even suggest a more rapid approach to exposure (i.e., flooding) – for example when the child's fear is circumscribed enough for all the relevant exposures to be accomplished in a single session; when the child or her family wishes to undergo a more rapid approach; and when gradual exposure is impractical due to geographical or time constraints.

Interoceptive exposures

This type of exposure is generally associated with symptoms of panic and is conducted when the child fears experiencing uncomfortable internal physiological sensations. For example, some children become very distressed when they experience dizziness, shortness of breath, heart palpitations, or sweatiness. These sensations can be aversive in and of themselves but they may also be associated with fears of crying in front of others, becoming ill, or dying. The exposure in this case is to induce on purpose the physiological sensations that the child fears; this is commonly done by having the child breathe quickly and deeply (hyperventilation), climb stairs (heart palpitations, sweatiness, shortness of breath), breathe through a straw (shortness of breath), spin in an office chair (dizziness), or sit up quickly after having sat with her head between her knees for a time (dizziness, change in blood pressure). Generally these exposures are fairly straightforward in their implementation, but it will be key for the clinician to make sure during assessment that the child actually fears the physiological sensations and not the external situation that caused them. Otherwise, if the situation is truly the trigger for anxiety, exposure would be better targeted toward that situation. Pincus, Ehrenreich, and Mattis (2008) offer a detailed discussion of interoceptive exposure.

Imaginal exposure

Imaginal exposure has three main applications: in directly targeting intrusive thoughts; in augmenting *in vivo* or interoceptive exposure; and in preparing for *in vivo* exposure. When imaginal exposure is used as a primary form of exposure, to address intrusive thoughts, particularly in dealing with OCD symptoms, the clinician begins by having the child describe the thoughts in as much detail as possible. Eliciting thoughts can be complicated by the child's embarrassment or anxiety about them, as well as on account of the child's developmental level. Once the thoughts have been identified, the clinician helps the child repeat the thoughts, orally or in writing, or listen to a recording of them – until his anxiety has diminished. The mode of exposure (e.g., oral vs. written) depends on which approach most closely replicates the child's symptoms and can be incorporated into a graduated fear hierarchy of the hierarchy. The clinician may need to assist the child by providing examples of common unwanted thoughts that may be similar to the child's. However, the clinician should be sensitive to the child's developmental level and not introduce content that would be inappropriate for the child. It is understandable for clinicians and parents to feel uncomfortable about encouraging children to repeat upsetting thoughts, particularly of a violent or sexual nature. The decision about what is appropriate for an exposure is based on the child's symptoms and how she describes them. Whatever thoughts the child is having, they need to be addressed, using the child's words, through exposure.

Imaginal exposure can also be used to augment *in vivo* exposures by addressing uncertainty or situations that cannot be directly confronted. For example, if a child is afraid that mummies will attack after he separates from his parents, *in vivo* exposure to separation could be enhanced through imaginal exposure to mummies' breaking into his room. Finally, if it is not possible to develop a tolerable, low-anxiety *in vivo* exposure that a child is willing to begin with, imaginal exposure can be used as a preliminary or as a first step.

Although it can be helpful, in our opinion imaginal exposure should be used infrequently for several reasons. First, many younger children, and even some adolescents, lack the cognitive control to fully engage in imaginal exposures for an extended period of time. Second, especially when children are not intrinsically motivated to reduce their fear and to engage in exposures, it could be difficult for the clinician to ensure that the child is fully participating in imaginal exposure: a child who outwardly appears to be concentrating may actually have turned his attention away from thoughts about the feared stimulus and is mentally avoiding the exposure altogether. Finally, children and adolescents whose abstract reasoning is less developed may be less able to connect the thought exercises of imaginal exposure to reality and to generalize the experience to their everyday life. Most importantly, in vivo exposures are typically more effective than imaginal exposures and should be used whenever possible.

Narrative exposure

Closely related to imaginal exposure is the use of narrative to create an exposure. Narrative exposure is generally conducted in the context of anxiety related to past events and trauma, specifically for post-traumatic stress disorder. The goal of exposure is to break the link between memories, thoughts, and reminders of the trauma on the one hand and anxiety, emotional distress, and avoidance on the other (see Deblinger and Heflin 1996). Exposure in this case proceeds by asking the child to write a narrative of the events (or to draw pictures that depict them, depending upon the child's developmental level), which effectively becomes the exposure that triggers the child's anxiety response. Therapy may proceed gradually up the hierarchy by asking the child to write progressively more detail and by elaborating upon the narrative. Latter steps of the hierarchy may be to ask the child to read the narrative aloud, and eventually to share it with others (as appropriate, given the circumstances of the past event). The goal in each exposure session is to ask the child to tolerate the anxiety that remembering the event arouses in her – tolerate it, that is, long enough for habituation to occur, which means gradually increasing the extent to which the child can tolerate memories of the event.

Exposure with response prevention

Nearly every child who experiences anxiety displays a set of safety behaviors – actions that, when performed, serve to "neutralize" or escape from the expected negative outcome. Response prevention – preventing the child from engaging in these safety behaviors when confronted with the feared situation – should be part of every form of exposure therapy; however, it is specifically associated with the treatment of obsessive compulsive disorder (OCD) (March and Mulle 1998). When a child with OCD experiences emotional discomfort and anxiety, he often responds with compulsions that serve to reduce his emotional tension. Exposure therapy proceeds by deliberately triggering the child's anxiety and then asking the child *not* to engage in the safety behavior that would otherwise reduce his distress, but wait instead for habituation to occur. In this way the child learns (i) that the anxiety can be tolerated and will eventually dissipate on its own, without the need for compulsive rituals and routine; and (ii) that negative events are unlikely to occur.

In children, it can be particularly difficult to identify safety behaviors. Some safety behaviors are fairly covert; such are crossing toes inside of shoes, making tongue movements inside of the mouth, saying prayers, and counting or performing other mental actions that are not directly observable. Further, children may initially be less motivated than their parents to engage in exposure therapy *without* the use of safety behaviors; thus they are not always motivated to *report* their safety behaviors. Some children have limited insight and are poor reporters of their own behavior, which makes their omission less intentional and more of an oversight. It will be important for the clinician to consult with the child's parents about known safety behaviors that they have observed, although the clinician should also rely on her own clinical observations. Does the child's anxiety and apparent distress match what would be expected for the current exposure and for what the child is reporting?

Developmental Considerations in Providing Competent Exposure Therapy to Children and Adolescents

As outlined above, successfully delivering exposure therapy requires competence in several specific areas; underlying each of these areas is a general competence in child development and developmental psychopathology. Working clinically with children is a complex task. Even children of similar ages will show varying levels of cognitive, social, and emotional development, which determine not only the child's ability to report internal experiences and emotions but also the way in which the clinician will interact with the child and the role of parents in therapy. Clinicians must also be effective in managing behavior and help children work through their reluctance to engage in exposure. Finally, children are embedded within family systems that function uniquely and often contain their own sources of stress (e.g., conflict, parental psychopathology, socioeconomic factors, etc.). Clinicians must be able to work with parents who often are themselves anxious and whose responses may be maintaining their child's anxiety (Young et al. 2013). Thus, having knowledge of developmental processes and experience in working with children and families is essential if one is to become competent in delivering exposure therapy to children and adolescents.

SUDs ratings

Accurately assessing a child's current level of anxiety during an exposure session is very important in determining when to end the exercise. The effect of ending the task before the child adequately achieves habituation is akin to that of behavioral avoidance in that the child's anxiety response may be negatively reinforced: she experiences a sudden reduction in her symptoms of anxiety by leaving the situation or by removing the feared stimulus, which may prompt future avoidance of similar situations for the purpose of gaining the same symptom relief. Younger children tend to be more concrete in their cognitive abilities and have less sophistication in their recognition and regulation of emotions. Hence SUDs ratings may differ according to developmental level. For example, asking younger children to accurately assess their own level of anxiety on a standard 0–10 scale may be too nuanced a task. Instead, asking younger children (approximately 7 years old and younger, though this will vary according to developmental level) to rate their anxiety using a "low, medium, high" scale or a "green, yellow, red" scale may be developmentally more appropriate and yield more accurate ratings. Some younger children, over the course of engaging in exposure therapy, learn that, when they report low SUDs ratings (even if these are not exactly true), the exposure task is concluded, which brings immediate relief from anxiety. Thus, when working with younger children, no matter whether the child is intentionally underreporting symptoms of anxiety or is developmentally not able to report symptoms accurately, the clinician may need to rely less on verbal reports of anxiety from the child. Instead, the clinician will rely more heavily on the parents' judgment of the child's anxiety, although she will pay careful attention to behavioral cues that the child exhibits. When in doubt, continue the exposure. There is no harm in extending an exposure even after the child's anxiety has subsided.

Adjusting parent involvement

The way in which the clinician involves parents will also need to be sensitive to a child's developmental level. The extent to which parents are involved as coaches will change as children's cognitive, emotional, and social development becomes more sophisticated. As a rule, exposure tasks need to be completed outside of therapy sessions (e.g., as part of homework). Younger children will be more dependent upon their parents than older children for the planning and implementation of these exposures; adolescents may even be somewhat independent. Nevertheless, due to the nature of anxiety and the natural tendency of anxious children to avoid their anxiety, even very mature adolescents may require some parental monitoring and reinforcement, which should ensure that exposures are conducted properly and on a regular basis. In order to balance the proper degree of parent involvement with patient autonomy, the clinician will need a firm understanding of child development in general, as well as the ability to assess developmental level and apply it to an individual client.

Choosing developmentally appropriate exposure tasks

The broader purpose in exposure therapy with children is ultimately to return a child to a more normative trajectory of development. Many anxious children avoid engaging in situations that would otherwise promote the acquisition of new skills and that are generally part of the developmental process of building competence, self-confidence, and autonomy in childhood. Engaging in exposure tasks will reduce a child's fear and anxiety, and it also presents opportunities for a child to gain experience and skill in new areas. As she is working toward competence, a clinician may ask herself: "What would I expect socially from a 14-year-old female? Is my client demonstrating behavior consistent with this developmental level? If not, how is anxiety playing a role, and how can I structure treatment so as to bring growth in these areas?" For example, exposure tasks for a child who is socially anxious with adults or authority figures may involve speaking to waiters or store clerks, practicing ordering her own food, asking adults for directions, and so on. For a teenager who struggles with similar fears, exposure tasks may involve inquiring about job applications, engaging teachers in conversation about grades, or speaking with a coach about missing practice. Thus, with a good knowledge of normative development and of the tasks that are generally mastered at particular stages of it, a clinician may choose exposures that have real-world significance for the child's daily functioning and that promote positive development.

Common Obstacles to Competently Delivering Exposure Therapy to Children and Adolescents

"A journey of a thousand miles begins with a single step": Getting started

We have already discussed the importance of thoroughly developing a fear hierarchy before beginning exposures. However, even presenting the concept of a fear hierarchy and beginning to discuss specific exposures can elicit anxiety and resistance from a child; parents are not immune to anxiety during this initial stage of therapy, either. Anxiety during this critical step – and how it is managed by the clinician – can set the stage for the rest of the therapy or can short-circuit it before it even begins.

When a child or a parent experiences significant anxiety about the process of exposure therapy itself, it can be helpful to emphasize the gradual way in which exposure will proceed. By design, exposure begins from the lowest fear in the child's hierarchy and progresses gradually, step by step, to the higher fears. Further, calling to mind an image of climbing up a downward-moving escalator may be helpful (be aware, however, that climbing up an escalator that goes down is decidedly counterculture, and most anxious children will not have broken such a rule – they will often laugh at the idea of it, though). Each step of the fear hierarchy is represented by a step on the escalator. The child begins by stepping onto the lowest step. As she steps up to the next step, however, the escalator has already moved down. The step that used to be rated as a 2 is now closer to a 1. As she takes another step up, the escalator has moved down yet again, and what was initially rated as a 3 is now experienced more like a 2, and so on. As the child progresses up her fear hierarchy, she is growing in confidence and ability, and the higher steps of her hierarchy are not so fearful anymore.

Leaving the comfort zone: Getting out of the office

Unlike many other modes of therapy, most exposures simply cannot be done in a traditional psychotherapy office setting. The most obvious reason for this appears in exposure for social anxiety: generally social exposure requires a public place, in which the child can interact with people other than just the clinician. Specific fears – such as of heights, elevators, animals – will likely require field trips out of the office, too. Exposure and response prevention for OCD will require seeking out triggers for a child's obsessions and compulsions. The competent clinician will be creative in finding and orchestrating effective exposures, often in real-life situations outside of the office.

For a clinician accustomed to more traditional modes of psychotherapy, this can be frustrating for several reasons. First, when the session is held outside of the office, a clinician may not be able to hold back-to-back, traditional 50-minute sessions; it takes extra effort and time to travel and set up exposures. Second, a good amount of pre-planning is necessary to arrange for effective exposures, and this, too, requires time and effort devoted to treatment planning – again, time spent outside of the traditional 50-minute session. Putting in this extra planning and energy may need to be actively modeled and encouraged by experienced mentors for clinicians who are learning exposure therapy; this will set a precedent for them. Further, compiling a list of activities that are commonly used for exposures, together with a number of places in which they can be accomplished, would reduce the amount of pre-planning that needs to be done. Finally, arranging in advance to meet a family at a particular location may help to make the session more efficient.

Pacing yourself

Once therapy is underway, finding the optimum pace at which to progress through the fear hierarchy can also be a common obstacle for clinicians new to exposure. Moving too quickly or too slowly are common mistakes. On the one hand, moving too quickly through the fear hierarchy may not allow for true habituation to occur at any one step; in this case the child will be facing fears that, in his hierarchy, are perhaps higher than he is ready for. When this happens, treatment dropout is more likely to occur. On the other hand, therapy that moves too slowly through the fear hierarchy can lead to boredom and discouragement with lack of progress. Further, each exposure session must follow the previous session closely enough in time so that habituation achieved in one session will carry over into the next, which leads to progressively lower SUDs ratings at the initiation of each successive session.

Sticking with the game plan

Once the clinician and the family have settled upon a good fear hierarchy and have identified a particular step of the hierarchy to target, we want to encourage the clinician to stick with the plan. It is quite natural for a weekly therapy session to begin with a "check-in," in which parents report on how the week went for their child and what difficulties she had. However, it is often very tempting for the clinician to then choose an exposure that will address these difficulties – even if it is not what the child has been working on over the past several sessions. Don't let the problem of the week alter the exposure plan. Doing so will likely slow overall progress; as we discussed previously, continuity between exposure sessions is necessary for habituation to carry over and to achieve progressively lower SUDs ratings. In addition, facing a brand new type of exposure every week will likely become overwhelming and discouraging for the child; on the contrary, it can be very motivating for a child to see steady progress from week to week on a single task.

When parents do come up with new concerns that are based upon recent behavior or events in the child's life, it may be enough to offer them some validation of their frustration, encouragement for their motivation and participation in therapy, as well as your commitment to returning to these issues when the time is right. The clinician may also take this opportunity to look back over the past several weeks of therapy and to highlight what progress the child has made on the current step of the fear hierarchy, expressing desire to continue working in that area so as not to lose ground.

Become a fearless leader

Ironically – but understandably – clinicians' own anxiety about conducting exposures stands perhaps as the greatest obstacle to successfully delivering exposure therapy. Many clinicians fear that the exposures will not be tolerated well by children or will cause them to become more anxious. On the other hand, clinicians may worry that exposures will cause a child to become obstinate, which may lead to a battle of wills within the therapy session – a scenario no clinician looks forward to. Compounding these worries is the common belief that asking children to engage in exposures will interfere with the clinician's ability to establish adequate rapport with the child. Still other clinicians fear that the parents of anxious children will not buy into the concept of exposure and will seek treatment elsewhere.

Each of these concerns is legitimate and constitutes a possible scenario with any given family. However, all of them are also manageable. Typically, anxious children are eager to please and will do well in therapy when given the support necessary to do so. Make therapy (even exposure therapy) fun! By being energetic and enthusiastic with parents and children alike, the clinician can create an atmosphere that is upbeat, engaging, and motivating. Many children enjoy the active nature of exposure therapy, and, if the clinician is able to put himself into the exposure and lead by example, many children who are at first reticent to begin will come along and will be engaged in the exposure. At the same time, being able to make mistakes (even to role-model making mistakes) and to make light of them with the child helps to keep the mood light.

When a child is reluctant or refuses to engage in an exposure during a treatment session, the clinician should not be afraid to back up, admit that perhaps treatment moved too quickly up the hierarchy, and find a way to break down the task into smaller steps. This will likely defuse the situation rather than make it escalate into a contest of wills. Parents often face similar situations at home while coaching the child to complete exposure homework assignments between sessions: they come for session the next week only to report that exposures went "horribly wrong" when the child's SUDs ratings went "through the roof" and he subsequently refused to proceed. This can happen early in the process of therapy, before children have had much opportunity to gain success and confidence with exposures, when parents are first learning to become effective coaches. Parents should be coached and clinicians may want to role-model creatively finding ways in which to break down the task into smaller, easier steps. Whether these challenges occur during the session or while completing homework assignments, it is important to expect the child to make a step forward in facing her fears and not allow continued avoidance. As always, liberal positive reinforcement – both verbal praise and tangible rewards – goes a long way in motivating children to participate.

Finally, we recommend that the reluctant clinician begin to reconceptualize exposure therapy. Without intervention, many children with an anxiety disorder would otherwise be at risk for missing important developmental experiences. Exposure provides children with "developmental guidance." Through exposure, the clinician is teaching the child new ways to interact with her world and how to bravely approach the things that cause fear, thereby promoting positive character development.

References

Abramowitz, Jonathan S., Brett J. Deacon, and Stephen P. Whiteside. 2011. *Exposure Therapy for Anxiety: Principles and Practice*. New York: Guilford Press.

Addis, Michael E., and Aaron D. Krasnow. 2000. "A National Survey of Practicing Psychologists' Attitudes toward Psychotherapy Treatment Manuals." *Journal of Consulting and Clinical Psychology*, 68: 331–9. DOI 10.1037/0022-006X.68.2.331

Beidel, Deborah C., and Samuel M. Turner. 2007. *Shy Children, Phobic Adults: Nature and Treatment of Social Anxiety Disorder* (2nd ed.). Washington, DC: American Psychological Association.

Deblinger, Esther, and Anne H. Heflin. 1996. *Treating Sexually Abused Children and Their Nonoffending Parents: A Cognitive–Behavioral Approach*. Thousand Oaks, CA: Sage.

Kendall, Philip C., Erika U. Brady, and Timothy L. Verduin. 2001. "Comorbidity in Childhood Anxiety Disorders and Treatment Outcome." *Journal of the American Academy of Child and Adolescent Psychiatry*, 40: 787–94. DOI: 10.1097/00004583-200107000-00013

Kendall, Philip C., Joanna A. Robin, Kristina A. Hedtke, Cynthia Suveg, Ellen Flannery-Schroeder, and Elizabeth Gosch. 2005. "Considering CBT with Anxious Youth? Think Exposures." *Cognitive and Behavioral Practice*, 12: 136–50. DOI: S1077722905800483

In-Albon, Tina, and Silvia Schneider. 2007. "Psychotherapy of Childhood Anxiety Disorders: A Meta-Analysis." *Psychotherapy & Psychosomatics*, 76: 15–24. DOI: 10.1159/000096361

Lang, Peter J. 1967. "Fear Reduction and Fear Behavior: Problems in Treating a Construct." In John M. Shlien (Ed.), *Research in Psychotherapy* (vol. 3, pp. 332–68). Washington, DC: American Psychological Association.

March, John S., and Karen Mulle. 1998. *OCD in Children and Adolescents: A Cognitive–Behavioral Treatment Manual*. New York: Guilford Press.

Ollendick, Thomas H., Lars Ost, Lena Reuterskiold, Rio Cederlund, Cristian Sirbu, Thompson E. Davis III, Matthew A. Jarrett. 2009. "One-Session Treatment of Specific Phobias in Youth: A Randomized Clinical Trial in the United States and Sweden." *Journal of Consulting and Clinical Psychology*, 77: 504–16. DOI: 10.1037/a0015158

Pincus, Donna B., Jill T. Ehrenreich, and Sara G. Mattis. 2008. *Mastery of Anxiety and Panic for Adolescents: Riding the Wave: Therapist Guide*. New York: Oxford University Press.

Seligman, Laura D., and Thomas H. Ollendick. 2011. "Cognitive Behavioral Therapy for Anxiety Disorders in Children and Adolescents." *Psychiatric Clinics of North America*, 20: 217–38. DOI: 10.1016/j.chc.2011.01.003

Valderhaug, Robert, K. Gunnar Gotestam, and Bo Larsson. 2004. "Clinicians' Views on Management of Obsessive–Compulsive Disorders in Children and Adolescents." *Nordic Journal of Psychiatry*, 58: 125–32.

Young, Brennan J., Dustin P. Wallace, Mark Imig, Lonnie Borgerding, Amy M. Brown-Jacobsen, and Stephen P. Whiteside. 2013. "Parenting Behaviors and Childhood Anxiety: A Psychometric Investigation of the EMBU-C." Manuscript submitted for publication.

15

Changing Maladaptive Behaviors, Part 2

The Use of Behavioral Activation and Pleasant Events Scheduling with Depressed Children and Adolescents

Sandra L. Mendlowitz

Introduction

The landscape for treating depression has been slowly shifting in recent years. While the efficacy of cognitive behavioral therapy (CBT) for depression – as well as for other internalizing disorders – has long been established in both adults and children (Beck, Rush, Shaw, and Emery 1979; Bhar and Brown 2012; Deckersbach, Gershuny, and Otto, 2000; Kazdin and Weisz 1998; Lewinsohn, Rohde, and Seely 1998), behavioral activation (BA) is emerging as an effective technique that is as successful as CBT (Butler, Chapman, Forman, and Beck 2006).

While there are some clinical variations in CBT, the critical components involve cognitive restructuring, problem solving, and anxiety management techniques. Developmental considerations are almost always made, as the concept of challenging maladaptive thoughts is developmentally challenging for youth. As in the treatment for adolescent depression study (TADS) (March and Vitiello 2009), CBT interventions for youth almost always involve social skills training, behavioral strategies, and concrete examples to help the client navigate through the therapy. A component analysis of CBT for depression demonstrates that it actually involves a large behavioral activation component. The utility of the cognitive component in CBT, however, has been questioned by a number of authors (Gortner, Gollan, Jacobson, and Dobson 1998; Hollan 2001; Jacobson, et al. 1996; Longmore and Worrell 2007). One of the main reasons for this challenge is that the introduction of the cognitive components of CBT often happens later in the process, when mood symptoms have already

Evidence-Based CBT for Anxiety and Depression in Children and Adolescents: A Competencies-Based Approach, First Edition. Edited by Elizabeth S. Sburlati, Heidi J. Lyneham, Carolyn A. Schniering, and Ronald M. Rapee. © 2014 John Wiley & Sons, Ltd. Published 2014 by John Wiley & Sons, Ltd.

improved. This trend has been noted across studies (Longmore and Worrell 2007). Further evidence for the importance of behavioral activation was brought by McManus, Van Doorn, and Yiend (2012), who examined two components of CBT – thought records and behavioral experiments challenging and changing the participant's beliefs – by using a single-session model. While both methods resulted in improvement, the behavioral experiment group obtained greater gains.

One of the most compelling pieces of evidence for the use of BA for depressed youth is from the TADS team (March and Vitiello 2009; Ritschel, Ramirez, Jones, and Craighead 2011; Treatment for Adolescents with Depression Study 2007). The study involved 432 moderately to severely depressed adolescents (12 to 17 years old) who were randomized into one of four conditions (placebo, fluoxetine, CBT alone, and CBT plus fluoxetine). In the initial phase of treatment the adolescents were taught about mood monitoring, pleasant activity scheduling, identification of cognitive distortions and thought challenges; optional strategies included relaxation strategies and mood regulation (Rhode, Reeny, and Robins 2006). In the next phase of treatment the adolescents were engaged in social skills training. While the final conclusion indicated that CBT plus medication was the most efficacious, results also suggested that TADS CBT was helpful in preventing relapse. Ritschel and colleagues (2011) noted that, unlike in traditional models of CBT, here there was a significant emphasis on the behavioral components of the CBT, which underscored the unique contribution of BA.

Foundations of Behavioral Activation

From a chronological perspective, behavioral therapies (BT) have earlier roots (Pichot 1989; Wolpe and Lazarus 1966) than cognitive therapies, which emerged in the early 1970s (Curran, Ekers, and Houghton 2011; Mahoney 1977). Wolpe (1958) was the pioneer of behavioral models of therapy. His techniques were developed from models of Pavlov's classical conditioning and were primarily focused on the treatment of anxiety disorders, where Wolpe successfully introduced the concept of systematic desensitization. Lazarus (1968) utilized these concepts and applied them to the treatment of depression (Curran et al. 2011). He noted that behavior therapists largely ignored the concept of depression. He, however, conceptualized depression as arising from a stimulus–response pattern. He theorized that depression was caused either by a lack of positive reinforcements or by reinforcements that had lost their effectiveness – a view shared by other behaviorists (Lazarus 1974).

Ferster (1973) and Lewinsohn (1974) both conceptualized depression in terms of positive and negative reinforcement, and this formed the basis of what is now called BA. Specifically, the underlying assumption is that, when depressed, the individual avoids positive events and thereby will experience few rewards or positive reinforcers (Ferster 1973). This results in a downward spiral, as the individual continuously removes him-/herself from perceived aversive situations and becomes more withdrawn and isolated. Consistent with this theory, Lewinsohn (1974) further suggested that a lack of positive rewards – in other words, fewer positive social interactions, due either to behavior or to the lack of social skills (Lejuez, Hopko, LePage, Hopko, and McNeil

2001) – maintains this depressive cycle and that an infusion of positively rewarding experiences was necessary to offset the cycle. He noted that skills learning was necessary to increase engagement. Lewinsohn proposed the use of pleasant events scheduling (PES), which was critical to BA: in PES positively rewarding activities were built into an individual's weekly schedule at hourly intervals, with the goal of increasing the opportunity for rewarding experiences (Martell, Dimidjian, and Herman-Dunn 2010).

In contrast, cognitive therapists conceptualize depression as emerging from maladaptive thoughts, whereby sufferers experience a negative view of the self, the external world, and the future (Beck et al. 1979; Kazdin and Weisz 1998). Depressed individuals select out negative stimuli and therefore their memory of events is biased toward negative patterns. Cognitive therapy (CT) focuses on the modification of faulty patterns or negative bias of thinking (Shaw 1977).

CBT techniques incorporate not only components involving the thinking process, such as distortions in thought, but also components related to cognition and behavior. Key to this perspective is the link between thoughts, emotions, and behaviors. CBT techniques involve more than a systematic modification of thought patterns; namely they also involve the concept of challenging the negative thoughts through behavioral experiments (McManus et al. 2012). CBT has been associated with a rapid response, both in adults (Longmore and Worrell 2007) and in children (McManus et al. 2012). The techniques have been widely adapted to many types of mental health problems, and there is a significant number of evidence-based protocols that have been developed for both adults and children (Klein, Jacobs, and Reinecke 2007; Treatment for Adolescents with Depression Study 2007).

While all of these therapies, which differ in their tenets, have demonstrated some effectiveness with respect to outcome, none is unique, except in its method of approach. While behavioral therapies focus on the learned experience, cognitive therapies focus on the influence of thoughts. All seek change through a modification of the way one perceives the environment. Hence an understanding of each of these types of interventions will yield a greater overall understanding of BA. Figure 15.1 draws a comparison between the four therapies described above: behavior therapy, cognitive therapy, cognitive behavioral therapy, and behavioral activation.

Key Features of Competencies

Several key areas of competence are required for the successful application of BA, including a thorough understanding of the theoretical underpinnings of BA and knowledge of how to conduct a BA assessment and subsequently apply the five core treatment components. Finally, appropriate understanding and use of PES remains a critical component of this competency.

Behavioral activation, defined

Behavioral activation is a type of behavior therapy for depression that targets the level of activity through focused activation strategies (Jacobson, Martell, & Dimijian, 2001; Sturmey, 2009). The theoretical underpinnings are borrowed from behavioral

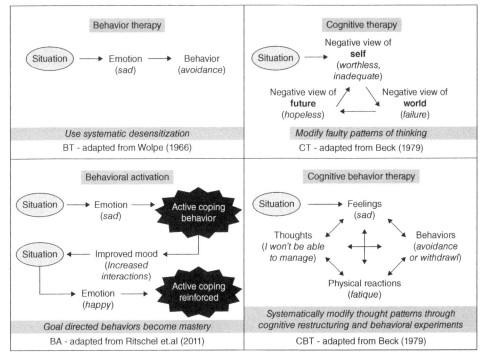

Figure 15.1   Comparison of models of depression. Adapted from Wolpe and Lazarus (1966); Beck, Rush, Shaw, and Emery (1979); and Ritschel, Ramirez, Jones, and Craighead (2011).

models of depression (Ferster 1973; Lewinsohn 1974). The general model suggests that low levels of positive experiences (rewards), coupled with high levels of negative experiences (perceived punishment), result in depressed affect. When BA is applied to depressed youth, it appears that children and adolescents experience depression because they focus on negative experiences rather than on rewarding or positive experiences. The model assumes that avoidance of activities interferes with the experience of positively reinforced situations (Kanter, Puspitasari, Santos, and Nagy 2012; McCauley, Schloredt, Gudmundsen, and Martell 2011). When positive reinforcement is blocked through avoidance and the individual's ability to experience pleasurable activities is hindered, depression can develop (Ritschel et al. 2011). Depressed individuals are more likely to attend to negative or aversive situations and to diminish their opportunities of engaging in pleasant activities that can result in positive reinforcement (Martell et al. 2010). They tend to use avoidant coping, which results in low positive reinforcement (Jacobson et al. 2001). Avoidance also limits the possible ways in which one could respond to a situation, creating additional stresses in an individual's life (Jacobson et al. 2001). Therefore the goal of BA is to help activate the person so that (s)he will be more likely to experience his/her behavior in ways that would be positively reinforcing and to re-engage in activities that (s)he once found pleasurable. This is largely accomplished through activity scheduling (Martell et al. 2010). (PES and activity scheduling are used interchangeably and will be explained below.)

Behavioral activation assessment
The process of BA assessment is one of reviewing the individual's situation and life events and his/her responses to the latter when depressed. Assessment typically involves a formal evaluation of depressive symptoms and the use of self-report questionnaires to measure mood (e.g., through an instrument like the Children's Depression Inventory: see Kovacs 1992). The use of objective measures is important, as the measurement obtained will serve as a baseline for measures of change after treatment. Less formal but imperative evaluations include: an understanding of daily activities (e.g., a daily activities list); activities currently avoided (number, intensity, patterns); any changes in activity levels (academic, family, peer-related, leisure); and immediate as well as long-term activities that the individual finds reinforcing. Assessment also includes an evaluation of potential triggers of depressive feelings, resultant behaviors, and consequences of these behaviors – both in the short and in the long term. These components are important in the development of appropriate and realistic – that is, obtainable – goals during the intervention phase.

Behavioral activation intervention
Jacobson and colleagues (1996: 297) identified five core elements of BA:

1.   monitoring daily activities and assessing the pleasure and mastery involved;
2.   assigning new daily activities to increase pleasure and mastery;
3.   imaginal rehearsal of activities before they are undertaken;
4.   problem solving any barriers to undertaking new activities;
5.   interventions to address social skills deficits such as assertiveness and communication training.

While core elements guide the principles of BA, activation is the most fundamental and important component (Antonuccio 1998; Bottonari, Roberts, Thomas, and Read 2008; Carvalho and Hopko 2011; Deckersbach et al. 2000; Gortner et al. 1998; Hollan 2001; Martell et al. 2010).

Pleasant events scheduling
Pleasant events scheduling is part of the weekly activity monitoring that is critical to successful implementation of BA. It is either a self-directed or therapist- or parent-assisted list of positive or reinforcing activities. While a validated scale has been created for adults (e.g., the pleasant events schedule: see MacPhillamy and Lewinsohn 1982), no empirically validated scale currently exists for children. Table 15.1 offers an example of a PES list.

   The schedule should include a column for the target activity, potential level of enjoyment (which can be adjusted during the course of treatment; using an intensity scale of 0–5 for young children and 0–10 for school-aged children or adolescents), previously enjoyed activities, and potentially enjoyable activities that the individual would consider a target goal. Given that individuals with depression have a bias toward negative thinking, it would not be unusual for a child or adolescent to underestimate how enjoyable an activity is; as such, using pre-post-ratings is important and will help provide evidence to challenge pessimistic attitudes (Friedberg and McClure 2002).

Table 15.1 Pleasant events list and rating.

Activity	Potential level of enjoyment 0–10	Used to enjoy	Would like to try
Playing video games	9	√	√
Reading a book	6		√
Playdate	8	√	√
Going to soccer	10	√	√
Watching football with my dad	5		√
Exercising at the gym with my friends	7		√
Going to a restaurant with my family	7	√	√
Going to the ice cream store	6	√	√
Shopping with my friends	10	√	√
Getting my homework assignments in on time	7		√
Watching my favorite TV show	7	√	√
Sitting with others at lunch	8	√	√

One method of helping a resistant child or adolescent participate in the process is to develop short-term achievable goals coupled with incentives for effort. Table 15.2 is an example of a PES log and Table 15.3 is another general type of activity log.

It is important that the person-specific pleasant events list is developed so as to be appropriate for the developmental stage and learning style of the child or adolescent (e.g., in how the target goals are set for activities, or in how information is recorded). Filling in this log should not become an onerous task for the child, since compliance is critical. It is also important that the activity should not inadvertently maintain avoidance patterns; so, for example, while reading a book may be a pleasurable activity, it has the potential to function as an escape mechanism – so this potential would need to be evaluated. Since depressed youth generally withdraw from activities, the PES is a way to assist them with engaging in rewarding experiences, increasing their level of activities, and helping to guard them against social withdrawal (Friedberg and McClure 2002).

Competence in Treating Anxiety Disorders and Depression

Below is the example of an individual case.

> Susan is a depressed and anxious 11-year-old. She stopped participating in after-school programs when her best friend changed schools. While she was quite willing to complete her anxiety-based CBT homework, she developed a strong resistance to engage in previously enjoyed sports activities, preferring to stay at home and read books. While she enjoyed reading, the activity served to isolate her from peers and to reinforce social withdrawal. A plan was developed to reintegrate Susan back into afterschool programming. Incentives were offered for completing activities and for providing pre-post ratings. Through increasing social interactions, Susan was more amenable to engaging in other activities.

Table 15.2 Pleasant events schedule (PES) and activity log for youth.[a]

ACTIVITY		DAY 1	DAY 2	DAY 3	DAY 4	DAY 5	DAY 6	DAY 7
	AM							
	AFT							
	PM							
	AM							
	AFT							
	PM							
	AM							
	AFT							
	PM							
	AM							
	AFT							
	PM							
	AM							
	AFT							
	PM							
	AM							
	AFT							
	PM							
	AM							
	AFT							
	PM							
	AM							
	AFT							
	PM							
	AM							
	AFT							
	PM							

[a]AM = morning; AFT = afternoon; PM = evening.
Rate the mood before and after the activity, on a scale of 0–10 where 0 = unhappy and 10 = very happy.
Indicate the amount of time spent in the activity: e.g., AM – mood = 5; amount of time = 20 mins.

It is important to understand that anxiety and depression tend to be comorbid disorders, especially in youth. Avoidance is a component of both anxiety and depression; although the reasons for the avoidance differ vastly in each condition, in both cases they are negatively reinforcing. In anxiety disorders, avoidance is used as a way to escape a feared situation and results in relief, thereby negatively reinforcing itself. For example, Susan is afraid that people would laugh at her speech, so she pretends she is ill and doesn't attend school. Her stomach aches disappear when

Table 15.3 General activity log for youth.

Time of day	Sunday	Monday	Tuesday	Wednesday	Thursday	Friday	Saturday
7:00	sleep	hockey practice		hockey practice	swim meet	hockey practice	sleep
7:30	sleep	hockey practice			swim meet		sleep
8:00	sleep		school	school			sleep
8:30	sleep	school	school	school	school	school	sleep
9:00	sleep	school	school	school	school	school	sleep
9:30	sleep	school	school	school	school	school	
10:00	sleep	school	school	school	school	school	
10:30		school	school	school	school	school	
11:00		school	school	school	school	school	
11:30		school	lunch	school	lunch	school	movies
12:00		lunch	lunch	lunch	lunch	lunch	movies
12:30	swim lessons	lunch	school	homework	school	lunch	movies
1:00		school	school	school	school	school	
1:30		school	school	school	school	school	sleep
2:00		school	school	school	school	school	sleep
2:30		school	school	school	school	school	guitar
3:00		school	school	school	school	school	
3:30		school		school	school		
4:00							
4:30		walk dog		homework	homework	TV	walk dog
5:00	dinner		math tutor	homework		TV	walk dog
5:30	homework		TV			PS3 with Matt	
6:00		dinner	dinner	dinner	dinner	PS3 with Matt	
6:30		homework	dinner	homework	dinner	PS3 with Matt	
7:00		homework	TV	homework	TV		dinner
7:30		homework	homework		TV		dinner
8:00			homework		homework		
8:30	guitar	guitar	guitar	sleep	guitar		guitar
9:00	homework	homework		sleep	guitar		
9:30	homework	homework		sleep			
10:00	homework			sleep			friends
10:30				sleep			friends
11:00				sleep	homework		
11:30			sleep	sleep	homework		
12:00	sleep	sleep	sleep	sleep	homework		

she is at home. In other words, when children remove themselves from fearful situations, their anxiety diminishes; hence they learn to avoid rather than face their fears. In contrast, avoidance in depression has more to do with removing an individual from the environment and its perceived difficulties. For example, Susan thinks her speech is not good and can never be as good as that of others, so there is no point in even trying to write the speech; hence she doesn't attend school, sleeps all day, but feels worse. In depression the avoidance does not result in relief, because the problems still exist; avoidance is negatively reinforced. Essentially, avoidance serves to allow the youth to maintain their depressed mood, as the avoidance leads to low mood, negativity, and loneliness.

In summary, the primary targeted behavior in both anxiety and depression is avoidance, although this behavior is manifested in very different ways in each disorder. In depression, BA targets the negatively reinforcing experience of depression by increasing the number of rewarding experiences. In anxiety, avoidance is addressed, in contrast, by confronting the feared situation.

Implementation of behavioral activation

It is important to underscore the key assumption of BA theory: depression is caused by situations (e.g., a family move, peer rejection, parental arguments); these are called "activating events." Since there is little – if any – positive reinforcement for these events, they increase one's vulnerability to depression. Avoidance develops as a way of escaping the activating events, but it is negatively reinforcing; and thus the pattern of inactivity is maintained – with its inherent fatigue, apathy, and loss of interest. PES is the approach used to increase activity levels (Jacobson et al. 2001; Lejuez et al. 2001; Martell et al. 2010). Increasing normal peer-related activities by diminishing social withdrawal is an important component of BA in youth (Friedberg and McClure 2002).

BA must be implemented in a stepwise approach in order for the client to achieve mastery. Breaking down goals (pleasant activities) into manageable steps is critical for self-reinforcement. The assignment of activities should be revised as needed, to confirm that they are achievable (Jacobson et al. 1996; Lewinsohn, Clarke, Hops, and Andrews 1990; Martell et al. 2010). If the child or the adolescent is extremely negative, motivators need to be addressed. Everyone is motivated by something; the key would be to determine what motivates that particular child. Very young children may be motivated by simple rewards (stickers, candy, etc.); teens may need other types of motivators. For example, use of electronics (amount of time and specific electronics) may be earned by engaging in agreed-upon activities.

Social skills training is an important component in the BA intervention for youth. A target goal for depressed youth frequently involves social interactions with peers. Social skills training can enhance positive peer interaction and is therefore clinically relevant. In order to bring about behavior change through a positively reinforcing activity, the youth must be viewed as responding in socially acceptable ways (Kazdin 1977). This can be problematic, as peer interactions are challenging for depressed children or adolescents. Educating youth through direct instruction, through role-play, or by problem-solving peer conflict and building in youth skills appropriate for social interaction – these two actions enhance the youth's confidence to engage in social interactions with peers (Friedberg and McClure 2002).

Competence in Treating both Children and Adolescents

Prior to the initiation of any therapy, a concise and detailed diagnostic assessment that includes self-report measures of depression is essential. In the case of youth, parental involvement in both assessment and intervention is critical. Unlike adults, youth are usually brought to treatment by their parents. While parents may not always know what their children are thinking, they are present to observe behavior and therefore can give the therapist valuable input regarding avoidant behaviors, responses to home-work, and degree of social interactions. They are also integral to the facilitation of behavioral activation; they help enhance the PES; and they provide coaching for youth, both during treatment and after its termination. The research literature has repeatedly demonstrated the profound effect that parents can have on the successful outcome of treatment (Lewinsohn et al. 1990; Mendlowitz et al. 1999; Wells and Albano 2005).

Parents play a vital role in the development of the youth's PES, especially when one is treating very young children, and they can have a profound effect on the successful outcome of treatment (Lewinsohn et al. 1990; Mendlowitz et al. 1999; Wells and Albano 2005). Parents may facilitate the recording of the information and may help create a list of pleasant activities, especially when these involve the family and play dates with peers or relatives. Depressed youth tend to express a negative bias toward unpleasant activities and need support in identifying pleasant events. These lists should be constantly revised as target goals are met. Support may be required until the youth begins to shift his/her cognitive bias toward pleasant activities. Additionally, parents may be required to facilitate activities for adolescents, for example by arranging to transport them to activities within and around the community – but also outside their local area.

Parents may also assist in the identification of social skills deficits that interfere with successful outcomes. As a welcome addition to what is achieved therapy, parents and siblings may help the depressed youth by role-playing and modeling participation in pleasant activities, so as to facilitate the learning of social skills (Hansen, MacMillan, and Shawchuck 1990). As noted, this self-monitoring task should be passed on to the youth, to help them develop independence and to instill confidence. Overall, parents can play a significant role in positive reinforcement from the provision of verbal encouragement, rewards, record keeping, and overall support.

Steps in behavioral activation with children and adolescents

The steps involved in BA therapy are: (1) understanding depression in the context of the BA model; (2) understanding activation, building a PES, developing an activity and mood log; (3) social skills and problem solving; (4) ongoing practice; (5) feedback and modification of activities; and (6) relapse prevention (Dobson et al. 2008; Lejuez et al. 2001; Martell et al. 2010; McManus et al. 2012; Ritschel et al. 2011; Trew 2011).

1. *Understanding depression in the context of the BA model* The role of avoidance in depression is not an easily understood concept. Laying the groundwork for any therapy is in itself a valuable tool for facilitating commitment and adherence

to the protocol, because the therapy is a collaborative approach between child or adolescent, parent (depending upon the age and developmental level of the youth), and therapist. Specific goals are outlined in the initial sessions. The framework of the sessions, of expectations, and of session outlines is reviewed – as well as the framework of homework expectations.

2. *Understanding activation, building a PES, and developing an activity and mood log: Providing an explanation of activity as a mediator of change* The purpose of activity – to increase energy levels, facilitate clear thinking, create opportunities for positive experiences, and provide ways to engage in situations – is discussed. Activities that both enhance and diminish mood are reviewed. Activities are planned and scheduled. PES is developed and self-monitoring techniques are illustrated. Figure 15.1, Table 15.1, Table 15.2, Table 15.3, and Figure 15.2 are examples of logs that can be utilized for both children and adolescents.

3. *Social skills and problem solving* Both social skills and problem-solving strategies facilitate positive social interactions and are important steps toward forming positive peer relationships. These relationships are critical in the maintenance of mood.

4. *Practice* Both in-session and assigned practicing of skills (i.e., in homework) are part of an ongoing process. Support, responsibility for practice, frequency, and monitoring are discussed. Practice is an opportunity to reinforce positive outcomes.

5. *Feedback and modification of activities* Communication between the therapist, the child or adolescent, and the parents is critical for overcoming any barriers in the target activities. The goal is to break negatively reinforced patterns of behavior. To achieve this, targets must be set and modified as needed, so that the target goal can be accomplished and positively reinforced.

6. *Relapse prevention* As in all therapies, prior to termination a review of triggers and effective strategies is made. Planned booster sessions are arranged.

Specific activation strategies outlined by Jacobson and colleagues (2001) are focused activation, graded task assignment, avoidance modification, routine regulation, and attention to experience. While these strategies were described for use with adults, they can also be useful in working with youth.

Given that depressed youth tend to avoid activities that may help them feel better, the process would be to identify what the youth previously enjoyed and to have them re-engage in those activities (this would be called focused activation). Such a process facilitates pleasure and breaks the cycle of negative reinforcement, because the individual achieves positive reinforcement through activity (see Figure 15.1). Working with both the youth and the parent to decide what activities would be best suited to initiate activation facilitates the process.

It is widely recognized that behavioral experiments are designed to be success-oriented. In view of this, activities should be designed to maximize success. Activities that are easy to engage in will provide positive reinforcement and will motivate the individual to eventually engage in more challenging activity steps. For youth, external rewards (e.g., parental praise, small gifts) are valuable motivators to encourage effort, especially when they feel challenged.

To explain an avoidance pattern to youth, especially young children who are experiencing depression, is not an easy task. However, this is an important concept for youth to understand as part of the mechanism of change. One method would be to define the child-specific pattern of avoidance that may be maintaining their mood. For example, the experience of being bullied at school leads to avoidance of peers, and hence to loneliness and low mood. Learning skills to cope with bullying, attending school, and participating in fun school activities will make it easier to attend school, make friends, and be happier.

> In our previous example, Susan had been the victim of bullying. When her best friend left the school, she feared her previous history of being bullied would recur. It was difficult for her to believe that she could engage in other positive peer relationships. The goal was to make her engage in activities where she could have positive peer interactions. Activities where she showed a high level of skill, coupled with social skills training, helped her to agree to participate in these activities. Once she engaged in them, the positive interactions reinforced ongoing participation, she eventually developed other peer relationships, and her mood improved.

Maintenance of routines and consistency, while an important strategy in BA, is also a healthy strategy for youth. Being able to anticipate situations is positively reinforcing to youth, because it enhances the person's capacity to reduce negative interactions.

As previously noted, depressed youth have an attentional bias to negative stimuli and, as a result, they engage in rumination that can interfere with perception of change. For example, a teen may claim that, in spite of spending time with his or her peers in the lunchroom and other places in the school, (s)he does not feel any change in his/her mood. In this scenario, the therapist would need to dismantle the situation to discover that, although the youth is present in the company of peers, (s)he continues to isolate him-/herself from peers – say, by not actively engaging in discussions. The task would then be to redesign the activity so as to include interaction with peers.

BA and CBT

While all of the aforementioned components are critical to the model of BA, there is some variation in the number of sessions and in the dissemination of the therapy. Moreover, the administration of therapy requires skill acquisition in order to be successful (Lejuez et al. 2001; Lewinsohn et al. 1990; Martell et al. 2010; Trew 2011). Although BA therapy is a very promising intervention with strong research evidence to suggest that it is effective, a closer examination of interventions (e.g., Ritschel et al. 2011) suggests that an integrated approach that includes both cognitive interventions and BA has been more successful than BA alone (Lejuez et al. 2001; Martell et al. 2010; McManus et al. 2012).

Figure 15.2 represents a model of integration of CBT and BA for children and adolescents. In Beck and colleagues' (1979) model of CBT there is a triad relationship (see Figure 15.1). These relationships are interconnected, so that changing any one of

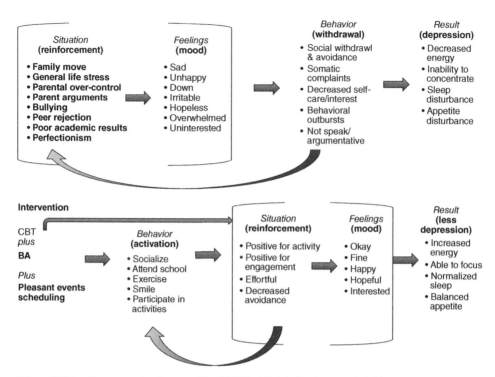

Figure 15.2 Conceptualization model of CBT with BA for depressed children and adolescents.

them changes the others. Depression develops from a set of dysfunctional or mistaken beliefs. Depression is maintained through negative views of the self, the world, and the future. In the BA model (Lewinsohn et al. 1998), depression arises from a lack of engagement in the environment (e.g., school, home) – a lack that, like in Beck's model, is also cyclical in nature. According to this model, depression can develop as a result of situational factors such as poor academic results, and is maintained through patterns of avoidance. Both CBT and BA strive to improve mood state by changing the patterns of behavior, which is facilitated through the learning of very specific skills. Through behavioral activation, the individual challenges inactivity in order to change his/her mood. Activity leads to more positive reinforcement and less depressive symptoms; an increase in positive emotions helps one shift to more helpful attitudes and beliefs (Lejuez et al. 2001), and therefore the integrated model has some useful perspectives on treating depressed youth.

Common Obstacles to Competent Practice and Methods to Overcome Them

As in any treatment intervention, the motivation for change is an important component. Finding this motivation may be difficult for the depressed child or adolescent. It has already been noted that parents play a significant role in treatment outcomes for youth. Generally speaking, the younger the children, the less autonomous they are in treatment;

therefore children require more parental involvement than adolescents – although parents do need to be involved at all stages of development.

So take a child who is depressed: how do you get him/her involved in BA, especially when (s)he may not be motivated to do anything?

1. Establish with the child or adolescent that they are following an activity plan, not an inactivity plan. This means that they will be required to follow the plan, not their mood. Any step forward is a step in the right direction. Creating small activities to initiate the start of the plan is critical.
2. Teach the parents not to engage in emotional responding. For example, when youth do not want to engage in an activity, they often resort to threatening their parents with self-harm or aggression. Parents often feel vulnerable; to activate a child who threatens self-harm or aggression or who does not feel motivated to move is counterintuitive. Parents then resort to becoming overprotective and overconcerned out of love, but they do not realize that they are enabling their child, which serves to increase the avoidant behavior. This is true for both anxiety and depression.
3. Always remember to keep steps manageable for both parents and youth. Change should always be incremental. Positively reinforcing both parents and youth for their efforts helps to motivate compliance.
4. Ask both the parent and the youth what they will achieve by engaging in the treatment. If the depressed youth responds with "nothing," work toward an understanding of potential change (benefits and lesser benefits), then help them to monitor changes in mood so that they may identify these benefits.

Conclusion

BA is an increasingly recognized treatment for depressed youth. Like in any treatment intervention, specific competencies are required in theoretical knowledge, and also an appropriate assessment and application of the technique. Graduated and developmentally sensitive approaches to treatment are necessary when adapting BA to children and adolescents. While there are obstacles involved in the use, for youth, of BA with parental involvement and proper therapist training, this represents a promising approach to treating depressive symptoms in youth.

References

Antonuccio, David O. 1998. "The Coping with Depression Course: A Behavioral Treatment for Depression." *The Clinical Psychologist*, 51: 3–5.

Beck, Aaron T., A. John Rush, Brain F. Shaw, and Gary Emery. 1979. *Cognitive Therapy of Depression*. New York: Guilford Press.

Bhar, Sunil S., and Gregory K. Brown. 2012. "Treatment of Depression and Suicide in Older Adults." *Cognitive and Behavioral Practice*, 19: 116–25.

Bottonari, Kathryn A., John E. Roberts, Sherilyn N. Thomas, and Jennifer P. Read. 2008. "Stop Thinking and Start Doing: Switching from Cognitive Therapy to Behavioral Activation in a Case of Chronic Treatment-Resistant Depression." *Cognitive and Behavioral Practice*, 15: 376–86. DOI: 10.1016/j.cbpra.2008.02.005

Butler, Andrew C., Jason E. Chapman, Evan M. Forman, and Aaron T. Beck. 2006. "The Empirical Status of Cognitve–Behavioral Therapy: A Review of Meta-Analyses." *Clinical Psychology Review*, 26: 17–31. DOI: 10.1016/j.cpr.2005.07.003

Carvalho, John P., and Derek R. Hopko. 2011. "Behavioral Theory of Depression: Reinforcement as a Mediating Variable Between Avoidance and Depression." *Journal of Behavior Therapy and Experimental Psychiatry*, 42: 154–62. DOI: 10.1016/j.jbtep.2010.10.001

Curran, Joe, David Ekers, and Simon Houghton. 2011. "Behavioral Activiation in the Treatment of Depression: Simon Houghton and Colleagues Explain How Different Forms of Behavioural Therapy Help People with Depression Cope with Their Condition." *Mental Health Practice*, 14: 18.

Deckersbach, Thilo, Beth S. Gershuny, and Michael W. Otto. 2000. "Cognitive–Behavioral Therapy for Depression: Applications and Outcome." *The Psychiatric Clinics of North America*, 23: 795–809.

Dobson, Keith S., Steven D. Hollon, Sona Dimidjian, Karen B. Schmaling, Robert J. Kohlenberg, and Robert J. Gallop. 2008. "Randomized Trial of Behavioral Activation, Cognitve Therapy, and Antidepressant Mediation in the Prevention of Relapse and Recurrence in Major Depression." *Journal of Consulting and Clinical Psychology*, 76: 468–77. DOI: 10.1037/0022-006X.76.3.468

Feldman, Greg. 2007. "Cognitive and Behavioral Therapies for Depression: Overview, New Directions, and Practical Recommendations for Dissemination." *The Psychiatric Cinics of North America*, 30: 39–50. DOI: 10.1016/j.psc.2006.12.001

Ferster, Charles B. 1973. "A Functional Analysis of Depression." *American Psychologist*, 28: 857–70.

Friedberg, Robert D., and Jessica M. McClure. 2002. *Clinical Practice of Cognitive Therapy with Children and Adolsecents: The Nuts and Bolts.* New York: Guilford Press.

Gortner, Eric T., Jackie K. Gollan, Neil S. Jacobson, and Keith S. Dobson. 1998. "Cognitive–Behavioral Treatment for Depression: Relapse Prevention." *Journal of Consulting and Clinical Psychology*, 66: 377–84.

Hansen, David J., Virginia M. MacMillan, and Carita R. Shawchuck. 1990. "Social Isolation." In Eva L. Feindler and Grace R. Kalfus (Eds.), *Adolescent Behavior Therapy Handbook* (pp. 165–90). New York: Springer.

Hollan, Steven D. 2001. "Behavioral Activation Treatment for Depression: A Commentary." *Clinical Psychology: Science and Practice*, 8: 271–4.

Jacobson, Neil S., Christopher R. Martell, and Sona Dimijian. 2001. "Behavioral Activation Treatment for Depression: Returning to Contextual Roots." *Clinical Psychology: Science and Practice*, 8: 255–70.

Jacobson, Neil S., Keith S. Dobson, Paula A. Traux, Michael E. Addis, Kelly Koerner, Jackie K. Gollan, Eric Gortner, and Stacey E. Prince. 1996. "A Component Analysis of Cognitive–Behavioral Treatment for Depression." *Journal of Consulting and Clinical Psychology*, 64: 295–304.

Kanter, Jonathan W., Ajeng J. Puspitasari, Maria M. Santos, and Gabriela A. Nagy. 2012. "Behavioral Activation: History, Evidence and Promise." *The British Journal of Psychiatry*, 200: 361–3. DOI: 10.1192/bjp.bp.111.103390

Kazdin, Allan E. 1977. "Assessing the Clinical or Applied Importance of Behavior Change Through Social Validation." *Behavior Modification*, 1: 427–52.

Kazdin, Allan E., and John R. Weisz. 1998. "Idenifying and Developing Empirically Supported Child and Adolescent Treatments. *Journal of Consulting Clinical Psychology*, 66: 19–36.

Klein, Jesse B., Rachel H. Jacobs, and Mark A. Reinecke. 2007. "Cognitive–Behavioral Therapy for Adolescent Depression: A Meta-Analytic Investigation of Changes in Effect-Size

Estimates." *Journal of the American Academy of Child and Adolescent Psychiatry*, 46: 1403–13. DOI: 10.1097/chi.0b013e3180592aaa

Kovacs, Marie. 1992. *Children's Depression Inventory*. New York: Multi-Health Systems.

Lazarus, Arnold A. 1968. "Learning Theory and the Treatment of Depression." *Behavioral Research and Therapy*, 6: 83–9.

Lazarus, Arnold A. 1974. "Multimodal Behavioral Treatment of Depression." *Behavior Therapy*, 5: 549–54.

Lejuez, Carl W., Derek R. Hopko, James P. LePage, Sandra D. Hopko, and Daniel W. McNeil. 2001. "A Brief Behavioral Activation Treatment for Depression." *Cognitive Behavioral Practice*, 8: 164–75.

Lewinsohn, Peter M. 1974. A Behavioral Approach to Depression. In Raymond J. Friedman and Martin M. Katz (Eds.), *The Psychology of Depression: Contemporary Theory and Research* (pp. 157–78). Washington, DC: Winston-Wiley.

Lewinsohn, Peter M., Paul Rohde, and John R. Seely. 1998. "Major Depressive Disorder in Older Adolescents: Prevalence, Risk Factors, and Clinical Implications." *Clinical Psychology Review*, 18: 765–94.

Lewinsohn, Peter M., Gregory M. Clarke, Hyman Hops, and John Andrews. 1990. "Cognitive–Behavioral Treatment for Depressed Adolescents." *Behavior Therapy*, 21: 385–401.

Longmore, Richard J., and Michael Worrell. 2007. "Do We Need to Challenge Thoughts in Cognitive Behavior Therapy?" *Clinical Psychology Review*, 27: 173–87. DOI: 10.1016/j.cpr.2006.08.001

MacPhillamy, Douglas J., and Peter M. Lewinsohn. 1982. "The Pleasant Events Schedule: Studies on Reliability, Validity, and Scale Intercorrelation." *Journal of Consulting and Clinical Psychology*, 50: 363–80.

Mahoney, Michael. 1977. "Reflections on the Cognitive–Learning Trend in Psychotherapy." *American Psychologist*, 32: 5–13.

March, John S., and Benedetto Vitiello. 2009. "Clinical Messages from the Treatment for Adolescents with Depression Study (TADS)." *American Journal of Psychiatry*, 166: 1118–23. DOI: 10.1176/appi.ajp.2009.08101606

Martell, Christopher R., Michael E. Addis, and Neil S. Jacobson. 2001. *Depression in Context: Strategies for Guided Action*. New York: W. W. Norton.

Martell, Christopher R., Sona Dimidjian, and Ruth Herman-Dunn. 2010. *Behavioral Activation for Depression*. New York: Guilford Press.

McCauley, Elizabeth, Kelly Schloredt, Gretchen Gudmundsen, and Christopher Martell. 2011. "Expanding Behavioral Activation to Depressed Adolescents: Lessons Learned in Treatment Development." *Cognitve and Behavioral Practice*, 18: 371–83.

McManus, Freda, Karlijn Van Doorn, and Jenny Yiend. 2012. "Examining the Effects of Thought Records and Behavioral Experiments in Instigating Belief Change." *Journal of Behavioral and Experimental Psychiatry*, 43: 540–7. DOI: 10.1016/j.jbtep.2011.07.003

Mendlowitz, Sandra L., Katharina Manassis, Susan Bradley, Donna Scapillato, Solvega Miezitis, and Brian F. Shaw. 1999. "Cognitive–Behavioral Group Treatments in Childhood Anxiety Disorders: The Role of Parental Involvement." *Journal of the American Academy of Child and Adolescent Psychiatry*, 38: 1223–9.

Pichot, Pierre. 1989. "The Historical Roots of Behavior Therapy." *Journal of Behavior Therapy and Experimental Psychiatry*, 20: 107–14.

Rhode, Paul, Norah C. Reeny, and Michele Robins. 2006. "Characteristics and Components of the TADS CBT Approach." *Cognitive Behavioral Practice*, 12: 186–97. DOI: 10.1901/jaba.2005.12-186

Ritschel, Lorie A., Cynthia L. Ramirez, Meredith Jones, and W. Edward Craighead. 2011. "Behavioral Activation for Depressed Teens: A Pilot Study." *Cognitive and Behavioral Practice*, 18: 281–99. DOI: 10.1016/j.cbpra.2010.07.002

Shaw, Brian F. 1977. "Comparison of Cognitive Therapy and Behavior Therapy in the Treatment of Depression." *Journal of Consulting and Clinical Psychology*, 45 (4): 543–51.

Sturmey, Peter. 2009. "Behavioral Activation is an Evidence-Based Treatment for Depression." *Behavior Modification*, 33: 818–29. DOI: 10.1177/0145445509350094

The Treatment for Adolescents with Depression Study (TADS). 2007. "Long-Term Effectiveness and Safety Outcomes." *Archives of General Psychiatry*, 64: 1132–4.

Trew, Jennifer. 2011. "Exploring the Roles of Approach and Avoidance in Depression: An Integrative Model." *Clinical Psychology Review*, 31: 1156–68. DOI: 10.1016/j.cpr.2011.07.007

Wells, Karen C., and Anne Marie Albano. 2005. "Parent Involvement in CBT Treatment of Adolescent Depression: Experiences in the Treatment for Adolescents with Depression Study (TADS)." *Cognitive and Behavioral Practice*, 12: 209–20. DOI: 10.1016/S1077-7229(05)80026-4

Wolpe, Joseph (1958). *Psychotherapy by Reciprocal Inhibition*. Stanford, CA: Stanford University Press.

Wolpe, Joseph, and Alan Lazarus. 1966. *Behavior Therapy Techniques: A Guide to the Treatment of Neuroses*. New York: Pergamon Press.

Further Reading

Clark, David A. 1995. "Perceived Limitations of Standard Cognitive Therapy: A Reconsideration of Efforts to Revise Beck's Theory and Therapy." *Journal of Cognitive Psychotherapy*, 9: 153–72.

Lewinsohn, Peter M., Richard F. Munoz, Mary Anne Youngren, and Antonette M. Zweiss. 1986. *Control Your Depression*. New York: Prentice Hall.

Miller, Lynn, Michael A. Southam-Gerow, and Robert B. Allin. 2008. "Who Stays in Treament? Child and Family Predictors of Youth Client Retention in a Public Mental Helath Agency." *Child and Youth Care Forum*, 37: 153–70.

Stark, Kevin. 1990. *Childhood Depression: School-Based Intervention*. New York: Guildford Press.

Wallis, Alison, Scott Milan, and Stephen Allison. 2012. "Behavioral Activation for the Treatment of Rural Adolescents with Depression." *The Austrialian Journal of Rural Health*, 20: 95–6. DOI: 10.1111/j.1440-1584.2012.01261.x

Watson, John B., and Rosalie Rayner. 1920. "Conditioned Emotional Reactions." *Journal of Experimental Psychology*, 3: 1–14.

Wierzbicki, Michael, and G. Perkarik.1993. "A Meta-Analysis of Psychotherapy Dropout." *Professional Psychology: Research and Practice*, 24: 190–5.

16

Managing Maladaptive Mood and Arousal

Donna B. Pincus, Ryan J. Madigan,
Caroline E. Kerns, Christina Hardway,
and Jonathan S. Comer

Introduction

Effective regulation of maladaptive mood and arousal is considered an essential skill for enhancing youth's resilience and fostering healthy developmental and mental health outcomes (Ciccetti, Ackerman, and Izard 1995; Eisenberg, Fabes, and Guthrie 1997). Learning to identify and regulate negative mood states is a critical skill for youth to develop in order to successfully navigate everyday, developmentally appropriate activities (Compas 1987). Youth with anxiety and depression often show difficulties with managing their maladaptive mood and arousal; thus it is not surprising that empirically supported treatments for internalizing disorders in youth focus largely on helping the youth to develop these skills (Suveg and Zeman 2004). As shown in Sburlati, Schniering, Lyneham and Rapee (2011), there are several empirically supported cognitive behavioral therapy (CBT) skills that specifically target children's and adolescents' maladaptive mood and arousal: (i) emotion identification, expression, and regulation; (ii) progressive muscle relaxation (PMR); (iii) applied tension; and (iv) breathing re-training. These techniques are included in numerous empirically supported treatment (EST) manuals for anxiety and depression in youth (Ollendick and King 2004). Any effective training of clinicians who will be implementing CBT with children and adolescents with internalizing disorders should incorporate specific training in the implementation of skills for managing maladaptive mood and arousal. In the present chapter each of these evidence-based skills for managing maladaptive mood and arousal are described one by one. For each skill, we describe key features of how a therapist would implement it competently, we address how it would be incorporated into anxiety and depression treatments, we make recommendations for developmentally appropriate adaptations, and we discuss how therapists can overcome common obstacles to its effective implementation.

Evidence-Based CBT for Anxiety and Depression in Children and Adolescents: A Competencies-Based Approach, First Edition. Edited by Elizabeth S. Sburlati, Heidi J. Lyneham, Carolyn A. Schniering, and Ronald M. Rapee. © 2014 John Wiley & Sons, Ltd. Published 2014 by John Wiley & Sons, Ltd.

Emotion Identification, Expression, and Regulation

Overview

Youth with internalizing disorders often exhibit difficulties identifying, expressing, and regulating their emotions. These difficulties may reflect developmentally appropriate cognitive and emotional limitations, as well as underlying deficits specific to the etiology of anxiety and depression. Building skill sets to deal with such difficulties constitutes an important developmental task for youth without psychopathology and is a critical part of CBT for youth with internalizing disorders. In consequence, competent CBT practice for youth internalizing disorders requires that therapists teach youth to identify, understand, accept, and express a variety of different emotions, as well as to monitor escalating negative emotions and subsequently engage in activities to regulate intense negative emotions (Sburlati et al. 2011). Not only are these skills themselves important components of CBT, but proficiency in these areas provides a foundation for additional CBT coping strategies such as cognitive restructuring, mood monitoring, developing trauma narratives, engaging in exposures, and so on. Therefore it is imperative that therapists are able to scaffold these skills, so that difficulties in processing and regulating emotions will not adversely affect skill acquisition and treatment engagement.

Emotion identification, expression, and regulation techniques are typically included in EST manuals for anxiety disorders in general (Kendall and Hedke 2006; Rapee et al. 2006); for panic disorder (Pincus, Ehrenreich, and Mattis 2008) and post-traumatic stress disorder (Cohen, Mannarino, and Deblinger 2006) in particular; and for major depressive disorder, too (Brent and Poling 1997; Lewinsohn, Clarke, Hops, and Andrews 1990; Curry et al. 2005). Session structures vary across manuals but typically involve a combination of individual (youth or parent alone) and family (youth and parent together) involvement, depending on developmental level, the nature of a youth's relationship with parents, and the stage of treatment. Parent involvement promotes parent emotion regulation skills, emotion regulation modeling, and parents' providing youth with supportive coaching. In addition, ESTs target emotion identification, expression, and regulation training through a combination of targeted treatment modules (see, e.g., "Identifying Anxious Feelings," in Kendall and Hedke 2006) and informal components of related treatment modules (for instance, emotion identification and expression may begin during early rapport building, as identified in Brent and Poling 1997; Cohen et al. 2006). Therapists who are less familiar with CBT may overlook these skill areas or may address them inadequately, either due to gaps in their knowledge of behavioral theory or as a result of their relying inflexibly on a particular treatment manual. Even seasoned therapists who typically address these areas might benefit from understanding additional ways to teach clients in greater depth emotion identification, expression, and regulation skills. Hence therapists must consider the specific techniques involved as well as the underlying principles of cognitive and emotional development (see Chapter 5), the nature of anxiety and depressive disorders, and the specific theoretical rationale for emotion identification, expression, and regulation skills (see Chapter 8 for the theoretical knowledge of anxiety and depressive disorders).

Key features of therapist competencies in emotion identification, expression, and regulation training

Training in *emotion identification and expression* teaches youth to understand the nature of emotions, identify signs or symptoms of specific ones, differentiate between them, and assess and rate the intensity of their own emotional experiences. *Emotion regulation* involves teaching youth to monitor the intensity of their emotions and subsequently engage in activities to moderate their emotions and behavior. Training methods include assessing youths' current abilities, didactic instruction via psycho-education, discussions, role-plays, games, modeling, therapist-directed coaching activities, contingency management, and homework assignments.

Emotion identification training begins during the assessment process, as youth start answering in-person interview and self-report questions regarding their presenting symptoms. Even at this early stage, therapists should attend to youths' familiarity and comfort with talking about their emotions. While some youth may have insight into, and feel comfortable reporting, their emotions, most – particularly when they are anxious or depressed – experience some difficulty discussing these symptoms. Conducting informal functional analyses can highlight whether these difficulties are due to underlying performance deficits or to skill deficits – categories that are described below.

Performance deficits may include underreporting due to lack of trust or experiential avoidance. Intense emotional arousal can impair youth's ability to process and express their emotions (for many youth, this arousal can be triggered by simply thinking or talking about their emotions). A therapist can identify when a performance deficit is present by looking at whether there is a discrepancy between the child's or adolescent's self-report (on a self-report measure) and his/her endorsement of symptoms in the clinical interview, where the youth is forthcoming on self-report measures but would underreport or become emotionally dysregulated. Under these circumstances, rapport building or therapist-guided distress tolerance activities may be necessary (e.g., the therapist facilitates distress tolerance by directing the youth to focus on neutral or emotion-incompatible activities). Skill deficits may include underlying cognitive or language difficulties that impair the processing and expression of one's emotional experiences. It can be helpful to compare how well youth report on other areas of their lives in order to form a baseline of cognitive or language functioning. When available, neuropsychological evaluations should be used to inform these treatment factors as well.

To assist in emotion identification training, therapists and youth should collaborate to identify which emotions the youth are already familiar with. This can be done through games or friendly competitions in which the youth are encouraged to identify as many emotions as possible in a few minutes. Therapists should then provide youth and caregivers with a rationale and background information about the nature of emotions, including the adaptive function of primary emotions (happiness, sadness, anger, fear). This helps to validate and normalize a client's emotional experience. It can often be helpful to describe emotions as "signals" analogous to a seatbelt alarm or a low battery light on an electronic device (e.g., "low-battery light signals the need to charge batteries, fear signals a danger, anger signals that something is unfair, happiness signals a desire to do something again, and sadness signals a need for help or a loss"). Incorporating the notion of "signals" helps youth to begin developing the language needed to understand and express their emotional experiences (e.g., I am angry because it feels unfair that you are making me go to school") (Madigan and Kurtz 2013). Once youth appear to grasp the adaptive functions of emotions, the discussion should incorporate the role of "false alarms" or maladaptive cognitions, emotions, and behaviors (the three-component-model of CBT). For example, youth could be taught to view their cognitions as triggers that send off a "false alarm" to our brains to make our bodies feel fearful physical sensations. In turn, these physical sensations can trigger us to feel alarmed and thus to avoid situations that are actually not dangerous or threatening. It is critical to teach youth the ways in which avoidance can only "re-ignite" the cycle, as the maladaptive thoughts get reinforced. Thus the "thoughts–feelings–behavior" components of CBT can be broken down for youth. It is typically helpful for the therapist to ask the child or adolescent to think of a maladaptive cognition that (s)he commonly has, and then for the therapist and client to actually draw out the three-component model by using blank circles that depict the cycle. In this way the three-component-model can be tailored to each client's situation.

Another core skill is identifying the physiological symptoms or sensations associated with specific emotions (e.g., "When I feel nervous my heart beats faster, my hands get sweaty, and I get the 'butterflies' in my stomach"). Developmentally appropriate explanations about the function of each symptom or sensation help to normalize clients' physiological sensations and can begin to correct related cognitive distortions. This is particularly important for youth with panic disorder or generalized anxiety disorder, who often experience a significant number of anxiety-related somatic symptoms. In depression, it may be helpful to identify sensations such as feeling "heavy," "weighed down," "numb" or "low energy." Using drawing or coloring activities, youth can identify which parts of their body are affected when they are feeling anxious or depressed (e.g., by using a blank outline of a person's body, the child can then draw a butterfly in the stomach, color in the lungs and heart, and so on).

Therapists must also be competent in teaching youth to differentiate between emotions. This can be done through "blending" activities in which secondary emotions are characterized by having components of the primary emotions. Younger clients may benefit from assigning colors to represent each primary emotion (e.g., happiness, sadness, anger, and fear), then "blending" colors to form more complex colors and emotions (e.g., mixing the feelings of nervous-blue with mad-red may form the secondary emotions of irritable or annoyed-purple; mixing the primary feelings of sadness and fear might form the secondary emotion of embarrassment). This scaffolding technique can also be implemented through activities such as making an "emotion soup" and a "feelings pizza" to represent and distinguish between primary and secondary emotions that may be occurring in the present or that have occurred in the past.

Emotional expression involves teaching youth to express what, why, and how intensely they are experiencing a specific emotion. To begin, therapists should teach youth to conduct behavioral chain analyses. This can be taught through interactive discussion, written activities, and role-play, or more concretely through interactive activities such as "matching" or making "emotion trains." For example, therapists should encourage youth to draw connections between situations, emotions, "signals," and behaviors (Madigan and Kurtz 2013). "Matching" activities can aid in this process by drawing two-step connections between situations and emotions to help children understand the kinds of situations that can lead to different emotions. "Detective" activities can be a fun and engaging way to begin teaching more complex behavioral chain analyses by filling in the gaps to hypothetical or client-specific examples. This can be particularly helpful for youth who experience difficulty identifying early symptoms of emotions and for youth whose internalized emotions may be masked by externalized emotions (e.g., reported anger at parents for making them go to school may be masking an underlying anxiety). By playing "detective" and working backwards from behaviors that occur at the end of a chain (these are often much easier for youth to identify), youth learn to recognize the key antecedent thoughts and emotions that led to the identified behavior. This skill will help youth identify emotional escalations leading to episodes of emotion dysregulation; and, if they can identify and intervene on the nervous, embarrassed, or sad thoughts and feelings, secondary outbursts of anger or panic may be more easily prevented.

For example, a sample conversation might look like this:

THERAPIST: We don't know what you were feeling or what happened to make you feel bad, but we do have some good evidence to use as detectives – you yelled at your parents and slammed the door. This behavior will go at the end of the train. What emotion(s) do these behaviors sound like they are coming from?

YOUTH: I don't know.

THERAPIST: Do people usually slam doors when they are feeling happy, mad, or nervous?

YOUTH: I don't know, mad or nervous?

THERAPIST: That sounds like a good guess to me. So, if feeling nervous signals something is dangerous and anger signals something is unfair, do you think your parents seemed dangerous or unfair in that moment?

YOUTH: Unfair, they are always unfair.

THERAPIST: Ok, so if something felt unfair it looks like you may have been feeling angry. This car will be anger.

THERAPIST: What felt unfair to you?

YOUTH: That my parents are always making me go to school which I hate because everyone laughs at me.

THERAPIST: So it sounds like school can make you feel nervous and your parents want you to go anyway? [*youth nods*] So, the first car on the train is the thought, "It's unfair that they are making me go someplace where I will be nervous and people will laugh at me?"

YOUTH: Yeah, they make me do that stuff all the time!

THERAPIST: Great detective work. So we figured out the cause of your yelling and slamming the door. The first car on the train was your thinking that your parents are being unfair for telling you to do something that makes you nervous. The second car is the emotion of anger or frustration. And the last car was yelling and slamming the door.

At this point the therapist may choose to continue "playing detective" and develop another "emotion train," sequencing the youth's preceding feelings of anxiety and embarrassment. The two trains or chains can then be linked together to form a larger behavioral chain. In either case, the therapist can help the youth use coping strategies to intervene or "break the train."

To improve emotion expression and ultimately emotion regulation, therapists must teach youth to rate and monitor the intensity of their emotions, so they can then take action to regulate these emotions before they are overwhelmed by them. To train youth to monitor the intensity of emotions, therapists should orient them to a developmentally appropriate rating scale (e.g., 0–10 scale, feelings thermometer, emotion-faces scale, etc.). Therapists and youth should collaborate to develop situation- and symptom-specific anchors at each level on the scale. Youths' prior behavioral and emotional difficulties should be anchored on the scale to highlight likely triggers of future emotion dysregulation. Symptom-specific anchors should also be assessed, in order to encourage youth to identify warning signs that they may become overwhelmed.

Emotion regulation strategies are designed to facilitate affective control to the degree required for the person to remain in control, have the use of other coping skills (Brent and Poling 1997), and be able to encode and comprehend new material during stressful treatment activities. Many CBT interventions designed to improve youth's overall ability to regulate their emotions and, ultimately, their symptoms of anxiety and depression require these youth to learn how to focus on, and tolerate, difficult emotions (e.g., through imaginal or situational exposure). However, it may also be necessary to teach youth to regulate their distress during acute moments of dysregulation, particularly early in the treatment (sometimes this is referred to as a "distress tolerance" skill) (Miller, Rathus, and Linehan 2007). These strategies are designed to divert the client's attention away from upsetting content and feelings by refocusing it on neutral or emotion-incompatible content. Youth should be encouraged to utilize these strategies when their emotions are either too intense to manage (e.g., they become too overwhelmed to cope adaptively) or when it is more appropriate for them to focus on their current environment (e.g., listening in math class, spending time with friends, trying to fall asleep). Many youth who come for treatment have become reliant on ineffective or maladaptive strategies for the regulation of their emotions. Given this, therapist-guided distress tolerance activities may be required to facilitate youths' emotion regulation while they learn to regulate them independently.

To assist emotion regulation training, therapists must provide a rationale for why and when it may be necessary to redirect their clients' attention to neutral or emotion-incompatible activities. This idea can be presented through a mental exercise analogy, where youth compare success in avoiding "thinking about a pink elephant" by "trying to stop thinking about it" with focusing on or engaging in another task. Activities designed to help youth regulate their emotions include maintaining a present focus (i.e., mindfulness) and distraction techniques (i.e., distress tolerance). These activities should be individualized to youth's abilities and common triggers. Therapists should start by identifying adaptive coping strategies already in place (e.g., playing video games or listening to music when upset). When emotions are particularly intense and difficult for youth to cope with, therapists should utilize activities that are more physical (e.g., going for a walk or jog, doing pushups, taking a shower). Cognitive strategies are also important, as they are more readily generalizable to a variety of contexts. Thought interruption and positive imagery can be taught to youth who are developmentally able to identify negative thoughts and subsequently refocus their attention to positive or incompatible coping thoughts and images (see Chapter 13 for a full coverage of these cognitive strategies). Activities designed to elicit incompatible emotions are also quite useful (e.g., watching a funny movie or you tube video, listening to pleasurable music, reciting one's favorite music lyrics or movie scenes).

Present-focused thinking (also known as a "grounding technique") involves refocusing a client's attention to what is going on around him/her at a specific moment. Depending on youth's comfort and stage of treatment, it may be counter-indicated to focus on certain trauma-related environmental stimuli. Cultivating present-focused thinking as a distress tolerance activity involves teaching youth to "scan their senses" (e.g., by asking themselves what they see, hear, feel, smell, and taste). As youth master present-focused thinking, therapists can begin directing them to focus on their thoughts and emotions. This will support subsequent cognitive restructuring (described in Chapter 12) and exposure tasks (described in Chapter 14) by enhancing youth's ability to focus more effectively on their negative cognitions and emotions, respectively. Therapists should continue to utilize these strategies until youth are reliably able to identify and regulate their emotions and tolerate exposure tasks.

Competence in treating anxiety disorders and depression

When working with depressed youth, emotion identification strategies should be woven into mood and activity monitoring. Clients can record daily "levels" of various emotions they experience, such as anxiety or sadness, by using a "feelings thermom-eter," which is a visual scale that depicts "amounts" of emotion on a graded scale from 0 to 8, for example, or on any other visual scale. As a homework assignment in both depression and anxiety treatments, clients are asked to record information about the daily fluctuations in their mood, as part of a weekly record of anxiety and depression. This weekly record is a chart that provides ample space for the client to specify the level of anxiety, anger, or sadness that they experienced each day of the week. Youth can then bring this mood-monitoring homework form to session, and therapists can utilize these data to gain important information on their clients' ability to identify and monitor the levels of emotion they experience. The emotion-monitoring form can also be used as a springboard for discussion, between the client and therapist, about the former's week, and can be utilized throughout therapy to assess whether the CBT techniques the client is learning result in an improvement of mood. Emotion identification training with depressed youth should also target somatic complaints specific to depression, which may vary considerably from those of anxiety.

When treating youth with panic disorder, it will be particularly important to ensure the that the client firmly understands the adaptive function of each physiological symptom of anxiety, as cognitive distortions around these symptoms (e.g., "my heart beating faster means I'm having a heart attack") often exacerbate and/or maintain panic-related symptoms. Youth with depression, trauma, and anxiety disorders will especially benefit from learning to track and regulate emotions, as gaining a sense of mastery over their emotions may enhance their compliance and motivation to engage in later exposure activities.

Emotion regulation skills can be tailored to children with anxiety specifically by talking about how emotions such as anxiety are natural, necessary, and harmless, and are experienced by everyone, across cultures. The therapist can discuss with the client ways in which anxiety can be helpful (e.g., in athletes performing in a competition, or in getting off the road if a car is approaching). The therapist might say: "So sometimes anxiety can be good and helpful because it protects you from danger, but sometimes anxiety is not helpful – when there is no real danger."

Competence in treating both children and adolescents

Teaching emotion identification, expression, and regulation to young children may require a more concrete approach than teaching these things to older children or adolescents. Young children may only be able to identify and comprehend a few basic emotional experiences (e.g., good–bad, happy, upset, scared, and the like). Therapists can help the young child find in magazines pictures of people who are experiencing certain types of emotions (e.g., happy people, sad people) in order to facilitate their acquisition of a feelings vocabulary. Therapists can also guide young children in making feelings identification cards that show pictures of children experiencing emotions. They can then help young children generate examples of situations where the child felt sad, angry, anxious, and so on. After young children learn to identify the basic emotions, therapists can work to teach them the concept of having control over changing one's emotions and the notion that emotional states can change – for example, "I was sad that someone broke my art project but then I felt happy when I realized that my friend wanted to help me make another one." In many cases, a child's development may call for a parent-based treatment approach. That is, elements of CBT may be too complex for young children to grasp, and therefore they may need to be implemented through therapist and parent coaching and contingency management (rewards). Parent coaching statements and rewards will become the proxy for implementing coping strategies and exposure activities (e.g., "It's time to use your brave thoughts to boss back anxiety and earn a reward for being brave"). Young children will likely benefit from concrete activities such as role-play, drawing, and playing games.

Many of the aforementioned strategies would be too concrete or developmentally inappropriate to use with older children or adolescents. Thus older children and adolescents might appreciate the use of analogies that help them understand the basis of emotions – for example a comparison of anxiety with an overly alert "watchdog," which is looking out for danger and whose job is to keep you safe, as described in Pincus and colleagues' (2008) manual for panic disorder treatment for adolescents. Nevertheless, many adolescents have never developed adaptive, healthy skills for managing emotions, and this may then lead to maladaptive coping strategies such as substance use or avoidant behaviors. Thus therapists should incorporate emotion education in a developmentally appropriate way into treatments for youth of all ages.

Common obstacles to competent practice and methods to overcome them

Unlike many adults, youth coming for treatment are not necessarily motivated for it and may be brought in by caregivers against their will. This often creates a level of resistance that must be addressed before treatment is possible. In some cases, youth are so distressed by talking and thinking about their emotions that they become too dysregulated to engage in certain treatment activities. Emotion regulation activities may first need to be facilitated largely by the therapist and caregivers. That is, rather than asking a client to perform a certain emotion regulation skill on his/her own (e.g., by saying "This might be a good time to use some positive imagery"), the therapist or caregiver may need to create a distraction for them (e.g., begin talking about something else, go for a walk with the client, give the client something to hold in his/her hands, or pull up a funny video to watch it together with the client).

Underlying skill deficits may also impede the client's ability to comprehend or master specific emotion identification, expression, and regulation strategies (e.g., a youth with receptive or expressive language disorders will need to have information presented differently). This may require the therapist to utilize graphic organizers or prompts (e.g., keeping an index card in his/her pocket, or having the parents present coping strategies through visuals or social stories). Whenever possible and acceptable, scaffolding skills through technology – smart phones, tablets, or computers – can help provide support and prompting; thus mood-tracking applications or programs could prompt the youth to engage in mood monitoring, in thought or emotion tracking, or in certain coping strategies when needed.

One common error therapists make is to teach emotion identification and expression insufficiently before they move on to other coping strategies. Some protocols call for therapists to spend one or two sessions addressing these skills. This should be done initially, or in conjunction with other coping strategies, until the client is able to accurately identify and discuss a variety of emotions, in session as well as in context (Cohen et al. 2006). Therapists must also be able to comfortably augment emotion regulation activities until youth are able to regulate their emotions independently. This requires that therapists have a firm understanding of the nature of emotions and emotion regulation and are able to pull emotion-regulation activities from their therapist "tool boxes." Additionally, youth with intense negative emotions often exhibit frustration, anger, and disruptive behaviors as a means of avoiding aversive stimuli. When these difficulties would otherwise prohibit treatment as usual, therapists must first address the problem behaviors and the masking emotions (often anger is masking underlying anxiety and/or depression).

Contingency management strategies or "behavior contracts" can be utilized in collaboration with youth and their caretakers, in order to replace the maladaptive strategies that should be avoided (say, aggression) with more adaptive strategies, which can be approached gradually ("I feel too scared to do it and need to take a break or do an easier task on the exposure hierarchy"). As this process will temporarily reinforce avoidance, it should only be used in cases where the client would otherwise avoid the situation completely, through maladaptive behaviors. It may also be necessary to utilize a response cost, where the youth receive tangible positive reinforcement for adaptive behaviors and lose privileges for operationalized maladaptive behaviors. When working with adolescents, it can be useful to set limits by using software and thus avoid unneeded physical conflict (e.g., turn the internet off or limit smart phone features by using "parental controls" rather than physically remove the video game console from an adolescent's bedroom).

Progressive Muscle Relaxation

Overview

Progressive muscle relaxation (PMR) is aimed at reducing muscle tension in clients and has been used in a variety of CBT interventions for the reduction of symptoms of anxiety and/or depression. Research suggests that PMR is an effective treatment for a variety of emotional and health-related problems in both adult and younger populations (Carlson and Hoyle 1993). Among younger children, PMR is one of several effective techniques for helping them calm themselves in the moment (Lohaus and Klein-Heßling 2003). Within the context of school, group instruction of PMR has been shown to reduce the aggression levels among elementary school students who were identified as suffering from emotional or behavioral disorders (Lopata 2003). PMR has been found to help adolescents suffering from depression and other stress-related emotional problems (Reynolds and Coats 1986). In this study, a 10-session treatment protocol was successfully implemented to help moderately depressed adolescents reduce their levels of depression to nonclinical levels. PMR has been used successfully to treat symptoms of asthma among female adolescents (Nickel, Kettler et al. 2005) and levels of anger among stressed male adolescents (Nickel, Lahmann et al. 2005). It is also considered an empirically supported treatment for helping children and adolescents cope with the anxiety and pain associated with painful medical procedures (Jay, Elliott, Katz, and Siegel 1987; Powers 1999). Thus PMR is very much a transdiagnostic skill, in that it has been shown to have utility in treatments that cut across various diagnostic categories. Therapists treating youth with anxiety, depression, or post-traumatic stress disorder might use PMR as one component of treatment.

Key features of therapist competency in conducting progressive muscle relaxation

To conduct progressive muscle relaxation with children and adolescents, the therapist should begin by telling the client that it is important to learn the difference between the way our body feels when it is tense and when it is relaxed. Explain to the client that having tense muscles can sometimes cue our brains that there is something to be afraid or worried about. Having awareness about the level of tension in our muscles and the ability to reduce tension can present many mental health benefits and can bring about feelings of contentment and confidence. Prior to conducing PMR, it is important to assess the client's level of relaxation on a 0–10 scale, for example (0 = very tense; 10 = very relaxed) in order to be able to better assess the success of the procedure. Explain to the client that, to begin this exercise, he or she should start to breathe in and out, focusing on the breath as it hits the back of the throat. Therapists can begin by teaching the breathing re-training exercises that are covered in this chapter, to help the client begin to relax. The overall purpose of this progressive muscle relaxation exercise – reduction of muscle tension – should also be explained. Therapists should let the client know that they will be leading him/her through a series of exercises that they will demonstrate in front of the client.

The exercises involve tensing and relaxing major muscle groups throughout the body with the aim of producing an overall state of bodily relaxation.

The therapist should tailor the PMR treatment to the developmental level and age of the client (see the section on competence in treating both children and adolescents in this chapter). First, ask the client to think of a place that feels most relaxing to him/ her (common responses are "my room," "the couch in my living room," or "on the beach"). The therapist should use this relaxing place as a starting point for beginning PMR. Ask the client to imagine being in his/her most relaxing place as (s)he takes deep, slow breaths. Therapists can add an imagery component by suggesting that the client think of the sounds and smells (s)he is experiencing while being, in his/her mind, in that relaxing place. As the therapist evokes this imagery, the client should be breathing slowly and sitting in a comfortable position. The therapist can state: "I am going to count from 10 to 1, and each time I count a number I want you to let yourself simply take deep breaths, in and out, while allowing yourself to become more and more relaxed; and when I get to 1, I want you to imagine that you are now in the place that is most relaxing and peaceful to you." Once the client appears to be relaxed, let him/her know that you are now ready to tense or relax muscle groups.

The first muscle group to be tensed is the hands. Ask the client to make fists with each hand and to squeeze each fist tightly, as if squeezing something in his/her hand. Therapists should say out loud: "Hold the tension in your hand for the count of three ... 1, 2, 3 ... feel the tension in your hands ... and release your fists/relax your hands." Ask the client to notice the difference between being tense and being relaxed. The therapist should wait approximately 15 seconds, then have the client repeat that exercise (tensing the fists) using a similar procedure as in the first trial. This exercise should be repeated altogether three times; this gives the client a chance to really experience and notice how (s)he can achieve a state of relaxation in his/her hands by tensing and holding the tension in the hands for at least three seconds, and then by relaxing the hands. Therapists who are implementing PMR should then proceed through the rest of the muscle groups using a similar tensing and holding, then letting go and relaxing procedure, allowing three trials per major muscle group. After the hands, the therapist can lead the client into tensing and relaxing the shoulders (by lifting the shoulders to the ears and then down again), the face (by tensing up the whole face and then letting go of the tension), the legs (by lifting each leg up, holding the tension, then relaxing), the arms (by holding the arms in front, tensing for three seconds, then relaxing). It is not necessary for therapists to rigidly adhere to one particular order for tensing and relaxing each muscle group; however, it is important to make sure you go through each muscle group with the client. Between muscle groups, the therapist should continue to refocus the client on his/her breathing.

In order to competently implement this procedure, therapists should speak in a calm, relaxing voice while they help the client learn PMR. Once the therapist has gone through all the major muscle groups with the client, (s)he should have the client try to tense his/her entire body for three seconds, then let go of the tension and relax. The client should appear to be extremely relaxed after learning this skill. To end the procedure, therapists should then let the client know that they will count from 10 to 1 and that, with each number, the client should take deep breaths and should allow him-/herself to become gradually more awake and open his/her eyes. When the client opens his/her eyes, the therapist should again assess his/her level of relaxation on a 0–10 scale (0 = very tense; 10 = very relaxed). At the end of the procedure, the therapist should check in with the client about his or her reaction to conducting PMR and use the suggestions listed in the "common obstacles" section to troubleshoot any important issues.

Competence in treating the anxiety disorders and depression

PMR can be utilized in treatments for both anxiety and depression in children. Given that both anxiety and depression can result in the disruption of children's healthy sleep patterns, PMR can assist both depressed and anxious clients with falling asleep at night. For children with generalized anxiety disorder or other anxiety disorders, relaxation strategies can help putting their minds and bodies at ease, to aid the process of going to sleep. For children with depression or anxiety, learning a concrete skill such as PMR can provide improved feelings of self-efficacy, increased control and awareness of one's body, and a tool for coping with stress. It is helpful to gauge clients' moods before and after PMR practice. Anxious clients often report that their moods improve when they become more relaxed. For clients with depression, therapists are typically trying to use behavioral activation strategies to help them become more engaged in their environment.

Competence in treating both children and adolescents

When one is treating young, preschool through school-aged children, it can be helpful to utilize more imagery while teaching them to progressively tense and relax their muscle groups. For example, instead of simply asking a child to tense his/her fists, the therapist could ask the child to imagine him-/herself squeezing lemons in each fist, to make a tall glass of lemonade. This use of imagery could help young children become more engaged in PMR. Similarly, when teaching a child to tense, then relax his/her neck muscles, the therapist could have the child imagine that (s)he is a turtle who first hides in his/her shell (bringing shoulders to the ears), then sticks his/her head out of the shell (shoulders drop). Total bodily tension can be taught by having children imagine that they are a strong tree, blowing in the wind, and in order to stay intact in the wind they have to tense up all of the branches (that is, all of their limbs) (Pincus 2012; Pincus and Otis 2001). For older children and adolescents, imagery can still be helpful; however, it should be developmentally appropriate, if they are to feel engaged in the procedure. Use of imagery that is too child-like for an adolescent could result in the adolescent being unmotivated to practice or use PMR; thus tailoring the imagery to the age and particular preferences of the client is very important.

Common obstacles to competent practice and methods
to overcome them

Some clients might report that they have a hard time using imagery to imagine themselves in a relaxing place. For these clients, it is possible to do PMR without imagery (just lead them through progressively tensing and relaxing their muscles without creating a relaxing scene that they are imagining). Other clients might benefit from the therapist creating the imagery for them (e.g., "Feel the breeze on your face as you sit on the beach ... feel the sand through your fingertips").

Some clients might report that they are being distracted from implementing PMR by maladaptive thoughts that are entering their mind. It is important to teach these clients not to judge themselves for having the thoughts, but to treat the thoughts like passing clouds – to notice them, without necessarily trying to change them. Instead, suggest that the client continually try to refocus his/her energy and attention on the muscle group that is being tensed and relaxed.

As PMR is a skill that requires practice, it is also possible that some children will report that they were too busy during the week to make time to practice their PMR. In these cases, it can be helpful to teach the PMR skill also to the parents and to suggest that the entire family create a time to conduct PMR together. It is helpful if a therapist can give the client a PMR script to practice with between therapy sessions. Some therapists might audio record their session, while the client is using a digital audio recorder. This recording can then be given to the client to listen to during the week. Other therapists have also relied upon previously published recordings of PMR for children that include imagery (Pincus and Otis 2001). If the therapist has provided for the client a pre-recorded session of PMR, the entire family can listen to it and practice together. It can be helpful if the therapist helps the child brainstorm barriers to practice, and also possible solutions. It is important that therapists emphasize how learning the skill of relaxation is like riding a bicycle: once the skill is mastered, it can be used with ease at many different moments in the child's life – before a test, to help with falling asleep, before a race, and so on.

Some clients might report feeling sore after implementing the procedure. Be sure the client is only repeating each muscle group three times and is tensing the muscle group for only three seconds. Therapists need to be sure that clients are not implementing the procedure incorrectly. If clients have a preexisting medical condition or an injury that prevents them from tensing and relaxing certain muscle groups, it is important to refrain from tensing this muscle group until the injury has healed.

Applied Tension

Overview

Applied tension (AT) is a technique that is utilized to prevent vasovagal syncope – that is, a sudden drop in blood pressure that leads to fainting – in individuals who participate in CBT targeting specific phobia, blood–injection–injury (BII) subtype (see, e.g., Öst and Ollendick 2001). While fainting is not typically associated with the body's physiological response to anxiety, it is estimated that up to 75 percent of the individuals diagnosed with BII phobia have a history of fainting at the sight of blood, needles, and/or during injections (Öst 1992). Due to the association between BII phobia and vasovagal syncope, applied tension is designed to counteract the vasovagal response that causes one to faint; and it does so by increasing blood pressure during exposure to phobic stimuli (Foulds, Wiedmann, Patterson, and Brooks 1990). Through this action, the AT technique allows clients to gain control over their physiological response, feel more confident in the presence of blood and needles, and successfully complete *in vivo* exposures.

AT has demonstrated efficacy at reducing or preventing the vasovagal response during the treatment of BII phobia in numerous studies with adult populations, and more recently with youth (Hellström, Fellenius, and Öst 1996; Mednick and Claar 2012). While this technique requires some practice if it is to be used independently, it can be implemented and mastered by clients in a relatively short period of time and has been successfully employed in single-session treatments for specific phobias (Öst, Svensson, Hellström, and Lindwall 2001).

Key features of therapist competency in conducting applied tension

Therapists who wish to use AT with young clients should be familiar with its rationale, be able to explain and model its use in the treatment session, and be adept at helping clients understand when and how to use AT in the course of *in vivo* exposures. Prior to training in AT techniques children or adolescents who faint frequently, it may be necessary for therapists to consult their client's pediatrician to determine if any medical conditions exist which may preclude the use of this method. Next, therapists should provide the client with a clear, developmentally appropriate physiological explanation of the vasovagal response that causes fainting. For example, they can explain that fainting is caused by a sudden drop in blood pressure and a subsequent decrease in the amount of blood available to the brain. Typically, when people faint, they fall to the floor, which helps their body regain blood pressure and sends blood back to the brain, so that they "wake up" and continue functioning. It can be explained that several situations or objects can trigger fainting and that seeing blood and getting an injection are a few of those triggers. Children and adolescents should be reassured that there is nothing truly harmful or life-threatening about fainting itself, but that it can be dangerous to fall as a result of fainting.

Additionally, it should be observed that simply having had a prior experience of fainting in the presence of blood or needles may strengthen or at least maintain clients' fear and avoidance behaviors related to these situations. Therapists can explain that, because these individuals faint when they "can't handle" the blood-related stimulus, they never allow themselves to habituate to the situation and learn that nothing truly terrifying happens as a result of seeing blood or receiving an injection. Prior to teaching the technique, therapists should also discuss the various symptoms that can be precursors to a fainting episode: lightheadedness, nausea, increased perspiration, blurry vision, and changes in hearing. These are especially important to assess and discuss in detail, because increasing clients' awareness of the particular symptoms they experience before fainting will eventually cue them to use applied tension to prevent this response.

Once their client has a firm grasp of the rationale behind AT, therapists should begin didactic instruction. First, they may model the procedure for the client to observe. In order to do so, therapists can sit in a chair facing their client and begin by tensing their arm muscles. This can be done by making fists and squeezing them tightly, while also contracting the biceps and forearm muscles. In order to simplify the procedure for young clients, it may be necessary to introduce each muscle group separately. Once therapists have modeled applying tension to the arm muscles, they can practice along with clients in 15–20-second trials, taking short breaks of 20–30 seconds between each trial. Clients should be told that, during each trial, they should continue applying tension until they feel a sensation of warmth in their head or face. During breaks, clients should be taught simply to discontinue applying tension rather than to relax their muscles. Once clients have successfully learned the procedure with their arm muscles, therapists can guide them through applying tension to the trunk and leg muscles in much the same way. Therapists should make sure to monitor their clients' breathing during applied tension and, if necessary, to remind their clients to breathe at a normal pace. It is not uncommon for youth to hold their breath when they first learn AT methods.

Because children and adolescents who learn AT are likely to eventually utilize this procedure while having their blood drawn or receiving an injection, it is important to teach children how to keep one arm relaxed while simultaneously tensing the other muscle groups. This can be difficult at first and will likely require practice to master. Initially it may be helpful to allow the child to move one arm while tensing the other muscles in the body, and then to gradually reduce movement in the arm until it hangs loose. It may also help to ask children to imagine one arm being made of "jello" while the rest of the body is made of steel. Following demonstration and joint practice of the procedure, therapists should assign regular practice as homework. It is also typically necessary for therapists to demonstrate applied tension to their clients' parents, so that the latter may be able to monitor practice at home. Parents should be warned that sometimes children may develop a headache after practice; if this should occur, it can be prevented in the future by reducing the number of trials or by applying a lighter degree of tension.

Before beginning *in vivo* exposures, therapists should review the applied tension techniques and remind their clients to begin using this method immediately upon the onset of pre-vasovagal sensations such as dizziness, lightheadedness, or changes in vision or hearing. Because therapists begin with exposures that are less likely to cause a vasovagal reaction, clients will have ample opportunities to practice AT before approaching situations that are more likely to result in fainting. During exposures, therapists should remain aware of clients' breathing and may need to remind them to breathe normally. Especially during early exposures, therapists can help by coaching children through the AT procedure, prompting them to take breaks between each trial and to begin applying tension once again after each break. As youth are increasingly successful at employing AT and gain momentum with this practice, therapists can gradually let their input and coaching fade away, allowing youth more independence as they confront their fears.

Competence in treating anxiety disorders and depression

AT is unique in that it is specifically designed to treat BII phobia, and therefore would not be routinely used to treat any other anxiety or mood disorder.

Competence in treating both children and adolescents

Because most of the research support for using AT has been demonstrated with adults and adolescents, evidence in the literature for its efficacy with very young children is lacking. This is not to say that the technique is necessarily counter-indicated with younger children. Rather, therapists should carefully consider the clinical, medical, and developmental implications before using it.

Common obstacles to competent practice and methods to overcome them

Youth often exhibit resistance to implementing these strategies during *in vivo* exposures, due to excessive fear of fainting. Because of this, it may be necessary to spend extra time engaging in cognitive restructuring and emotion regulation strategies. Since there is a small chance that youth may in fact faint, cognitive restructuring should specifically target catastrophic thoughts about "how bad" it would really be, what would happen if fainting did occur, and how the client would cope with it effectively even if fainting did happen (see Chapter 12 for more details on cognitive restructuring).

Breathing Re-training

Key features of therapist competencies in implementing breathing re-training

Breathing re-training is aimed at countering anxiety-related hyperventilation or overbreathing, which some individuals with panic disorder experience. Breathing re-training is commonly implemented within CBT for panic disorder with or without agoraphobia; but it can also be used in treatments for other internalizing disorders, when shallow or quick breathing causes panic-like symptoms. It has also been utilized to help youth cope with the anxiety and pain associated with stressful medical procedures.

The primary task of the therapist who implements breathing re-training is to help the client learn how to slow down and deepen his/her breathing so as to moderate the amount of oxygen inhaled (Pincus et al. 2008). As a first step, before beginning to teach a client to conduct breathing re-training, it is helpful to demonstrate how physiological sensations can impact anxiety levels. This can be accomplished by explaining the fact that panic attacks are the result of the occurrence of both physical sensations and fear of these sensations, and that this co-occurrence can operate in a vicious cycle, whereby the fear of the sensations can actually increase their intensity. It is also important to review with the client the various triggers that may prompt panic sensations. One such trigger might be a maladaptive thought such as: "If my heart races while I'm in school, I won't be able to handle it"; another trigger might be a behavior, for instance avoidance of feared situations; and the third possible trigger is a physical sensation (e.g., being warm), which can also trigger panic-like sensations.

After describing the link between physical sensations and anxiety, as well as the triggers that can lead to those physical sensations, the therapist ought to describe and model for the child or adolescent how these physical sensations occur. In this manner, the therapist would explain how overbreathing (taking rapid, short breaths and exhaling very hard, at about three times the normal rate) causes one's body to get rid of more carbon dioxide than usual – which, although not dangerous, can produce disturbing physical sensations. The therapist can model this by having the client stand up and instructing him/her to conduct an overbreathing exercise along with the therapist: both would take rapid short breaths together and would exhale very hard and quickly. After the client finishes, have the client describe what types of physical sensations he/she is having. It is important to point out that there are similarities in physical sensations between exercises such as this one (which lowers carbon dioxide levels) and symptoms experienced during panic. Before teaching a client a new way to breathe, it is important to set the client up with a good rationale for learning this skill. One possible way this might be done is as follows:

> People with anxiety problems often overbreathe, or take rapid, short breaths, without being aware of doing so. Breathing is normally under the body's automatic control, but we can actually exert voluntary control over our breathing, as we do when we swim. Emotions can also affect our breathing rate. Can you think of an emotion you could experience that might cause you to breathe more rapidly? Since we know that overbreathing can trigger subtle changes in our carbon dioxide levels and that these changes can trigger panic-like sensations, I would like to teach you a way to become more aware of your breathing – and then to change your breathing patterns. When you overbreathe, you can actually see that you are using your chest muscles instead of your abdominal muscles. [*Therapist should role-play overbreathing and should have the client watch to see what part of the therapist's body is moving rapidly (the chest).*] Sometimes chest breathing can cause your chest to feel tight, or can cause chest pain or tense muscles. Sometimes chest breathing can even trigger panic-like feelings. So it is important to learn to change your breathing pattern so that you can diminish the chances that these sensations trigger panic.

As with any specific CBT technique, once the client understands the rationale for learning breathing re-training, (s)he will be much more likely to be motivated to learn and utilize this skill. To teach breathing re-training to a client, it is important to break it down into two major skills. The first skill is the *breathing component*, which is comprised of two parts: (i) learning to monitor and change the way one breathes (switching from chest breathing to abdominal breathing) without trying to change the rate of breathing; and (ii) learning to change the rate of one's breathing (slowing breathing down). Once the client masters these parts, (s)he can then learn the next major skill, which is the *meditational component*. In this component clients learn to focus their attention on breathing and to slow down their thoughts.

Therapists need to be able to model appropriate diaphragmatic breathing. They should do this by having the client watch and imitate as the therapist places one hand on his/her chest and the other on his/her stomach, just above the navel. The therapist should show the client that his/her stomach – not chest – should be moving up and down as (s)he breathes in and out. It is very helpful if therapists give the client some basic instructions for implementing breathing re-training. They should instruct the client to relax for a few seconds prior to beginning, while breathing at the normal rate. Then they should instruct the client to place one hand on the chest, the other on the diaphragm. Each time the client breathes in, (s)he should count, either out loud or in the mind, beginning with "1"; and each time the client exhales, (s)he should think or say "relax." Clients should continue doing this until they reach a count of 10, and then they should start again from "1," practicing for approximately 10 minutes. Therapists can demonstrate all this using the words "one (breathe in), relax (breathe out)." Clients should be encouraged to practice this skill as homework, every day.

Once the client has mastered diaphragmatic breathing, the therapist can teach him/her how to slow the rate of his/her breathing. This should be done by explaining that changing the rate of counting will assist the client to slow his/her breathing rate. Therapists should then demonstrate this process and how counting at gradually slower rates during diaphragmatic breathing can help slow down their breathing. The client should then practice this exercise for at least a few minutes, in the therapist's presence. Therapists should provide guidance and correction if the client is not implementing the skill correctly. They should point out that the goal is to slow the rate of breathing gradually, so as to reach an average rate of 8–10 breaths per minute (i.e., approximately three seconds per inhaling, three seconds per exhaling).

Throughout these breathing exercises therapists should encourage clients to focus only on their breathing. They should also remind clients that the skill of breathing re-training is like riding a bicycle: it becomes habitual with practice. The meditational component of breathing re-training can be helpful in assisting clients to focus more deeply on their breathing, without being distracted by passing thoughts. Clients should be taught how to gently notice thoughts as they pass through their minds, but to refocus attention on their breathing. Initially it is important for clients to practice in quiet, distraction-free, peaceful spaces that are conducive to relaxation. Therapists should remind clients that, once they master the skill of breathing re-training, they can conduct this exercise in more challenging surroundings (while watching television, standing in line, in class, in the supermarket, etc.).

When the client has had an opportunity to practice breathing re-training as homework, therapists should check in with him/her to find out whether any difficulties arose during practice and, if they did, to help troubleshoot them (see the section on common obstacles to competent practice in this chapter, and also Chapter 11, which deals specifically with homework-related competencies).

Competence in treating the anxiety disorders and depression

Learning how to become aware of one's breathing, how to slow it, and how to use meditational strategies can be very helpful not only for clients with panic disorder, but also for clients with other anxiety disorders, such as generalized anxiety disorder, or for clients with other internalizing disorders, such as depression. Learning to conduct breathing re-training is not difficult and clients can develop feelings of self-efficacy as they begin to practice and master this skill. Clients who have depression may feel irritable or sad, or may have low energy levels. Learning the skill of meditation can be helpful for children or adolescents who are depressed. However, these clients may find it more difficult to concentrate on breathing, or to manage maladaptive thoughts that make focusing on breathing hard. Such clients might benefit from monitoring their mood both before and after the breathing re-training practice, to see whether they notice any improvements in their mood after taking time to focus on the skill. Parents of children who are depressed might also be taught the skill, as breathing re-training often results in feelings of relaxation and well-being.

Competence in treating both children and adolescents

The skill of breathing re-training can be taught to children, adolescents, and adults. The meditational component, however, can be more difficult to teach to a very young child, who may not yet grasp the concept of "noticing thoughts in one's mind." With young children, it can be helpful if therapists teach the diaphragmatic breathing skill first to the child, and then also to the parent. Children might enjoy practicing the skill with their parents, and therapists should suggest this as an option for practice. Adolescents, on the other hand, are often able to learn all of the components of breathing re-training – diaphragmatic breathing, slowing breathing, and the meditational component. Adolescents might prefer to have more independence in their practice schedule at home. Therapists can also ask adolescents whether they prefer to teach their own parents, during the session, how to conduct breathing re-training (which should give the therapist an opportunity to see how well the client has digested the material), or whether they would rather have the therapist teach the parents this skill. In some cases, especially with older adolescents, it may be most appropriate to teach the adolescent the skill alone in session. Given that breathing re-training is such a concrete skill, it is often one that children report they enjoy learning, and they notice when they can implement the skill with more ease.

Common obstacles to competent practice and methods to overcome them

Therapists should be prepared that some clients will have trouble implementing and learning this skill, or practicing it on their own. If a client has trouble implementing breathing re-training, have him/her imagine that his/her lungs are like balloons, and that, as (s)he breathes in, the balloon inflates. You can also have the client push out his/her stomach before taking a breath, or placing a light book on his/her stomach, so as to be able to visualize the book going up and down as (s)he breathes. Another technique is to have the client lie on his/her stomach, head resting on his/her arms. All of these techniques make it more difficult for chest breathing to take place.

At times, therapists may have to respond to clients who complain that they have difficulty thinking exclusively about their breathing when they conduct the breathing re-training exercise. In such cases it is important for therapists to encourage clients not to get angry or upset with themselves, but rather to notice these thoughts and gently refocus their attention back to the exercise. Therapists should encourage clients to continue to practice the skill of breathing re-training, and their ability to focus attention should improve considerably.

Therapists ought to have a number of techniques they can suggest if the client is having difficulties with diaphragmatic breathing. They could refer the client back to the importance of learning about one's breathing patterns and changing them, if that client is particularly resistant to learning the skill. The therapist could also help clients who have trouble slowing down their breathing by suggesting that they do it more gradually (e.g., by counting at a gradually slower rate). It is also very possible that therapists will hear from clients who describe having difficulties with the meditational component of breathing re-training. They could advise that these clients practice breathing re-training first thing in the morning, while they are still sleepy, or that they lower the lights in the room while they practice, or that they practice with soft, relaxing music in the background. Therapists can also encourage clients to practice throughout the day and to begin to notice when they might be naturally starting to do more diaphragmatic breathing.

Conclusion

Learning skills for managing maladaptive mood and arousal are critical for children's healthy development and protect against the development of psychopathology. All of the skills reviewed in this chapter can be useful for therapists to utilize with youth who experience difficulties in managing negative emotions that are often part of everyday life; but they might be especially hard for youth with anxiety or depression to manage effectively. Each of the skills reviewed in this chapter can be adapted for use with both young and older children and adolescents, and we have illustrated this throughout. In addition, we have provided information about how each skill could be applied to clients with anxiety or depression. Through clinical experience and practice, beginning therapists will develop the necessary key competencies for implementing emotion identification, regulation, and management skills, applied tension, breathing re-training, and progressive muscle relaxation with clients and for tailoring these skills to the needs of each client. By receiving training in these techniques, therapists will be well equipped to teach these skills to the children, adolescents, and families who can benefit most from them.

References

Brent, David, and Kimberly Poling. 1997. *Cognitive Therapy Treatment Manual for Depressed and Suicidal Youth.* Pittsburgh, PA: University of Pittsburgh, Services for Teens at Risk.

Carlson, Charles R., and Rick H. Hoyle. 1993. "Efficacy of Abbreviated Progressive Muscle Relaxation Training: A Quantitative Review of Behavioral Medicine Research." *Journal of Consulting and Clinical Psychology*, 61: 1059–67. DOI: 10.1037/0022-006X.61.6.1059

Ciccetti, Dante, Brian P. Ackerman, and Carroll E. Izard. 1995. "Emotions and Emotion Regulation in Developmental Psychopathology." *Development and Psychopathology*, 7: 1–10.

Cohen, Judith A., Anthony P. Mannarino, and Esther Deblinger. 2006. *Treating Trauma and Traumatic Grief in Children and Adolescents.* New York: Guilford Press.

Compas, Bruce E. 1987. "Stress and Life Events during Childhood and Adolescence." *Clinical Psychology Review*, 7: 275–302.

Curry, John F., Karen C. Wells, David A. Brent, Gregory N. Clarke, Paul Rohde, Anne Marie Albano, … John S. March. 2005. *Treatment for Adolescents with Depression Study (TADS) Cognitive Behavior Therapy Manual: Introduction, Rationale, and Adolescent Sessions.* Durham, NC: Duke University Medical Center, The TADS Team.

Eisenberg, Nancy, Richard A. Fabes, and Ivana K. Guthrie. 1997. "Coping with Stress: The Roles of Regulation and Development." In Sharlene A. Wolchik and Irwin N. Sandler

(Eds.), *Handbook of Children's Coping: Linking Theory and Intervention* (pp. 41–70). New York: Plenum Press.

Foulds, Jonathan, Klaus Wiedmann, James Patterson, and Neil Brooks. 1990. "The Effects of Muscle Tension on Cerebral Circulation in Blood-Phobic and Non-Phobic Subjects." *Behaviour Research and Therapy*, 28: 481–6.

Hellström, Kirstin, Jan Fellenius, and Lars G. Öst. 1996. "One versus Five Sessions of Applied Tension in the Treatment of Blood Phobia." *Behaviour Research and Therapy*, 34: 101–12. DOI: 10.1016/0005-7967(95)00060-7

Jay, Susan M., Charles H. Elliott, Ernest Katz, and S. Stuart E. Siegel. 1987. "Cognitive–Behavioral and Pharmacologic Interventions for Children's Distress during Painful Medical Procedures." *Journal of Consulting and Clinical Psychology*, 5: 860–5. DOI: 10.1037/0022-006X.55.6.860

Kendall, Philip C., and Kristen A. Hedke. 2006. *Cognitive Behavioral Therapy for Anxious Children: Therapist Manual* (3rd ed.). Ardmore, PA: Workbook Publishing.

Lewinsohn, Peter M., Greg N. Clarke, Hyman Hops, and Judy Andrews. 1990. Cognitive–behavioral treatment for depressed adolescents. *Behavior Therapy*, 21(4): 385–401. DOI: 10.1016/S0005-7894(05)80353-3

Lohaus, Arnold, and Johannes Klein-Hessling. 2003. "Relaxation in Children: Effects of Extended and Intensified Training." *Psychology & Health*, 18: 237–49. DOI: 10.1080/0887044021000057257

Lopata, Christopher. 2003. "Progressive Muscle Relaxation and Aggression among Elementary Students with Emotional or Behavioral Disorders." *Behavioral Disorders*, 28: 162–72.

Madigan, Ryan J., and Steven M. S. Kurtz. 2013. *Teacher–Child Interaction Training: A Modular Approach to Emotion Regulation*. Unpublished manuscript.

Mednick, Lauren M., and Robyn L. Claar. 2012. "Treatment of Severe Blood-Injection-Injury Phobia with the Applied-Tension Method: Two Adolescent Case Examples." *Clinical Case Studies*, 11: 24–34. DOI: 10.1177/1534650112437405

Miller, Alec L., Jill H. Rathus, and Marsha Linehan. 2007. *Dialectical Behavior Therapy for Suicidal Adolescents*. New York: Guilford Press.

Nickel, Cerstin, Christian Kettler, Moritz Muehlbacher, Claaas Lahmann, Karin Tritt, Rainhold Fartacek, and Marius K. Nickel. 2005. "Effect of Progressive Muscle Relaxation in Adolescent Female Bronchial Asthma Patients: A Randomized, Double-Blind, Controlled Study. *Journal of Psychosomatic Research*, 59: 393–8. DOI: 10.1016/j.jpsychores.2005.04.008

Nickel, Cerstin, Claas Lahmann, Karin Tritt, Thomas H. Loew, Wolfhardt K. Rother, and Marius K. Nickel. 2005. "Short Communication: Stressed Aggressive Adolescents Benefit from Progressive Muscle Relaxation: A Random, Prospective, Controlled Trial." *Stress and Health: Journal of the International Society for the Investigation of Stress*, 26: 169–75. DOI: 10.1002/smi.1050

Öst, Lars G. 1992. "Blood and Injection Phobia: Background and Cognitive, Physiological, and Behavioral Variables." *Journal of Abnormal Psychology*, 101: 68. DOI: 10.1037/0021-843X.101.1.68

Öst, Lars G., and Thomas H. Ollendick. 2001. *Manual for One-Session Treatment of Specific Phobias*. Unpublished manuscript.

Öst, Lars G., Lisa Svensson, Kerstin Hellström, and Robert Lindwall. 2001. "One-Session Treatment of Specific Phobias in Youths: A Randomized Clinical Trial." *Journal of Consulting and Clinical Psychology*, 69: 814. DOI: 10.1037//0022-006X.69.5.814

Ollendick, Thomas and Neville King. 2004. "Empirically Supported Treatments for Children and Adolescents: Advances towards Evidence-Based Practice." In Paula M. Barrett and Thomas H. Ollendick (Eds.), *Handbook of Interventions that Work with Children and Adolescents: Prevention and Treatment* (pp. 3–26). West Sussex, England: John Wiley & Sons.

Pincus, Donna B. 2012. *Growing Up Brave: Expert Strategies for Helping Your Child Overcome Fear, Stress and Anxiety.* New York: Little, Brown.

Pincus, Donna B., and J. D. Otis. 2001. *I Can Relax: A Relaxation CD for Children* (Audio compact disc). Boston, MA: Psychzone.

Pincus, Donna B., Jill T. Ehrenreich, and Sara G. Mattis. 2008. *Mastery of Anxiety and Panic for Adolescents: Therapist Guide.* New York: Oxford University Press.

Powers, Scott W. 1999. "Empirically Supported Treatments in Pediatric Psychology: Procedure-Related Pain." *Journal of Pediatric Psychology*, 24: 131–45. DOI: 10.1093/jpepsy/24.2.131

Rapee, Ronald M., Heidi J. Lyneham, Carolyn A. Schniering, Viviana Wuthrich, Maree Abbott, Jennifer Hudson, and Ann Wignall. 2006. *The Cool Kids Child and Adolescent Anxiety Program Therapist Manual.* Sydney: Centre for Emotional Health, Macquarie University.

Reynolds, William M., and Kevin I. Coats. 1986. "A Comparison of Cognitive–Behavioral Therapy and Relaxation Training for the Treatment of Depression in Adolescents." *Journal of Consulting and Clinical Psychology*, 54: 653–60. DOI: 10.1037/0022-006X.54.5.653

Sburlati, Elizabeth S., Carolyn A. Schniering, Heidi J. Lyneham, and Ronald M. Rapee. 2011. "A Model of Therapist Competencies for the Empirically Supported Cognitive Behavioral Treatment of Child and Adolescent Anxiety and Depressive Disorders." *Clinical Child and Family Psychology Review*, 14, 89–109.

Suveg, Cynthia, and Janice Zeman. 2004. "Emotion Regulation in Children with Anxiety Disorders." *Journal of Consulting and Clinical Psychology*, 33: 750–9.

Further Reading

Francis, Sarah E., Peter G. Mezo, and Stephanie L. Fung. 2012. "Self-Control Training in Children: A Review of Interventions for Anxiety and Depression and the Role of Parental Involvement." *Psychotherapy Research*, 22: 220–38. DOI: 10.1080/10503307.2011.637990

Gilroy, Lisa J., Kenneth C. Kirkby, Brett A. Daniels, Ross G. Menzies, and Iain M. Montgomery. 2003. "Long-Term Follow-Up of Computer-Aided Vicarious Exposure versus Live Graded Exposure in the Treatment of Spider Phobia." *Behavior Therapy*, 34: 65–76. DOI: 10.1016/S0005-7894(03)80022-9

Klein-Heßling, Johannes, and Arnold Lohaus. 2002. "Benefits and Interindividual Differences in Children's Responses to Extended and Intensified Relaxation Training." *Anxiety, Stress and Coping: An International Journal*, 15: 275–88. DOI: 10.1080/1061580021000020734

Lohaus, Arnold, Johannes Klein-Heßling, Claus Vögele, and Christiane Kuhn-Hennighausen. 2001. "Psychophysiological Effects of Relaxation Training in Children." *British Journal of Health Psychology*, 6: 197–206. DOI: 10.1348/135910701169151

Rausch, Sarah M., Sandra E. Gramling, and Stephen M. Auerbach. 2006. "Effects of a Single Session of Large-Group Meditation and Progressive Muscle Relaxation Training on Stress Reduction, Reactivity, and Recovery." *International Journal of Stress Management*, 13: 273–90. DOI: 10.1037/1072-5245.13.3.273

Shapiro, Jennifer R., Emily M. Pisetsky, Wen Crenshaw, Shanna Spainhour, Robert M. Hamer, Maureen Dymek-Valentine, and Cynthia M. Bulik. 2008. "Exploratory Study to Decrease Postprandial Anxiety: Just Relax!" *International Journal of Eating Disorders*, 41: 728–33. DOI: 10.1002/eat.20552

Taylor, Daniel J., and Brandy M. Roane. 2010. "Treatment of Insomnia in Adults and Children: A Practice-Friendly Review of Research." *Journal of Clinical Psychology*, 66, 1137–47. DOI: 10.1002/jclp.20733

17

Problem-Solving Skills Training

Ana M. Ugueto, Lauren C. Santucci,
Lauren S. Krumholz, and John R. Weisz

Introduction

Originally described by D'Zurilla and Goldfried (1971), problem solving is one of the most common and versatile treatment approaches used to help children overcome anxiety and depressive disorders (Chorpita and Daleiden 2009). Children with depression and anxiety often have difficulty solving problems and usually give up easily, or they apply one overlearned behavioral strategy to resolve a problem. When the problem persists, they may feel that problems are impossible to solve – or, more specifically, impossible *for them* to solve. Depressed children who have a negative or *depressogenic* cognitive style (Gladstone and Kaslow 1995; Jacobs, Reinecke, Gollan, and Kane 2008) may not recognize that having problems is part of life and is "normal." Instead they may see everyday or common problems as something that is happening to them alone, and they may think: "Why does bad stuff only happen to me?" Similarly, anxious youth with a cognitive bias toward threat interpretation (see Vasey and MacLeod 2001 for a review) may see the world as a dangerous place, where they must avoid any possible perilous situation to stay safe. Finally, children with traumatic stress may have learned maladaptive behaviors as a way to cope with uncontrollable traumatic experiences and, subsequently, use these same behaviors to manage difficult social situations and emotional dysregulation (Cohen, Mannarino, and Deblenger 2006).

Teaching youths that problems are universal and should be expected is fundamental in training children and adolescents to use problem solving. Problem solving helps youth inhibit the tendency to react impulsively (e.g., by running away) or act passively (e.g., by waiting for the situation to resolve itself, or for someone else to fix it). Learning how to solve problems, through the generation and evaluation of solutions, helps counteract rigid thinking associated with anxiety and depressive disorders and teaches children how to use a specific strategy to increase cognitive flexibility and

Evidence-Based CBT for Anxiety and Depression in Children and Adolescents: A Competencies-Based Approach,
First Edition. Edited by Elizabeth S. Sburlati, Heidi J. Lyneham, Carolyn A. Schniering, and Ronald M. Rapee.
© 2014 John Wiley & Sons, Ltd. Published 2014 by John Wiley & Sons, Ltd.

to gain a broader perspective on events. Problem solving can be used to help youth solve a variety of problems, whether academic (e.g., poor grades), social (e.g., bullying), familial (e.g., negotiating with parents) or related to activating events (e.g., divorce of parents), treatment goals (e.g., making friends), and moods (e.g., feeling bored). When youth are able to recognize a problematic situation, apply the sequential problem-solving method, and successfully solve a problem, they may feel empowered and be more likely to use the skill to solve future problems. Problem solving helps children break abstract and overwhelming problems into concrete and solvable parts.

The following sections of this chapter were based on a selection of cognitive behavioral therapy (CBT) treatment manuals for anxiety (Kendall and Hedke 2006; Rapee et al. 2006), trauma (Cohen et al. 2006), and depression (Brent and Poling 1997; Clarke, Lewinsohn, and Hops 1990; Curry et al. 2005), as well as on the clinical experiences of the authors (e.g., Chorpita and Weisz 2009). For the purposes of this chapter, children and adolescents are collectively referred to as "children" or "youth."

Key Features of Problem-Solving Competencies

When you teach children problem solving, it is important to teach them that problems are part of life, that everyone has them, and that one can learn how to cope or solve problems effectively. Problems can be small (e.g., forgetting homework) or large (e.g., fight with a boy-/girlfriend), and may be fixed quickly (e.g., by apologizing to a friend) or may take time to solve (e.g., studying daily for an upcoming test). Regardless of type or size, any problem that is within the control of the youth can be solved by using a sequential approach. The CBT approach to problem solving typically involves five steps:

1. identifying and defining the problem;
2. generating a list of possible solutions;
3. evaluating the strengths and weaknesses of each possible solution;
4. choosing a solution;
5. using the solution and determining whether the problem was solved or whether another solution is needed to solve it.

In step 1 – identifying and defining the problem – it is critical that children choose a problem that is within their ability to solve; trying to solve a problem that it outside of one's control will only lead to feelings of frustration, helplessness, and hopelessness. Therapists should help them determine whether they can change the situation or need instead to change their reaction when the situation cannot be changed (Rapee et al. 2006). For example, youth may not be able to change the divorce of their parents, but they may be able to change their emotional reaction to the divorce. Therapists should educate children that changing one's reaction to a situation is something that is within one's control, even if the situation itself cannot be altered.

Once an appropriate problem has been selected, the problem should be defined in specific and concrete terms. Problems that are too vague (e.g., "I hate school") or too ambiguous (e.g., "School is boring") will be difficult to solve because they do not define the exact problem or identify the goals of problem solving. Additionally, it will be difficult to generate alternative solutions if the problem is not defined clearly. If a youth defines a problem too broadly, the therapist should ask questions in order to better understand and to help the child refine the problem. Take the example of "I hate school." Using Socratic questioning, the therapist can guide the child to reframe the problem thus: "I failed my science test and need to get a passing grade on the next test."

In step 2 – generating a list of solutions – the therapist should help the youth think of as many alternatives as possible. During this phase, encourage the child to think creatively. Quantity, not quality of solutions is the goal, as brainstorming is a way to stimulate cognitive flexibility (Curry et al. 2005). If the child is having difficulty brainstorming ideas, the therapist may offer some suggestions to stimulate the child's thoughts; the greater the number of ideas, the greater the likelihood of finding an effective solution. In order to increase the number of alternatives, combinations of ideas also are encouraged. For example, a youth may list "Ask questions in class" and separately list "Go to afterschool tutoring." These solutions can be combined into an additional one, "Ask questions in class and go to after-school tutoring," which would be a third solution. Remember, too, that ideas should not be criticized or ruled out from the start; any solution the child describes should be listed, even if it seems implausible (e.g., "Study every day after school for five hours"), ridiculous (e.g., "Break into school and steal the test"), or antisocial (e.g., "Cheat off another student"). The inclusion of unrealistic or ridiculous solutions makes the task more fun and more engaging for the child, and encourages the child to think more creatively, "outside the box," about possible solutions. In fact, if the child does not generate such a solution, the therapist should volunteer one, to demonstrate that any solution that comes to mind should be listed, regardless of how outrageous it might be. In our experience, children are usually thinking of such solutions even if they do not say them aloud to the therapist; so, if the therapist articulates an outlandish solution, the child may then do the same. Evaluation of the merits of each possible solution should be withheld until the next step.

In step 3 – evaluating the strengths and weaknesses of each possible solution – each solution is scrutinized as to its unique advantages and disadvantages for solving the problem. Children should think about, and predict, the utility of each solution and then list as many "strengths and weaknesses," "pros and cons," "positive and negative consequences," or "good and bad reasons" as they can. If youth are having difficulty generating the advantages and disadvantages of a given solution, therapists can query the youth, or even suggest possible benefits and limitations, to ensure that the evaluation is a fair appraisal of the solution. Moreover, therapists should encourage children to think of both short- and long-term consequences of the solution. This is particularly important for solutions that are implausible, ridiculous, or antisocial. For example, a child who lists "Cheat off another student" would also have to list the advantages (e.g., "Wouldn't have to study," "Would probably get a better grade") and the disadvantages (e.g., "Would get expelled if I were caught," "The other student may not know more than I do," "Would never learn the material which I may need some day"). If the evaluation does not accurately reflect the strengths and weaknesses of a solution, youth will be at a disadvantage when they have to select one solution to try to solve the problem.

In step 4 – choosing a solution – children must choose the solution they think will best solve the problem. Ideally, they would choose the solution with the most advantages and fewest disadvantages, and thus the one most likely to actually solve the problem. To help the child choose the most effective solution, the therapist and the child can list the solutions in the order of their likely success, from highest to lowest. This technique helps the child pick the most preferred solution, while it also guides the child's next steps should the first solution prove ineffective. However, some children may feel strongly about a solution that the therapist does not favor. In these instances, youth should be allowed to choose the solution they want to use without any criticism from the therapist. For example, a child may choose "Study with a friend," while the therapist thinks "Ask questions in class and go to after-school tutoring" would be a more successful solution. In this case, the therapist should defer to the child, who may then learn something useful after implementing the solution. Also, to facilitate use of the solution, the chosen solution may need to be broken down into smaller steps (Rapee et al. 2006). For example, "Study with a friend" might involve asking a friend to study together, setting up a study schedule, bringing books and other materials to the study session, and studying for two hours. It is important for the therapist to explain to the child that there is no one "correct" or "perfect" solution; most problems may be addressed adequately in a number of different ways, and choosing a solution that is "good enough" is better than doing nothing and simply waiting for the problem to subside, or for someone else to solve it (Curry et al. 2000).

In step 5 – using the solution and determining whether the problem was solved or whether another solution is needed to solve it – children are encouraged to implement the solution and determine its effectiveness for solving the problem. Without this step, youth may continue implementing an ineffective solution without thinking about why it failed and without choosing another one, which may work better. Usually children are not able to implement the solution during a therapy session, so the therapist should assign step 5 as homework and review it with the child at the next session. If the child implements the solution and this does not produce the desired effects, the child should repeat step 4 and choose the next best solution. If the child had ranked the possible solutions in step 4 (as described above), (s)he can then try the second solution on the list; and, if that does not work, the third, the fourth, and so on – until a solution successfully solves the problem. When the first solution does not solve the problem as expected, youth with anxiety and depression may feel helpless and ineffective. It is important to reiterate to them that problem solving is a learning process and that it is impossible to predict all the consequences of a solution before it is implemented.

Competence in Treating Anxiety Disorders and Depression

Anxiety

Problem solving is a particularly important skill in the context of anxiety treatment, as anxious youth tend to rely on unhelpful strategies, such as escape or avoidance, to manage fear (American Psychiatric Association 2000; Dadds and Barrett 2001). Problem solving can be a helpful tool when a child is confronted with an anxiety-provoking situation, as happens during *in vivo* exposures (Kendall et al. 2005). In such a situation, anxious youth may overestimate the likelihood that something scary or dangerous will happen and may underestimate their ability to cope in case "something" occurs, which may ultimately lead them to avoid (or try to avoid) the situation (Dadds and Barrett 2001). Going through sequential problem solving may help the child plan in advance how to handle an anxiety-provoking situation (e.g., by thinking positive thoughts and then by "riding the wave of anxiety"), how to choose a less challenging exposure when what was planned feels too difficult for the time being (e.g., by saying hello to one stranger instead of saying hello to two strangers), or how to know what steps to take if his/her mind goes blank in the face of anxiety (e.g., take a deep breath). In the case of traumatic stress, children may have a limited repertoire of responses when dealing with interpersonal situations and may cope with anger or withdrawal. Thus, problem solving may help youth manage strong emotions in a more prosocial manner (Cohen et al. 2006).

When teaching sequential problem solving to anxious youth, therapists should consider that children may be reluctant to solve their own problems when these are related to fears. Additionally, youth with anxiety may have difficulty defining clearly what problem to solve. For example, a child might say "I hate swimming class," which may lead to solutions such as "bring a friend" or "try out another sport," when in fact the child dislikes swimming class because he misses his mother and worries that something bad will happen to her when she is not with him. So it is important that the therapist use Socratic questioning to identify the real problem (e.g., "I'm afraid something bad will happen to my mom when I am at swimming class"). Furthermore, if the therapist sets a goal with the child by discussing what the latter hopes to achieve through problem solving and by making this achievement into a goal, the therapist should also ensure that the goal is realistic for the child. For example, if a socially anxious child tends to blush when speaking to others, the goal "Don't turn red" may not be realistic. A better goal may be instead this: "Keep talking to a friend even when I start turning red."

When generating solutions, it is important to allow "bad ideas," or the unhelpful solutions that the child currently engages in, to make it onto the list (e.g., "Stay home from school the day I have to give a book report"). However, given that youth with anxiety tend to rely on escape or avoidance to manage negative emotions, the therapist should encourage the child to generate other possible solutions as well. Similarly, if the list includes solutions that involve avoiding a feared situation, use the evaluation step to consider the weaknesses of such solutions. While a "pro" of avoidance may be "I wouldn't feel anxious if I stayed home from school," the "cons" may include long-term consequences such as "I would never learn that I can handle it," or "I won't get over my fears." If a child chooses an avoidant solution to practice, the therapist should refrain from criticizing the choice and, instead, allow the child to implement the solution and then evaluate the results. During the evaluation stage, the child may uncover for himself or herself why this avoidant choice is not the best option (see section "Common obstacles to competent practice and methods to overcome them"). Sequential problem solving helps to break down overwhelming situations into problems that can be solved. When large problems are broken down, anxious youth have an opportunity to increase their sense of self-efficacy and to gather evidence that contradicts their anxious thoughts and feared outcomes.

Depression

Problem solving is an integral component of depression treatment (Chorpita and Daleiden 2009); it is the key strategy for depressed youth to employ in the face of situations that cause distress. Symptoms associated with depression, such as low energy or fatigue, a sense of helplessness and hopelessness, and suicidal ideation can interfere with a child's or adolescent's ability to effectively solve problems (Stark, Streusand, Arora, and Patel 2012). These symptoms often lead to maladaptive behavioral tendencies related to problem solving: avoidance of activities due to the energy and effort that must be exerted to engage in problem solving; tendency to attempt only one – overlearned – behavioral strategy; difficulty generating beneficial solutions; tendency to give up quickly if the desired outcome is not achieved; impulsive suicide attempt when no other solution can be fathomed (Abela and Hankin 2008). These tendencies express and support the depressed youth's belief that (s)he is unable to successfully manage life stressors. Therapists can help depressed children break this vicious cycle by teaching them problem solving, while remaining aware of the common difficulties that interfere with a depressed youth's ability to effectively apply this approach. Therefore therapists must carefully consider factors that could affect depressed children's acquisition and application of the problem solving approach. These factors encompass negative thoughts, feelings, and behaviors that characterize depressive disorders, which should be addressed by therapists before, during, and after teaching this skill. Prior to initiating problem-solving steps, therapists may need to address interfering feelings (e.g., depressed or irritable mood) and behaviors (e.g., social withdrawal and lethargic behavior) through mood boosting activities; or they may need to address interfering thoughts about the problem – or about one's ability to solve the problem (e.g., "I can't do anything right") – through cognitive restructuring.

When helping depressed youth identify and define a problem, therapists should be aware of possible cognitive distortions related to all-or-nothing thinking (e.g., "If I don't get 100 percent on the test, I'm a failure") and exaggeration (e.g., "Nothing ever works out for me"), which may become apparent and may interfere with this step. In addition, depressed youth may benefit from breaking a problem into smaller parts in order to feel more hopeful about being able to solve it. Examples of problems that may occur for depressed youth are low mood, interpersonal conflict, academic failure, social isolation, suicidal ideation, and thinking that one is not good (smart, funny, attractive, or athletic) enough. When generating a list of possible solutions, therapists may initially need to provide increased support to depressed children in order to help them brainstorm a variety of solutions. It is especially important that solutions not be evaluated at this point, in part because of the tendency of depressed youth to criticize their own ideas. When evaluating the strengths and weaknesses of each solution, therapists should ensure that there is careful consideration of its advantages and disadvantages, since depressed youth are more likely to focus on the potential disadvantages of each solution. In contrast, for children who list suicide as a possible solution and only see the advantages of self-harm, the disadvantages need to be considered and discussed thoroughly. To increase the sense of mastery and agency, therapists should encourage youth with depression to select the solution of their choice to implement, except in cases where the solution involves self-harm (e.g., suicide or non-suicidal self-injury). Children should also be reminded that sometimes multiple solutions must be tried before the outcome they desire is achieved. Therefore it can be beneficial for youth to create a backup plan involving several additional solutions in case the initial one did not work. After therapists have taught problem solving, they should encourage children continuously to use this approach through therapeutic homework assignments and opportune moments in session.

Successfully solving a problem can increase a youth's sense of competence about being able to manage problems that arise as a normal part of the developmental process. In addition, effectively solving a specific problem can lead to enhanced mood, at least temporarily. Most importantly, each problem that depressed children effectively solve provides evidence contradicting the belief that they are hopeless or helpless. And for youth at risk of suicide, problem solving helps them re-evaluate the consequences of an impulsive and life-threatening act, think of alternatives that may be more effective, and try something other than self-harm (Brent and Poling 1997). Thus problem solving should be incorporated into the treatment of depression for youth because it is a key ingredient in alleviating depressive symptoms and building a more positive sense of self.

Competence in Treating both Children and Adolescents

Children

Problem solving can be a useful tool when planning for the life events that children may encounter – such as starting school, attending camp for the first time, getting in a fight with a friend, moving to a new town, or the birth of a sibling. Already a relatively concrete skill, sequential problem solving can be made even more developmentally appropriate for children by using child-friendly language to describe the process, presenting the skill in an engaging manner, providing scaffolding such as visual cues and writing down the five steps, and encouraging caregiver involvement.

Language such as "what's the problem," "think of solutions," "pick one," and "try it" may be helpful for children. Additionally, visual cues with smiling and frowning faces can be used as headings to signify the strengths and weaknesses of each solution. Acronyms like "RIBEYE" (Relax, Identify the problem, Brainstorm solutions, Evaluate solutions, say Yes to one solution, and Encourage child to try solution: see Curry et al. 2005: 79) and "STEPS" (Say what the problem is, Think of solutions, Examine each one, Pick one and try it out, and See if it worked: see Weisz, Thurber, Sweeney, Proffitt, and LeGagnoux 1997), or a mnemonic like "The Five Ps of Problem Solving: Problem, Purpose, Plans, Predict and pick, and Pat yourself on the back": see Stark et al. 2007, pp. 33–5) can make it easier for youth to remember and implement all of the problem-solving steps. Therapists can also suggest possible solutions for young children, who may have difficulty generating ideas independently.

To introduce the skill, choose a silly or fun problem to solve. For example, tell the child he or she has to move a piece of paper from one side of the room to the other without getting out of his or her chair. Potential solutions might be making the paper into a ball and throwing it across the room, or creating a paper airplane and sailing it to the other side. Then, after evaluating the strengths and weaknesses of each solution, the child gets to pick one and try it out in session. Alternatively, the therapist can present the child with a cartoon image of a dog who appears sad, on one side of a fence, and a bone wrapped in a bow, on the other side of the fence. Using this image as an example, the therapist can walk through the problem-solving steps to help the dog get its bone. Once familiar with the problem-solving process, children can discuss problems in their own life.

Instructing the caregiver in the use of sequential problem solving may facilitate the use of this skill outside of therapy. If possible, the child should teach the caregiver the steps to problem solving and should show the caregiver how to apply these steps to a particular problem – perhaps the silly problem presented to the child initially. Once the caregiver knows the sequential problem-solving steps, (s)he can support the child in the use of this skill by gently reminding the child when and how the skill can be used, and, if needed, by helping the child apply these steps to problems as they arise. In addition, the caregiver can be encouraged to give praise for the application of this skill, in order to promote its use. Caregiver involvement can be particularly helpful for younger children who may have difficulty completing homework, identifying appropriate problems, or remembering the sequence of steps. Behavioral rehearsal, both in and out of session, will help promote generalization of this tool to the child's life.

Adolescents

In order to competently teach adolescents to use problem solving, therapists should make adaptations that are developmentally (e.g., cognitively, emotionally, and socially) appropriate. Although the core components of problem solving are the same across developmental levels, therapists will need to make adjustments in the *way* problem solving is taught. Adolescents with lower cognitive functioning may benefit from the use of concrete strategies for problem solving, initially with more frequent support from therapists and caregivers. Adolescents with limited social maturity may need more assistance in generating prosocial solutions and in evaluating how others would respond to their solutions; some help in the area of perspective-taking skills may be welcome. The types of problems that adolescents face will likely differ in content from the types of problems experienced by children. For example, adolescents may struggle with developing and navigating romantic relationships, desiring more independence from their caregivers, questioning their sexual orientation, and experimenting with drugs and alcohol. While these are common developmental challenges, they can generate problems for the adolescent that can be addressed through problem solving. Before helping adolescents apply problem solving to distressing situations in their own lives, therapists should provide adolescents with engaging examples of problems to be solved that are common for youth of the same age (e.g., an adolescent girl who feels self-conscious because other classmates are spreading a rumor that she is promiscuous; or an adolescent boy who is insulted by older boys in the locker room for being small). Encouraging the active participation of adolescents in applying problem solving is beneficial: such participation helps them establish increased autonomy, empowers them, and equips them to solve problems independently. While some caregivers may be helpful and supportive of the adolescent where this skill is concerned, therapists should carefully consider to what extent caregivers should be involved; and this should be done on the basis of the developmental level of the teen as well as on the dynamic of the adolescent–caregiver relationship (e.g., the therapist should ask him/herself: "Would the caregiver's presence facilitate or antagonize the adolescent?" If the latter, that would result in further conflict with caregivers).

Example 17.1 Adolescent with depression

David is a 15-year-old boy diagnosed with major depressive disorder. He arrives at the session upset about not making the basketball team at his school.

1. Identifying and defining the problem:
   I am feeling sad because I did not make the team.
2. Generating a list of possible solutions:
   A. *Play video games.*
   B. *Do nothing and wait for sadness to go away.*
   C. *Change my thinking.*
   D. *Sign up for another afterschool activity.*
   E. *Transfer to a different school and try out for the basketball team there.*
3. Evaluating the strengths and weaknesses of each possible solution:
   Solution A: *Play video games.*
   - **Pros**: Video games are fun. I will get better at playing them.
   - **Cons**: It's not possible to play video games all day. I will probably still feel sad when I'm not playing them.

   Solution B: *Do nothing and wait for sadness to go away.*
   - **Pros**: This will be easy. I don't have to do anything.
   - **Cons**: It may take a long time to stop feeling sad. I might get bored doing nothing.

   Solution C: *Change my thinking.*
   - **Pros**: This is quick. I know how to do it. It can help me feel better.
   - **Cons**: It can be hard to figure out more positive thoughts.

   Solution D: *Sign up for another afterschool activity.*
   - **Pros**: I'll still get to do something I like after school. I could meet new people.
   - **Cons**: It might not be as fun as basketball. If I have to try out again, I may not make it.

   Solution E: *Transfer to a different school and try out for the basketball team there.*
   - **Pros**: I get to play on a basketball team.
   - **Cons**: I'll have to make all new friends. I might not make the team at that school. I might not like my new teachers.
4. Choosing a solution:
   I'll combine solutions C and D. I'll change my negative thoughts to more positive thoughts, and I'll join the track team because anyone can join, and I already have a few friends on the team.
5. Using the solution and determining whether the problem was solved, or whether another solution is needed to solve the problem:
   The solution worked! I changed my thought from "I'm not good at basketball" to "I am good at basketball. I just didn't play my best during tryouts." Also, I joined the track team. I am enjoying being on the team, and my new thoughts are helping me feel better about myself.

Common Obstacles to Competent Practice
and Methods to Overcome Them

Therapists often face difficulties teaching children to successfully use sequential problem solving on their own. Sometimes youth will be so upset by a problem that they cannot calm down enough to learn or apply the problem-solving method; in these situations, therapists should allow children to express their frustrations and feelings, to use another coping skill (e.g., relaxation), and then to begin the problem-solving approach once they are less emotional and more rational (Curry et al. 2005). In order to facilitate the child's use of problem solving, the therapist can first teach the child the sequential steps with the help of a fun problem (e.g., keep a balloon in the air without using your hands). This allows the youth to focus on learning the steps instead of focusing on the problem. Then the therapist can select a common problem typical for children, like forgetting a homework assignment, to show how the steps can be used in a different way. Finally, the therapist should encourage the child to select a real-life problem. If the youth says that he or she does not have any problems, the therapist can tell the child that problems can be small, everyday problems and remind the child of a problem previously mentioned in session. Once the therapist has taught the child problem solving, (s)he should look for opportunities to reinforce this skill in session. Common examples include using problem solving if a child is not doing the therapy homework or is losing it, does not want to participate in a particular therapeutic exercise, or no longer wants to attend therapy. Additionally, therapists should use problem solving whenever a crisis arises. For example, if a youth comes into session upset about a fight with a friend, a grade on an assignment, or an upcoming tryout for a team or play, the therapist can suggest using problem solving. Likewise, if a caregiver complains that the child was suspended from school for aggressive behavior, the therapist can use problem solving with that child, to make him/her think of alternative behaviors that would not lead to punishments. Finally, it is important that the therapist's approach be Socratic: the act of querying should help the child identify the problem more specifically and the questions themselves should make him/her think of possible solutions, or of advantages and disadvantages of possible solutions; the therapist should not tell the child what solutions to list, what the pros and cons of each solution are, or what solution to choose, and (s)he certainly should not guarantee that any solution will be 100 percent effective. Therapists should also anticipate specific problems that may arise in relation to each of the five steps.

The most common obstacles for step 1 are that the problem is not solvable by the youth and/or is too large in scope. Take the example of the daughter of a deployed military solider who tells the therapist: "My dad is fighting in Iraq and I want him to come home." This is certainly a problem that the child cannot solve. In this situation, the therapist should explain to the child that some situations are such that we cannot change or solve them no matter how much we would like to, and that in these special situations we can only change what is in our control. The therapist can then ask the child how she feels about her father being deployed and identify these feelings (e.g., sad mood, missing father) as a problem that can be solved.

In step 2 typical therapist mistakes include not letting a youth list antisocial, implausible, or ridiculous alternatives out of fear that the child would choose one of these ineffective solutions. Allowing children to list antisocial solutions proves to the child that *any* solution may be listed for consideration. Remember that all possible solutions will be evaluated in step 3; but solutions that are not on the list cannot be evaluated. For example, if a therapist is working with a child who often hits his younger brother when he is annoyed, and the child does not list that behavior, the therapist would be wise to suggest it. This way the advantages and disadvantages of each approach, including the child's typical antisocial one, can be considered and evaluated, and this will make it less likely that the child actually will select an antisocial solution. Another common mistake is that therapists do not suggest possible solutions when youth are having difficulty brainstorming alternatives. When children can only generate one or two solutions, the therapist should suggest alternatives or use a Socratic approach to help them generate more ideas. Furthermore, therapists should suggest some outlandish ideas themselves, to illustrate that the goal is to think of as many solutions as possible, regardless of how effective they may be. This approach usually gets youth laughing and stimulates more solutions.

A frequent obstacle in step 3 is that the child does not list all possible strengths and weaknesses of the solutions and does not evaluate the *unique* advantages and disadvantages of each. If children keep listing the same or generic pros ("It would help me solve the problem") and cons ("I wouldn't get into trouble") for each solution, therapists should encourage them to think about positive and negative aspects of a particular solution that the other solutions do not have. The more the youth can see the differences between the solutions, the easier it should be for them to choose one.

In step 4 therapists often have difficulty when a child wants to choose a solution that the therapist does not believe will be most effective, especially one that may even reinforce avoidant or antisocial behavior. If this happens, therapists can review the strengths and weaknesses, emphasizing the negative aspects of the chosen solution and the positive aspects of other, more desirable ones. However, if the child still prefers the less effective solution, the therapist should allow the child to implement it, unless it involves self-harm. If the chosen solution does not solve the problem, the therapist should discuss the failure of the solution with the child at the next session. This discussion can lead to the re-evaluation of the chosen solution, the reconsideration of the other solutions, the generation of more solutions, and the selection of a new solution that may be more likely to solve the given problem. Additionally, if the therapist is concerned about the child implementing a less effective solution and then having to wait several days to discuss the outcome with the therapist, the therapist can have the child choose in advance a second solution, which the child can implement if the first does not solve the problem. An additional obstacle often encountered in step 4 is that therapists fail to help youth break the solution into smaller steps before implementing it, which may result in difficulty initiating the solution.

Therapists should review step 5 in the next session, to discuss how well the solution worked. Failure to do so will make it less likely that youth will use problem solving in the future. During the review, the therapist can praise the child, highlight how this skill helped, or, when the solution did not solve the problem, discuss the limitations of the solution and remind the child to try another one if the first was unsuccessful. When the first solution is not successful, the therapist should encourage the youth to try another one immediately instead of waiting for several days to speak with the therapist. When discussing the problem initially, the therapist and the child can identify a solution, and then identify one or more backup solutions in case the first solution does not work (for details about ranking solutions, see steps 4 and 5 in the section "Key Features of Problem-Solving Competencies"). An unsuccessful solution should not be viewed as a failure but, instead, as an opportunity to try another solution.

Problem solving is a highly versatile skill and one of the most common ones used in CBT to treat children with anxiety and depression. In a review of evidence-based treatments, problem solving came up as the fifth and the ninth most common coping skill taught to youth with depression and anxiety, respectively (Chorpita and Daleiden 2009). Children with internalizing disorders have difficulty solving problems and often act impulsively or passively when faced with distress. Youth can learn the five sequential steps – identifying a problem, generating a list of possible solutions, evaluating the strengths and weaknesses of each one, choosing a solution to implement, and finally implementing it and determining whether the problem was solved or whether another solution is needed – as a part of learning how to effectively solve problems that impact their functioning. Learning problem solving increases children's cognitive flexibility and behavioral repertoire, counteracts perceptions of helplessness and hopelessness, and enhances self-efficacy. Children and adolescents with depression and anxiety disorders can learn alternatives to avoidance, passivity, and other maladaptive strategies. By using developmentally appropriate adaptations, the five steps of problem solving can be employed by youth of all ages in solving a variety of stressors.

While problem solving is a prominent component in the treatment of depression and anxiety, it is also used in the treatment of externalizing problems such as oppositional behavior, delinquency, truancy, substance abuse, and attention deficit hyperactivity disorder (ADHD) (Chorpita and Daleiden 2009). Problem solving can be taught in order to help children control their aggressive behavior (e.g., Kazdin, Siegel, and Bass 1992) and is also included in behavioral parent training (e.g., Sanders 1999). With adolescents, problem solving is the key feature of effective negotiation and compromising with friends, caregivers, and authority figures (Clarke et al. 1990; Curry et al. 2005). Regardless of the symptoms or disorders being treated, problem solving is a systematic technique that slows impulsive behavior and allows children to convert what feels like a conundrum into a solution. With coaching and practice, youth can learn to apply problem solving to a myriad of situations or conflicts and can learn, in effect, how to become their own therapist.

References

Abela, John R. Z., and Benjamin L. Hankin (Eds.). 2008. *Handbook of Depression in Children and Adolescents.* New York: Guilford Press.

American Psychiatric Association. 2000. *Diagnostic and Statistical Manual of Mental Disorders* (4th ed. rev.). Washington, DC: Author.

Brent, David., and Kimbery Poling. 1997. *Cognitive Therapy Treatment Manual forDepressed and Suicidal Youth.* Pittsburgh, CA: University of Pittsburgh, Services for Teens at Risk.

Chorpita, Bruce F., and Eric L. Daleiden. 2009. "Mapping Evidence-Based Treatments for Children and Adolescents: Application of the Distillation and Matching Model to 615 Treatments from 322 Randomized Trials." *Journal of Consulting and Clinical Psychology,* 77: 566–79. DOI: 10.1037/a0014565

Chorpita, Bruce F., and John R. Weisz. 2009. *Modular Approach to Therapy for Childrenwith Anxiety, Depression, Trauma, or Conduct Problems (MATCH-ADTC).* Satellite Beach, FL: Practice Wise.

Clarke, Gregory, Peter M. Lewinsohn, and Hyman Hops. 1990. *Leader's Manual for Adolescent Groups: Coping with Depression Course.* Portland, OR: Kaiser Permanente Center for Health Research.

Cohen, Judith A., Anthony P. Mannarino, and Esther Deblinger. 2006. *Treating Trauma and Traumatic Grief in Children and Adolescents*. New York: Guilford Press.

Curry, John F., Karen C. Wells, David A. Brent, Gregory N. Clarke, Paul Rohde, Anne Marie Albano, … John S. March. 2005. *Treatment for Adolescents with Depression Study (TADS) Cognitive Behavior Therapy Manual: Introduction, Rationale, and Adolescent Sessions*. Durham, NC: Duke University Medical Center, The TADS Team.

D'Zurilla, Thomas J., and Marvin R. Goldfried. 1971. "Problem Solving and Behavior Modification." *Journal of Abnormal Psychology*, 78: 107–26. DOI: 10.1037/h0031360

Dadds, Mark R., and Paula M. Barrett. 2001. "Practitioner Review: Psychological Management of Anxiety Disorders in Childhood." *Journal of Child Psychology and Psychiatry*, 42: 999–1011.

Gladstone, Tracy R. G., and Nadine J. Kaslow. 1995. "Depression and Attributions in Children and Adolescents: A Meta-analytic Review." *Journal of Abnormal Child Psychology*, 23: 597–606. DOI: 10.1007/BF01447664

Jacobs, Rachel H., Mark A. Reinecke, Jackie K. Gollan, and Peter Kane. 2008. "Empirical Evidence of Cognitive Vulnerability for Depression among Children and Adolescents: A Cognitive Science and Developmental Perspective." *Clinical Psychology Review* 28: 759–82. DOI: 10.1016/j.cpr.2007.10.006

Kazdin, Alan E., Todd Siegel, and Deborah Bass. 1992. "Cognitive Problem-Solving Skills: Training and Parent Management Training in the Treatment of Antisocial Behavior in Children." *Journal of Consulting and Clinical Psychology*, 60: 733–47. DOI: 10.1037/0022-006X.60.5.733

Kendall, Phillip C., and Kristina A. Hedke. 2006. *Cognitive Behavioral Therapy for Anxious Children: Therapist Manual* (3rd ed.). Ardmore, PA: Workbook Publishing.

Kendall, Phillip C., Jennifer L. Hudson, Muniya Choudhury, Alicia Webb, and Sandra Pimentel. 2005. Cognitive–Behavioral Treatment for Childhood Anxiety Disorders. In: Euthymia D. Hibbs and Peter S. Jensen (Eds.), *Psychosocial Treatments for Child and Adolescent Disorders: Empirically Based Strategies for Clinical Practice* (2nd ed., pp. 47–73). Washington, DC: American Psychological Association.

Rapee, Ronald M., Heidi J. Lyneham, Carolyn A. Schniering, Viviana Wuthrich, Maree Abbott, Jennifer Hudson, and Ann Wignall. 2006. *The Cool Kids "Chilled" Adolescent Anxiety Program Therapist Manual*. Sydney, Australia: Centre for Emotional Health, Macquarie University.

Sanders, Matt R. 1999. "The Triple P: Positive Parenting Program: Towards an Empirically Validated Multilevel Parenting and Family Support Strategy for the Prevention of Behavior and Emotional Problems in Children." *Clinical Child and Family Psychology Review*, 2: 71–90. DOI: 10.1023/A:1021843613840

Stark, Kevin, Sarah Schnoebelen, Jane Simpson, Jennifer Hargrave, and Rand Glenn. 2007. *Treating Depressed Children: Therapist Manual for "ACTION."* Ardmore, PA: Workbook Publishing.

Stark, Kevin, William Streusand, Prerna Arora, and Puja Patel. 2012. "Childhood Depression: The ACTION Treatment Program." In Philip C. Kendall (Ed.), *Child and Adolescent Therapy Fourth Edition: Cognitive–Behavioral Procedures* (pp. 190–233). New York: Guilford Press.

Vasey, Michael W., and Colin MacLeod. 2001. "Information-Processing Factors in Childhood Anxiety: A Review and Developmental Perspective." In Michael W. Vasey and Mark R. Dadds (Eds.), *The Developmental Psychopathology of Anxiety* (pp. 253–77). New York: Oxford University Press.

Weisz, John R., Christopher A. Thurber, Lynne Sweeney, Valerie D. Proffitt, and Gerald L. LeGagnoux. 1997. "Brief Treatment of Mild to Moderate Child Depression Using Primary and Secondary Control Enhancement Training." *Journal of Consulting and Clinical Psychology*, 65: 703–7. DOI: 10.1037/0022-006X.65.4.703

18

Social Skills Training

Lauren S. Krumholz, Ana M. Ugueto, Lauren C. Santucci, and John R. Weisz

Introduction

Learning to develop and maintain healthy interpersonal relationships is a critical developmental task for children and adolescents (here referred to as "youth"). Youth with anxiety and depression often have interpersonal difficulties, which may reflect limited understanding of social skills, problems with applying the skills in everyday life, or a combination of the two. These difficulties may arise in part because anxious and depressed youth often withdraw socially or react maladaptively, thus limiting their opportunities to learn and practice social skills and to establish healthy relationships. Anxious and depressed youth may increasingly face peer rejection and may experience vulnerability to bullying. Fortunately social skills can be learned and improved through practice.

Social skills training (SST) can be an important component of comprehensive cognitive behavioral therapy (CBT): it enriches interpersonal connections, which can matter so much to girls and boys with internalizing disorders and problems. SST typically addresses *interpersonal engagement, building and maintaining friendships, communication and negotiation, assertiveness,* and *dealing with bullying* (Sburlati, Schniering, Lyneham, and Rapee 2011). These components are included in evidence-based treatments (EBTs) for social phobia (Beidel, Turner, and Morris 1998), post-traumatic stress disorder (Cohen, Mannarino, and Deblinger 2006), transdiagnostic anxiety disorders (Rapee et al. 2006), and major depressive disorder (Clarke, Lewinsohn, and Hops 1990; Curry et al. 2003).

CBT methods of SST include psycho-education, therapist modeling, interactive discussions about hypothetical and real-life examples, behavioral rehearsal, imaginal and *in vivo* exposures, and homework assignments. These methods can be used in group, individual (caregiver or child), and joint caregiver–child sessions. Ideally, SST

Evidence-Based CBT for Anxiety and Depression in Children and Adolescents: A Competencies-Based Approach,
First Edition. Edited by Elizabeth S. Sburlati, Heidi J. Lyneham, Carolyn A. Schniering, and Ronald M. Rapee.
© 2014 John Wiley & Sons, Ltd. Published 2014 by John Wiley & Sons, Ltd.

is tailored to each youth's needs (e.g., specific knowledge deficits or performance issues), as informed by a social skills assessment (e.g., through interviews and observation). Throughout treatment, therapists should provide continual feedback and reinforcement to nurture young clients' acquisition and use of the skills. In the next section we describe training in five key social skills, drawing from the aforementioned EBTs and our own clinical and research experience.

Key Features of Interpersonal Engagement Skills

Interpersonal engagement skills training improves youngsters' ability to navigate social interactions using developmentally appropriate verbal and nonverbal behavior. This training can be useful for anxious and depressed youth in general, but it may be particularly valuable for youth with social phobia. Training focuses on using body language and voice quality, reading social cues, performing greetings and introductions, starting and maintaining conversations, listening and remembering what others have said, and joining and leaving group conversations (Beidel et al. 1998; Rapee et al. 2006). Methods for teaching these skills include didactic instruction, modeling, and behavioral rehearsal.

Therapists should begin by providing youth and their caregivers with a rationale as to the importance of interpersonal engagement skills (e.g., these skills help kids form friendships and have positive interactions with others); then they should describe which skills will be targeted. Therapists should also explain the need to *practice* social skills. In addition to noting that everyone can benefit from practice and that this is a good way to receive feedback about your strengths and areas for improvement, therapists may ask youth for examples of skills they have learned through practice (e.g., riding a bike, playing an instrument) – thus illustrating that learning interpersonal skills is like learning other skills youth have already mastered.

To help young clients better comprehend social cues and use body language and voice quality effectively, therapists should discuss nonverbal behavior that helps people communicate (e.g., facial expressions, eye contact, physical proximity). It can be beneficial to model inappropriate social behavior (e.g., frowning, looking and standing away from the conversational partner), and have youth identify nonverbal errors. Then therapists can model appropriate nonverbal behavior and request feedback, including asking which of the two people portrayed in the examples most kids would prefer to talk to, and why. Additionally, Weisz and colleagues recommend video-recording youth while they are presenting both a "negative" and a "positive" self. This video is then viewed with the youth to facilitate a discussion of differences in presentation style (Weisz, Thurber, Sweeney, Proffitt, and LeGagnoux 1997).

Assisting youth to perform greetings includes teaching them such simple skills as saying "hello" in a pleasant, audible voice and looking at the person when they speak. Another core skill is initiating and maintaining conversations; this involves knowing when to start a conversation (e.g., when first introduced to someone, when seeing a familiar person), how to start a conversation (e.g., smile, comment on something you have in common) with different types of people (e.g., strangers, familiar others), and how to choose an appropriate conversational topic. "Safe" conversational topics for youth include current events, school activities, and common interests (e.g., music and sports). Maintaining conversations involves asking open-ended questions ("What are you doing this summer?"), giving another person time to respond, and recognizing when and how to change topics (e.g., when there is a pause in conversation, use a transitional statement: "Another thing I wanted to talk about is…"). Because anxiety and depression can negatively impact concentration, training should also include practice in listening and remembering information (e.g., a person's name and hobbies) during conversations. To train youth to join and leave group conversations, therapists should use role-plays of relevant real-world scenarios (e.g., joining adolescents at a lunch table, or walking away from children playing kickball).

Additional interpersonal engagement skills (e.g., giving and receiving compliments, talking on the telephone) can also be taught, depending on a youth's particular areas of difficulty. During interpersonal engagement skills training, therapists should first model the skills and then have children engage in behavioral rehearsal, both in session and through therapeutic homework, while continually providing praise for effort and constructive feedback to help shape skill development.

Key Features of Friendship Skills

Friendship skills encompass ways to build and maintain healthy friendships (e.g., Beidel et al. 1998). Friendship skills are often taught to youth with social phobia or depression, and to others who have withdrawn from social interactions. Training in friendship skills involves discussing suitable places to meet friends, inviting children to social activities, reading social cues to gauge someone's level of interest, maintaining consistent contact with friends, and communicating about how to treat others in friendships. Teaching friendship skills in a group format allows group members to work together, contribute their ideas, and role-play skills with others.

When discussing where to meet friends, therapists should encourage brainstorming of different places and activities and should create a list of options. If needed, therapists can make suggestions (e.g., school) and youth can elaborate (e.g., on the school playground, or in art class). Other possible options are community centers, places of worship, and extracurricular programs.

Skill in inviting others to join activities must be complemented by skill in (i) reading social cues and using realistic appraisal of whether the other person is interested; (ii) identifying simple joint activities (e.g., going to a movie); and (iii) using interpersonal engagement skills (e.g., smile, eye contact) to extend an invitation. It is useful to role-play how to extend an initial invitation (e.g., "Want to shoot hoops later?") and to help children determine another person's interest level through nonverbal (e.g., facial expression) and verbal cues. Given that depressed and socially anxious youth often misinterpret cues and assume others are not interested, therapists should listen for overly negative or unrealistic interpretations of others' neutral behavior and, if needed, help youth make more realistic appraisals. Instruction will also be needed in how to proceed depending on the other person's response (e.g., if the response is affirmative, schedule a time for the activity; if it is neutral, ask at a later time; if it is negative, leave that person alone and consider asking someone else). It is beneficial for youth to discuss and practice how they would accept and decline invitations from others in a prosocial manner.

For training in maintaining friendships, therapists should remind their clients that, after *making* a friend, they need to take steps to *maintain* the friendship. Therapists can then teach skills for sustaining friendships (e.g., staying in regular contact, helping friends when they need support, letting friends have other friends), while also eliciting ideas from youth about how to maintain relationships.

Following discussions of these friendship skills, behavioral rehearsal is needed. Therapists can model how to invite someone to join in an activity; then they can encourage youth to role-play scenarios generated by the therapist (e.g., "When inviting your chemistry lab partner to get ice-cream, you say…") and by themselves. Discussing and role-playing problematic social situations with friends can help facilitate skill application. After behavioral rehearsal, therapists should offer praise and corrective feedback and should request constructive comments from the youth participating in each role-play (e.g., ask each child what went well during the role-play: "Good job smiling and asking me to the game" – and what could be improved: "It would be helpful if you looked me in the eyes"). Homework assignments (e.g., inviting someone to an activity this week) will help youth practice these skills.

Peer generalization activities, which involve arranging interactions between youth learning social skills and socially adept peers, also provide opportunities to practice friendship and interpersonal engagement skills (see Beidel et al. 1998 for a more detailed description).

Key Features of Communication and Negotiation Skills

Youth with anxiety and depression may have difficulty communicating, negotiating, and building lasting relationships. Communication includes sending information to others (e.g., by speaking) and receiving information from them (e.g., by listening). Youth can be taught specific strategies to improve communication skills and to become a clearer speaker and a more active listener (Clarke et al. 1990; Curry et al. 2003; Rapee et al. 2006). Failure to say what you mean with accuracy, or to hear what others say without judgment, leads to communication failure and conflict. When conflict arises, youth should be taught to listen carefully, in order to understand others' points of view. Listening does not mean that you *agree*; it simply means that you *hear* what the person is saying. To illustrate the rules of communication, we will use the example of Hannah telling Kate that she interrupts her. While the speaker (Hannah) is talking, the listener (Kate) should not ignore, interrupt, or give advice. Instead, Kate should try to understand Hannah's feelings and point of view while being patient and respectful. Once Hannah is finished, Kate should respond by restating what Hannah said and summarizing how Hannah feels (e.g., "It sounds like you feel disrespected when I interrupt you"). Then Kate can explain her perception of the situation by describing how she feels (e.g., "I was excited to tell my story"), how she reacted (e.g., "I didn't realize I interrupted you. I thought you were done talking"), and what happened – without giving an opinion (e.g., "I started telling my story before you finished"). After both parties share their experiences, Kate may offer to change her behavior (e.g., "I'll try not to interrupt you") or Hannah may suggest how Kate's behavior could change (e.g., "Please try not to interrupt me"). This is but one example; therapists should encourage their young clients to practice communication skills using their own local idioms. By communicating clearly, youth can more effectively inform others of their feelings about an activating event, which may lead to behavior change as well as to fewer future conflicts.

Negotiation and compromise are critical to any relationship, whether between family members, friends, or romantic partners. Therapists should teach youth that the key to compromising is listening when there is conflict, identifying its source, and using problem-solving to resolve it (Clarke et al. 1990; Curry et al. 2003). The reader can consult the problem-solving chapter (Chapter 17) for a description of the five basic steps. When interpersonal disputes are being negotiated, each person involved should participate in solving the problem. For example, if an adolescent wants a later curfew, both the adolescent and caregiver should volunteer possible solutions. Additionally, Clarke and colleagues (1990) recommend that each person mark solutions with a plus or minus sign, to identify which ones are unanimously agreeable. Next, each person should identify strengths and weaknesses in every solution and whether or not (s)he favors it; and each person should be positive and fair in his/her assessment. The two parties must then agree on a solution, which, for one or both, will mean compromising. For instance, the adolescent may want curfew extended by an hour and the caregiver may not wish to extend curfew at all, but they agree to an extended curfew of 30 minutes. Finally, once a solution is reached, the exact details should be written in a contract (Clarke et al. 1990) that states what each person is expected to do, what will happen if either person defaults, and what length of time the agreement is for. Neither party can change the contract until it expires, as it may take time for the agreement to work. A contract for an extended curfew may read:

> Alisha's curfew is 10:30 p.m. on weekends. If she arrives at 10:31 p.m. or later, she can't go out the next weekend. If not home by 10:45 p.m., Mom will call her cell phone to see where she is. If Alisha keeps her curfew for one month, Mom will consider extending her curfew.

Negotiation and compromise are particularly relevant to adolescents seeking greater independence (e.g., when they want to borrow the family car), but may also be applicable to younger children (e.g., when they want to spend the night at a friend's house).

Key Features of Assertiveness Skills

Depressed and anxious youth often have trouble acting assertively – for example, refusing unreasonable or unwanted requests, asking others to change their behavior, or interacting with authority figures (e.g., teachers, coaches, parents). Instead they may react passively – for instance by believing that others are taking advantage of them, by feeling powerless to change their situation, and by avoiding confrontation – or aggressively – for example, by believing that others are trying to take advantage of them and confronting them directly, lashing out physically or verbally. In contrast, assertive youth stand up for themselves by expressing their thoughts and feelings in an appropriate way, which does not harm or violate the rights of others and is consistent with their culture and context. The CBT approach to assertiveness (e.g, Beidel et al. 1998; Clarke et al. 1990; Curry et al. 2003; Rapee et al. 2006) often involves teaching steps like these:

1. Recognize your emotion in the situation.
2. Recognize the emotions of others in the situation *and* let them know you understand how they feel.
3. Tell others how you feel about the situation using "I" statements that avoid criticizing other people (e.g., "I think/don't think," "I feel/don't feel," "I want/ don't want," "I agree/disagree") (Curry et al. 2003).
4. Practice giving brief, honest, tactful feedback when denying a request, asking for some course of action, correcting others' misperceptions, or offering an alternative solution.

Therapists should also help young clients pay attention to their nonverbal behaviors (how they look and present themselves to others) when acting assertively. Youth should stand up straight, with shoulders back, maintain eye contact, and speak in an audible, firm, and pleasant voice, so that others can hear and understand what they are saying. Therapists should be aware of cultural differences and avoid teaching behaviors that may come across as rude or disrespectful instead of assertive. In addition, therapists should emphasize the importance of safety in the context of assertiveness training (e.g., a child in an abusive situation should not be told to be assertive).

Therapists should provide thorough practice of both verbal and nonverbal assertive behaviors. This can begin with having youth list situations in which they feel taken advantage of (e.g., kids cutting in line, or a friend asking to copy homework) and then having them role-play each, starting with easier ones. Youth can role-play with the therapist, with other adults at the clinic, with parents, siblings, and therapy group members. Clarke and colleagues (1990) describe a technique called "assertive imagery," in which adolescents take a mental photograph of a situation they want to change and then convert that photograph into a movie in which they act assertively and others respond in the desired manner. Role-playing a challenging scenario is a way to gain experience as well as confidence.

Assertiveness training often may need to be combined with realistic appraisals, since the youth' distorted interpretations of how others perceive them could interfere with their willingness to exhibit assertive behavior. For example, socially anxious children often fail to act assertively because they think others will not like them if they stand up for themselves or make a demand. Thus young clients may need guidance from therapists for changing overly negative and unrealistic appraisals into more accurate and realistic ones during assertiveness training.

Key Features of Dealing with Bullying Skills

Bullies often target youth who are anxious or submissive or whose reaction makes the bully feel powerful. Assertiveness skills are an important first step in reducing peer victimization. At times, however, enhanced assertiveness is not enough, and youth with anxiety and depression will need additional strategies. Moreover, being assertive in situations of physical bullying could provoke an escalation in violence. Thus, for physical aggression, youth should speak to an authority figure they trust, who can implement environmental changes. The strategies below – as outlined in Rapee et al. (2006) – are most appropriate for teasing or verbal aggression:

1. Help the youth identify someone to talk to about what is happening and how (s)he feels.
2. Encourage the youth to stay close to safe people – for instance, trusted peers or teachers – so as to reduce the likelihood of bullying and increase the likelihood that the bully will be caught. Identify times during the day when the youth is more isolated or away from authority figures (say, on the school bus, at lunch, in recess between classes) and brainstorm ways to expand the audience. If the bully speaks loudly, (s)he may have a greater chance of being caught. Therefore brainstorm how to get the bully to raise his/her voice (e.g., "I didn't catch that. Could you say that one more time?" or gesturing toward his/her ear to suggest the child did not hear what was said) and then role-play these new responses.
3. Teach unexpected ways to respond to bullies. For example, rather than retreating or becoming defensive, angry, or fearful, help the youth identify "clever come-backs" (Rapee et al. 2006), remain calm and uninterested, or ignore the bully's comments. In session, ask the youth to recall situations where bullying occurred, brainstorm what (s)he could have said or done differently, and consider how the bully might have responded. Then rehearse these strategies and decide which of them may be most effective in future encounters.

Caregivers should also be taught skills to help their children deal with bullying. Caregivers can learn ways to support the development, rehearsal, and implementation of the preventative and alternative responses described above; they can be a resource for their child by talking about the bullying, helping to plan ways for the child to be near peers and teachers throughout the day, and so on. In cases of physical aggression, caregivers should seek assistance from the school.

With the rise in technology use among youth, cyber-bullying is an increasingly prevalent form of peer-victimization. Cyber-bullying differs from more traditional bullying in that the perpetrator can remain largely anonymous, bullying can occur any time, and derogatory messages or rumors can be widely and rapidly distributed. Many of the skills reviewed apply to youth who experience cyber-bullying. Specifically, rather than responding with anger or defensiveness – which may perpetuate bullying – these youth should ignore the message or otherwise not respond. They should also keep evidence of cyber-bullying (e.g., save texts or emails, take screenshots of social media sites) in case this information needs to be shared with authority figures. Any threats of violence, sexually explicit messages, or child pornography should be carefully considered, and therapists should consult the ethical code or guidelines of their local professional body and relevant legislation in order to determine how to proceed.

Competence in Treating Anxiety Disorders and Depression

Anxiety

Anxious youth may be particularly vulnerable to impairments in social skills (Kingery, Erdley, Marshall, Whitaker, and Reuter 2010). These social skills deficits may derive from avoidance of social situations – due for instance to fear of negative evaluation, or to fear of doing something embarrassing – which limits social learning opportunities (Rubin and Burgess 2001). Other anxious youth may show maladaptive interpersonal behavior in an effort to protect themselves from perceived threat; so for instance a boy with post-traumatic stress might lash out against peers viewed as threatening (Marsee, Weems, and Taylor 2008). Both social avoidance and hostility can prevent anxious youth from acquiring social skills, while simultaneously supporting the belief that social situations are risky and hard to navigate. In some cases, anxious youth may *know* social skills but not *apply* them due to interfering anxiety: they would become paralyzed by fear when meeting new people (Kingery et al. 2010). Despite the cause of interpersonal difficulties, anxious youth will likely benefit from SST.

Since symptoms associated with anxiety (e.g., misconstrual of the danger of social situations and heightened physiological arousal) can inhibit interpersonal behavior, therapists often need to adapt SST to address the needs of anxious youth. These youth frequently overestimate the likelihood of negative events and underestimate their ability to cope if a negative event were to occur (Dadds and Barrett 2001). Therefore it is important to inquire about children's negative predictions (e.g., "What are you afraid is going to happen?") and then, following the application of each skill, ask whether these predictions came true. Trying out new skills – such as inviting someone for a play date, acting assertively, or confronting bullies – may be particularly anxiety provoking. In building these skills, it is important to use a graduated approach with anxious youth. It may be helpful to construct a fear hierarchy of behaviors in different situations to guide progression through SST. If elevated levels of anxiety persist even after behavioral rehearsal or real-life application of skills, a graduated exposure perspective would suggest that the rehearsal or application may not have lasted long enough to lead to reduced anxiety. Hypothetical scenarios can be designed and sequenced for repeated behavioral rehearsal until habituation is achieved. Anxious youth may also have social interaction habits that make them less appealing to others (e.g., timidity, submissiveness, poor eye contact). These habits can be targeted for practice as part of rehearsing improved nonverbal interaction skills.

Including caregivers in SST can support treatment gains, particularly for younger anxious children (Barrett 2000). Caregivers' usual reactions to their children's anxiety can range from being overly empathic and protective to being highly intolerant and critical. Since the preferred approach to helping youngsters manage anxiety and improve social skills is not necessarily intuitive, therapists may need to model recommended ways of interacting with anxious youth during SST (e.g., they may show enthusiasm for treatment, use differential attention to reinforce bravery, praise the child's efforts and accomplishments, accept and tolerate the child's distress). Caregivers may benefit from knowing which skills their child is learning and practicing; that knowledge will enable them to support the child with encouragement, praise, and feedback on use of the skills. Caregivers may also need to learn how to manage their own emotional reactions to the child's distress and to accept that there will be mistakes and setbacks on the child's path to acquiring improved social skills and greater independence in applying these skills.

Depression

Youth with depression frequently experience interpersonal problems that seem to be reciprocal and transactional, in that impaired social relationships can lead to depression and depression can negatively impact relationships with others (Pilowsky 2009; Rudolph, Flynn, and Abaied 2008). Social skills deficits can also result from limited social interaction, which may stem from low energy, fatigue, or feelings of hopelessness (Rudolph, Hammen, and Burge 1994). Some depressed youth under-stand effective social skills, but may find that their depression interferes with applying them in everyday life (Stark et al. 2008). Irritability, which can accompany depression, may lead to conflict-laden relationships and eventual isolation. The accumulation of negative interactions can exacerbate depressed youth' negative beliefs about self (e.g., "I'm unlikeable") (Rudolph et al. 2008). SST may help address depression by enhancing both interpersonal relationships and self-perceptions.

Therapists should be attuned to common difficulties for depressed youth and adjust SST accordingly. When depression includes distorted thoughts (e.g., "No one likes me") and negative core beliefs (e.g., "I'm ineffective"), youth should be encouraged to gather contradictory evidence (e.g., "Megan seemed to like talking to me," "I got Max to help with our group project"). Rigid, all-or-nothing thinking (e.g., "I'm right and he is totally wrong" or "If I give in now, I'll never get what I want") may require modification. In these and other situations, therapists may need to use cognitive restructuring to address unhelpful thoughts and negative core beliefs before and during SST. Interpersonal engagement skills may be particularly helpful for socially isolated youngsters. In presenting the rationale for SST to depressed youth, therapists can rightly emphasize that improving social skills helps combat depression because engaging in positive activities with others is mood boosting. Moreover, liking and being liked by others helps people feel happier. Because depression often entails magnifying negative events, overgeneralizing predictions of undesirable outcomes, incorrectly taking personal responsibility for negative events, minimizing positive events and attributes, and giving up at the first sign of difficulty or failure, therapists need to prepare depressed youth to persist in using their skills, even when the evidence of success is mixed and the desired outcomes are not imme-diately accomplished. This is especially true in complex social situations, in which others' responses are difficult to predict or control (e.g., even after an assertive response, a bully may continue bullying).

Incorporating caregivers into SST can help facilitate and maintain treatment gains, especially for younger children. Caregivers may find their depressed children difficult to be with when they are sad or irritable, and may respond in negative ways. Therapists can help caregivers understand factors (noted earlier) that impede the development of children's social skills. Caregivers should encourage their children's use of social skills (e.g., during home practice) and provide positive reinforcement for practicing learned skills, with the objective of building self-efficacy related to interpersonal behavior. In addition, caregivers can help their children challenge negative automatic thoughts that interfere with the use of improved social skills.

Competence in Treating both Children and Adolescents

Children

Identifying anxious and depressed children's areas of difficulty with the performance of effective social skills and intervening at a young age can help minimize the build-up of negative sequelae associated with social isolation, conflictual relationships, and bullying. When assessing a child's social skills and the factors that interfere with their effective use, therapists should rely heavily on information provided by caregivers and on direct observation, because children may not fully understand, or be able to articulate, their challenges in the social domain.

Therapists should consider children's developmental level in the realms of cognitive, emotional, and social functioning in order to fit the intervention to their abilities. Younger children and children with lower cognitive functioning will likely benefit from simpler explanations of treatment procedures and activities and from ample modeling from therapists. SST also needs to be adjusted to children's attention span (e.g., there should be frequent breaks for those with difficulties in sustaining attention). Children with underdeveloped emotional skills may benefit from learning emotion identification (i.e., how to correctly label feelings and differentiate between varying levels of emotional distress) and emotion regulation (e.g., relaxation) prior to starting SST. Children who are socially immature may require highly explicit instruction in social skills before engaging in role-play.

More generally, therapists can employ the following recommendations to match children's developmental stage during SST. Children will benefit from concrete, active, and engaging approaches to learning and applying social skills. For example, when teaching young children about social cues such as facial expressions, therapists can have them cut out magazine pictures of people showing different emotions (Beidel et al. 1998). Children will need opportunities for behavioral rehearsal with different types of people (e.g., clinic receptionist, other children, family members) to increase generalization and real-world applicability of the skills. It also is important to start with easier scenarios, so that children experience success, which can build their confidence to try more difficult role-plays. Therapists should be aware of common social dilemmas for children and should solicit input about challenging social situations, so role-plays can be tailored to address children's key issues (e.g., the child is excluded by others on the playground). In addition, therapists should understand how social difficulties are manifested by children of various ages. For example, peer aggression in the preschool years tends to involve brief episodes, but in middle and later childhood aggression is more likely to involve repeated and prolonged victimizing of particular children (Kochenderfer and Ladd 1997; Monks, Ruiz, and Val 2002). To enhance children's motivation to participate in SST activities, therapists may need to implement a reward system for their effort. Rewards should be proportional to the task (e.g., stickers for engaging in role-plays) and meaningful to the child.

Therapists should flexibly match the amount of caregiver inclusion in treatment with the maturity of the child and the nature of the caregiver–child relationship. Younger children may benefit from more caregiver involvement, as they frequently require caregivers' assistance in practicing interpersonal skills. Therapists should work with caregivers to design opportunities for children to develop friendships and use the skills they learned (e.g., organize play dates and trips to places where children often gather, such as parks). Therapists can also teach caregivers techniques to enhance their children's acquisition and use of social skills (e.g., reducing reassurance, building children's independence, encouraging and praising children's use of skills, and ensuring completion of therapeutic homework).

Adolescents

When working with adolescents, therapists should teach and adapt skills to the developmental – cognitive, emotional, social – level of the teen. Even adolescents with reasonably effective emotion regulation skills and capacity to change their behavior may have difficulty learning and implementing new social skills. Additionally, some youth may be reluctant to discuss problems related to interpersonal skills or bullying for fear of embarrassment, while socially immature adolescents may find role-playing silly and may have difficulty practicing specific behaviors without laughing. On the other hand, socially mature adolescents may find certain therapeutic activities to be overly childish, if these are not presented in a developmentally appropriate manner.

Although the core components of each social skill are the same for children and adolescents, therapists should adjust to each individual how the skills are taught and should tailor examples to the problems the adolescent is facing or may experience. As adolescents begin dating, working as an employee, playing on a sports team, running for student body office, or pursing their own interests in music, art, and technology, they will need to learn appropriate ways to voice their opinion, stand up for their rights, and not let peers (e.g., romantic partners, co-workers, team members) or authority figures (e.g., teachers, parents, coaches, bosses) take advantage of them. Relationships with friends become more complex during adolescence, and individuals who were once friends may become enemies. Additionally, dating, attending unchaperoned parties, fitting in or being "cool," and desiring more independence take on greater importance. Therapists should view these challenges as opportunities to teach adolescents how to defend themselves from bullies, negotiate for greater responsibilities and privileges with authority figures, say "no" to unwanted offers of drugs, alcohol, and sexual advances in a firm, assertive manner, and compromise with friends and romantic partners to solve small disagreements and avoid greater conflicts. Therapists can frame the skills and related behaviors as a way for adolescents to more effectively advocate for themselves and their needs, and as skills to be used with a variety of people in a multitude of situations. When role-playing, the adolescent client can first act as the peer she is having difficulty with, while the therapist acts as the client, modeling how the adolescent could respond. Next the roles can be reversed, so that the teen client practices acting as herself/himself. In these role-plays, therapists should be careful to not agree or "give in" to the client or offer to change behavior too quickly, as another person is unlikely to do so.

Common Obstacles to Competent Practice and Methods to Overcome Them

Understanding obstacles that can interfere with SST is crucial to effectively teaching social skills to youth with depression and anxiety. One set of obstacles can derive from failure to conduct a thorough assessment designed to inform treatment planning. A comprehensive assessment involves multiple methods (e.g., observation, interviews, and validated questionnaires) and informants (e.g., child, caregiver, and teacher) focused on the youth's current functioning and abilities (Whitcomb and Merrell 2013). Collecting information from independent observers may be especially important in the assessment of social skills, as skills may differ across settings and youth may have limited insight into their own behavior. The social skills assessment should reveal the youth's strengths and most severe problems and areas of functional impairment. For example, a boy with social phobia who is bullied may have a great sense of humor, but significant difficulty staying close to others to maintain an audience – a helpful strategy for dealing with bullying. In this case, treatment should help him manage anxiety in social situations prior to targeting skills for dealing with bullying. Assessment of functioning and abilities should occur throughout treatment to evaluate progress and to guide treatment. Furthermore, therapists must be aware of a family's cultural background and appreciate contextual factors that are salient for a youth (e.g., cultural, ethnic, gender, and religious issues). For example, teaching an Orthodox Jewish adolescent girl to shake hands with a man could violate cultural rules about appropriate touch between men and women.

Additional obstacles can stem from insufficient collaboration among therapists, youth, and caregivers. Through close collaboration and a strong working relationship, therapists can identify interpersonal skills deficits and design treatment to maximize success. Therapists should move at the child's pace, striking a balance between challenging the youth to use the learned skills and understanding the difficulties that this may present. A climate of openness to feedback will help caregivers and youth feel more comfortable discussing setbacks in treatment, how the youth is progressing, and which skills require additional practice.

Another obstacle is the therapist's hesitation to model interpersonal skills and to have children engage in role-plays. While didactic presentations and interactive discussions about social skills are important, therapists must also ensure that young clients have ample opportunities to observe and practice social skills. Therapists may hesitate because they are reluctant to increase their clients' anxiety, or they may feel unprepared to manage distress from youth and caregivers during role-plays or exposure tasks. Learning to appreciate the rationale and empirical foundation of these techniques and understanding long-term gains that result from short-term distress during these activities can help to assuage therapists' hesitancy.

Failure to adequately include caregivers in treatment is an additional obstacle. Therapists should take steps to ensure appropriate caregiver involvement. Inquiring about barriers to involvement and initiating joint problem solving to address those barriers can increase caregiver participation (e.g., when caregivers have busy schedules, therapists can try to remain flexible as to when they are available to meet). Ideally, caregivers will learn the same skills as their children, in order to act as coaches, encouraging and reinforcing children's application of social skills at home, at school, and in the community. Ongoing communication between youth and caregivers about the skills being learned and how practice is working can help caregivers play a crucial role and help youth take ownership of the skills.

Another obstacle involves children's lack of motivation to participate in SST. As noted earlier, therapists should make learning social skills fun, engaging, and interactive and should provide encouragement and labeled praise for effort (e.g., "Great job looking me in the eyes and smiling when you said hello"). When youth resist role-playing, therapists can use humor and funny situations (e.g., the therapist can first demonstrate the wrong way to join a group and then give each child a "scripted" personality for a role-play) or can have the whole group complete the first several role-plays together. Young people's desire to actively participate in SST can also be increased by tying the skills to their goals for therapy (e.g., "Today we are going to talk about how to start conversations with people; this will help you make new friends like you said you wanted when we first started meeting"). Some youngsters may also benefit from a reward system designed to enhance motivation.

Finally, one of the most common obstacles is the difficulty generalizing learned social skills and extending them to new people and new situations. The goal of generalization must be actively targeted by therapists. If youth are not progressing in the generalization of skills, therapists need to carefully consider the source of interference. Has the therapist arranged for ample opportunities for the child to practice the skills with different people in various situations? Has the youth received corrective feedback following behavioral rehearsal? Are cognitive distortions preventing the successful application of skills? Is the youth afraid that, even if (s)he exhibits good interpersonal skills, (s)he will not achieve the desired outcomes? The most frequent reason for the limited generalization of skills is a lack of practice outside of therapy sessions. Home practice assignments are key. If these assignments are not completed, therapists should openly discuss with caregivers and youth the factors interfering with practice and should work to find solutions. It can also be helpful for therapists to start with smaller homework requests and gradually increase them as youth successfully complete assignments. Including SST can be critical to success in CBT for anxious and depressed youth, as it builds skills that generate powerful payoffs in the social world of young people.

References

Barrett, Paula M. 2000. "Treatment of Childhood Anxiety: Developmental Aspects." *Clinical Psychology Review*, 20: 479–94.

Beidel, Deborah C., Samuel M. Turner, and Tracey L. Morris. 1998. *Social Effectiveness Therapy for Children: A Treatment Manual*. Unpublished manuscript.

Clarke, Gregory, Peter M. Lewinsohn, and Hyman Hops. 1990. *Leader's Manual for Adolescent Groups: Coping with Depression Course*. Portland, OR: Kaiser Permanente Center for Health Research.

Cohen, Judith A., Anthony P. Mannarino, and Esther Deblinger. 2006. *Treating Trauma and Traumatic Grief in Children and Adolescents*. New York: Guilford Press.

Curry, John F., Karen C. Wells, David A. Brent, Gregory N. Clarke, Paul Rohde, Anne Marie Albano, … John S. March. 2003. *Treatment for Adolescents with Depression Study (TADS) Cognitive Behavior Therapy Manual: Introduction, Rationale, and Adolescent Sessions*. Durham, NC: Duke University Medical Center, The TADS Team.

Dadds, Mark R., and Paula M. Barrett. 2001. "Practitioner Review: Psychological Management of Anxiety Disorders in Childhood." *Journal of Child Psychology and Psychiatry*, 42: 999–1011.

Kingery, Julie N., Cynthia A. Erdley, Katherine C. Marshall, Kyle G. Whitaker, and Tyson R. Reuter. 2010. "Peer Experiences of Anxious and Socially Withdrawn Youth: An Integrative Review of the Developmental and Clinical Literature." *Clinical Child and Family Psychology Review*, 13: 91–128.

Kochenderfer, Becky J., and Gary W. Ladd. 1997. "Victimized Children's Responses to Peers' Aggression: Behaviors Associated with Reduced versus Continued Victimization." *Development and Psychopathology*, 9: 59–73.

Marsee, Monica A., Carl F. Weems, and Leslie K. Taylor. 2008. "Exploring the Association between Aggression and Anxiety in Youth: A Look at Aggressive Subtypes, Gender, and Social Cognition." *Journal of Child and Family Studies*, 17: 154–68.

Monks, Claire P., Rosario O. Ruiz, & Elena T. Val. 2002. "Unjustified Aggression in Preschool." *Aggressive Behavior*, 2: 458–76.

Pilowsky, Daniel J. 2009. "Depression: Causes and Risk Factors." In Joseph M. Rey and Boris Birmaher (Eds.), *Treating Child and Adolescent Depression* (pp. 17–22). Philadephia, PA: Lippincott Williams & Wilkins.

Rapee, Ronald M., Heidi J. Lyneham, Carolyn A. Schniering, Viviana Wuthrich, Maree Abbott, Jennifer Hudson, and Anne Wignall. 2006. *Cool Kids Child and Adolescent Anxiety Program Therapist Manual*. Sydney: Centre for Emotional Health, Macquarie University.

Rubin, Kenneth H., and Kim B. Burgess. 2001. "Social Withdrawal and Anxiety." In Michael W. Vasey and Mark R. Dadds (Eds.), *The Developmental Psychopathology of Anxiety* (pp. 407–34). New York: Oxford University Press.

Rudolph, Karen D., Megan Flynn, and Jamie L. Abaied. 2008. "A Developmental Perspective on Interpersonal Theories of Youth Depression." In John R. Z. Abela and Benjamin L. Hankin (Eds.), *Handbook of Depression in Children and Adolescents* (pp. 224–49). New York: Guilford Press.

Rudolph, Karen D., Constance Hammen, and Dorli Burge. 1994. "Interpersonal Functioning and Depressive Symptoms in Childhood: Addressing the Issues of Specificity and Comorbidity." *Journal of Abnormal Child Psychology*, 22 (3): 355–71.

Sburlati, Elizabeth S., Carolyn A. Schniering, Heidi J. Lyneham, and Ronald M. Rapee. 2011. "A Model of Therapist Competencies for the Empirically Supported Cognitive Behavioral Treatment of Child and Adolescent Anxiety and Depressive Disorders." *Clinical Child and Family Psychology Review*, 14: 89–109.

Stark, Kevin D., Jennifer Hargrave, Brooke Hersh, Michelle Greenberg, Jenny Herren, and Melissa Fisher. 2008. "Treatment of Childhood Depression: The ACTION Treatment Program." In John R. Z. Abela and Benjamin L. Hankin (Eds.), *Handbook of Depression in Children and Adolescents* (pp. 224–49). New York: Guilford Press.

Weisz, John R., Christopher A. Thurber, Lynne Sweeney, Valerie D. Proffitt, and Gerald L. LeGagnoux. 1997. "Brief Treatment of Mild-to-Moderate Child Depression Using Primary and Secondary Control Enhancement Training." *Journal of Consulting and Clinical Psychology*, 65: 703–7.

Whitcomb, Sara A., and Kenneth W. Merrell. 2013. *Behavioral, Social, and Emotional Assessment of Children and Adolescents* (4th ed.). New York: Routledge.

19

Modifying the Family Environment

Polly Waite, Monika Parkinson, Lucy Willetts, and Cathy Creswell

Introduction

Studies that have evaluated family-based CBT interventions have not provided compelling evidence that the inclusion of families improves treatment outcome for children and young people by comparison with individual child-focused treatments (Creswell and Cartwright-Hatton 2007); however, the very fact that most young people live with their family and rely on it for their basic needs to be met suggests that families should be taken into consideration in some respect when treating the child or young person. Accordingly, evidence-based treatments for anxiety and depression in young people have typically recommended the involvement of families in treatment; but the degree to which they are involved and the nature of this involvement varies. In some cases parental involvement may be focused on facilitating treatment for the young person (e.g., by bringing him/her to treatment sessions and by encouraging him/her to complete home tasks), but in other cases family factors may play a role in the maintenance of the disorder, hence the treatment may be more efficient and effective if these factors are addressed as part of the treatment.

This chapter describes different ways clinicians may target potential family-maintenance factors, using a range of techniques drawn from evidence-based treatment programs and from our own clinical practice. We will begin by describing a model for understanding possible family-related cognitive and behavioral pathways to the development and maintenance of anxiety and depression in children and young people. We will then outline specific therapist competencies for working with families, before referring to how families have been involved within specific interventions for anxiety disorders and depression in children and young people. Finally, we will discuss decision-making considerations about who should be involved in treatment and common obstacles to overcome in treatment.

Evidence-Based CBT for Anxiety and Depression in Children and Adolescents: A Competencies-Based Approach,
First Edition. Edited by Elizabeth S. Sburlati, Heidi J. Lyneham, Carolyn A. Schniering, and Ronald M. Rapee.
© 2014 John Wiley & Sons, Ltd. Published 2014 by John Wiley & Sons, Ltd.

The Role of the Family Environment in Anxiety and Depression in Children and Young People

Although the role of the family environment in the development and maintenance of anxiety and depression in children and young people is not fully understood, research evidence to date suggests an interplay between a number of different factors, which include genetics, the young person's temperament, and environmental factors. Environmental factors that are particularly amenable to intervention are parental expectations, beliefs, and behaviors around and in response to the child. Figure 19.1 shows a model for understanding potential cognitive and behavioral parenting pathways to anxiety and depression in children and young people, adapted from Creswell, Murray, James, and Cooper (2011). The model suggests that anxiety or depression in children and young people may be maintained by particular parental beliefs, expectations, and behavioral responses as well as by wider parental practices, which may themselves be reinforced by the young person's anxious or depressive responses. Furthermore, parental psychopathology may both elevate, and be elevated by, an increased level of these cognitive and behavioral responses among parents and their children.

One example, outlined in the model, is a scenario where a parent may have overly high expectations of his/her child that lead to criticism, conflict, and low levels of praise (Cole and Rehm 1986). Such responses may then reinforce the young person's negative self-belief and withdrawal, thus creating a bigger discrepancy between parents' expectations and the young person's performance. Alternatively, if a parent holds low expectations, for example, of his/her child's ability to cope with challenge, this may lead to parental over-involvement and reduced encouragement (Creswell, Apetroaia, Murray, and Cooper 2012). These responses may cause a young person

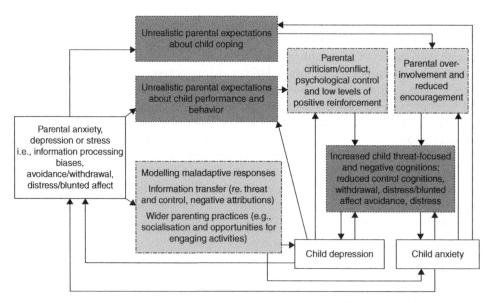

Figure 19.1 Cognitive and behavioral parenting pathways to child anxiety and depression. Adapted from Creswell, Murray, James, and Cooper (2011).

to have a low sense of mastery and highlight potential threats in the environment, thus maintaining anxiety and confirming the parent's beliefs and expectations.

In addition to parental responses to the child, parental behaviors around the child may also serve to maintain the young person's symptoms of anxiety and depression. For example, parental modeling of maladaptive responses, such as inhibited behaviors (Murray et al. 2008), avoidance of problem-solving behaviors, or withdrawal from pleasant activities (Goodman and Gotlib 1999) may promote similar responses among children and young people. Similarly, parental narrative styles may transfer information that highlights possible dangers or reinforces avoidance of potential challenge (e.g., Barrett, Rapee, Dadds, and Ryan 1996).

Key Features of Competencies

The above model has implications for how therapists work clinically with families of children and young people with anxiety and depressive disorders in order to improve efficiency and outcomes from treatment. In line with this model, Sburlati, Schniering, Lyneham, and Rapee (2011, p. 94) outline the following specific CBT techniques for working with families: (i) parent emotion management; (ii) parent expectations management; (iii) family communication and conflict resolution; (iv) parental intrusiveness and overprotection management; (v) parental contingency management; and (vi) parent modeling of adaptive behavior. We will now describe each of these techniques in greater detail, highlighting the theory and research behind each one, describing how therapists can implement these techniques and, finally, providing case examples that aim to highlight how a therapist could make use of these techniques when working with child and adolescent anxiety and depression.

Parent emotion management

It is well established that parents of children and young people with anxiety have higher rates of anxiety and depressive disorders than parents of young people who are not anxious (e.g., Cooper, Fearn, Willetts, Seabrook, and Parkinson 2006; Last, Hersen, Kazdin, Orvaschel, and Perrin 1991), and that lifetime prevalence rates of depression in parents of children and young people with depression are considerably higher than in parents of young people who do not have depression (e.g., Asarnow, Goldstein, Tompson, and Guthrie 1993). Furthermore, parental anxiety and depression have been found to be associated with poorer treatment outcomes for children and young people with anxiety (e.g., Cobham, Dadds, and Spence 1998; Cooper, Gallop, Willetts, and Creswell 2008; Southam-Gerow, Kendall, and Weersing 2001), while remission in depression in mothers has been found to have a positive impact on their child's psychiatric symptoms (including depression) and functioning (e.g., Birmaher 2011; Weissman et al. 2006; Wickramaratne et al. 2011).

There are a number of reasons that may account for poorer treatment outcomes for children and young people in the context of parental emotional difficulties, including shared stressful life events (e.g., Hammen et al. 1987) and genetic factors (e.g., Eley et al. 2011); but here we have focused on those cognitive and behavioral factors that are amenable to therapeutic change. As suggested in Figure 19.1 and illustrated in Case 19.1a, anxiety and depression in parents are hypothesized to make them behave in a way that may maintain their child's problem. Examples of such behavior are taking over, enabling the child to avoid a situation, disengaging from the young person and from the family, and modeling maladaptive responses. These responses may be accounted for by parents' negative expectations about the child (e.g., "she'll freak out," "he's not going to be able to cope," or "she's going to fail") or by parents' ability to alter or cope with the situation ("unless I get involved, they won't be able to cope," "there is nothing I can do," or "I can't bear it").

If the anxiety or depression experienced by the parent is clinically significant, that parent may be keen to seek individual therapy to address his/her own concerns. However, many individuals with significant mental health difficulties wait a considerable amount of time before seeking help through clinical services (e.g., Hollander 1997; Stobie, Taylor, Quigley, Ewing, and Salkovskis 2007); this is likely to relate to a range of factors, including fear of or shame about revealing one's experiences to others. Therefore the child's or young person's clinician may have an important role in enabling the parent to make sense of his/her symptoms and to understand their impact on the child, in challenging any associated beliefs that may be unhelpful

---

Case 19.1a   Background to Joshua

Georgia was the mother of two sons. Her younger son, 8-year-old Joshua, was referred to the clinic for separation anxiety and generalized anxiety. Joshua had difficulty going to school as he struggled to part from his mum at the school gate in the morning and worried about being away from her during the day in case something bad happened to her. Georgia responded to Joshua's separation anxiety by taking him into the class each day, sorting out his coat and bag for him and waiting with him until the class was ready to start. Joshua also experienced anxiety during the school day about a variety of everyday issues: struggling with his work, forgetting his school lunch money, and being teased by another child. Georgia frequently went into school and tried to resolve these issues on Joshua's behalf. At home, Joshua found it difficult to go upstairs without his mum or brother, as he worried something might get him. Bedtimes were also a problem and Georgia was finding it increasingly difficult to get Joshua to go to sleep without her being there to reassure him.

During sessions with Georgia it became clear that she experienced a great deal of anxiety about her children and worried that harm might come to them. She described how it was difficult for her to allow them to go out of her sight without experiencing worry and intrusive images of something bad happening to them. She found that she could only manage the worry by phoning to check they were okay or by keeping the boys in her sight, even when they were playing in the back garden. She also refused invitations from friends to go out in the evening, as she worried that, if she went out and left the boys with a babysitter, something terrible could happen without her being there to protect them.

Case 19.1b   Working with Joshua's mum around her own emotions

Joshua's mum, Georgia, worked with the therapist to better understand her own cognitions, feelings, and behaviors and together they were able to *map out how these were contributing to Joshua's anxiety. Through psycho-education and by carrying out a survey* of other parents, the therapist successfully taught Georgia that these kinds of worries and images, while distressing, are normal and experienced by everyone. She had already come to the conclusion that her phone calls were exacerbating the problem, and so the therapist and Georgia designed a *behavioral experiment* that Georgia then undertook, in which Joshua went to a friend's house and she did not phone to check on him. As a result, she learned that nothing bad happened, that she could cope without phoning, and that over time her anxiety diminished. In turn, this had a positive effect on Joshua's anxiety, as it increased his confidence that he could cope with being away from his mum without her making contact, and it set him an example of ways to manage fears and worries.

---

in relation to the child's treatment progress, in addressing issues around stigma and blame, in providing information about services and the process of therapy, and in supporting the parent in the referral process.

In cases where symptoms are not at a clinically significant level, *parent emotion management* (Sburlati et al. 2011) can be used throughout treatment (e.g., Rapee et al. 2006), to enable parents to learn the same CBT strategies that are taught to the young person. By using the example of Joshua and his mother Georgia, Case 19.1b illustrates strategies that a therapist could use to address parental emotions.

Parental expectations management

The expectations that parents place on their children can impact on parental behavioral responses and ultimately on the young person's self-perception. Parents of children and young people with depression are more likely to have unrealistically high expectations of their children (Cole and Rehm 1986) and are less likely to provide positive reinforcement, or they reserve positive reinforcement for high achievements (Cole and Rehm 1986; Pineda, Cole, and Bruce 2007). High parental criticism and hostility, emotional over-involvement, and a lack of warmth have been observed in families of children and young people with depression (e.g., Asarnow et al. 1993; Goodman and Gotlib 1999), and young people with depression consistently report less support, warmth, and closeness from parents (Greenberger, Chen, Tally, and Dong 2000). In the context of depression in children and young people, these parental expectations and behaviors are likely to compound the young person's difficulties. For children and young people with anxiety, it is hypothesized that low parental expectations, for example, about the child's ability to cope may lead parents to reinforce their child's avoidant and over-dependent behaviors, maintaining the young person's anxiety (e.g., Creswell et al. 2011; Hudson and Rapee 2004).

The main features of parental expectations management strategies include therapists' identification of areas where parental expectations are unrealistic (e.g., either too high or too low/anxious), and working with parents to find a more balanced and empathic approach. For children and young people with both anxiety and depression, this may first involve psycho-education with the family about the influence of symptoms of anxiety and depression on the young person, in order to help parents develop realistic expectations. This may be followed by discussion and formulation designed to develop a shared understanding of the potential cycles in which parental expectations and responses may maintain the young person's anxious and/or depressed cognitions and behaviors, and vice versa. Parents are thus helped by therapists to identify and try out different responses to their child, in order to test alternative expectations and appraisals of their child's behaviors. Case 19.2a illustrates several strategies that therapists may use to help parents manage their expectations of their child.

Case 19.2a   Sophie's background and helping her parents to manage expectations

Fifteen-year-old Sophie was referred by her general practitioner to the local child and adolescent mental health service after her mother reported that she "couldn't cope with her anymore." Sophie had become withdrawn and quiet but also very irritable at times. She had stopped seeing friends and going to her usual afterschool clubs and would often spend hours in her room, avoiding the rest of the family and avoiding her usual activities and chores. When Sophie did spend time with the family, it often resulted in arguments, especially with her mother and younger brother. Sophie also started avoiding doing her schoolwork, and she would get very upset with her parents when they commented on this. It became clear after a detailed assessment that Sophie was depressed and had been feeling progressively worse over the past six months. The family had experienced a number of stressful events prior to Sophie's mood change and, in addition, Sophie's boyfriend had recently ended their relationship. Sophie's mum also had a long history of depression, which was currently controlled with medication. Sophie's father suffered from periods of intense anxiety and saw himself as "a bit of a perfectionist."

In the initial treatment sessions, the therapist aimed to *develop a shared understanding* of Sophie's difficulties, with both Sophie and her parents. It became clear that the family experienced regular conflict about small matters and there were difficulties in being able to see others' points of view. Sophie and her parents avoided open and honest discussions and seemed to engage in a lot of "mind-reading without listening," which tended to result in misunderstandings and stressful interactions. For example, Sophie's father thought that Sophie just didn't care about her schoolwork, so he reminded her regularly about her recent low grades as a way of trying to motivate her to work harder. He actually thought she was very bright and capable and didn't understand why she wasn't applying herself more. Sophie assumed that her father thought she was stupid and lazy and felt criticized whenever he mentioned her grades. She was convinced that he thought she was "a waste of space." Sophie would become angry and snap back at her father, which usually escalated into arguments. It was also evident that the family was overwhelmed by many practical problems that were not being addressed, and this added to the stress and regular family conflict.

The therapist first *established a list of agreed goals* with the family. Everyone was encouraged to agree to an order of *priority for these goals*. Both Sophie and her parents identified several shared goals, including the goal of "everyone getting along more" as an important area to work on, and Sophie wanted her parents to "stop being on her back all the time." The therapist *provided psycho-education about depression* and associated symptoms and the role of stress as a risk and maintaining factor in depression. The therapist emphasized the debilitating nature of depressive symptoms and suggested that Sophie may be struggling with her usual set of activities and responsibilities due to these symptoms. This helped the parents to *lower their expectations* of Sophie's behavior. The therapist *modeled patient and active listening* and summarized everyone's experiences and possible maintenance cycles through the use of *simple maintenance diagrams* on a flipchart. It was helpful for the family to see how small misunderstandings or times when they didn't listen to each other and made assumptions often led to bigger arguments and seemed to make Sophie feel more "useless," depressed, hopeless, and withdrawn from the family.

In a separate session with Sophie's parents, the therapist revisited the topics from the previous session and encouraged the parents to further discuss family interactions and how these may impact on Sophie's mood. This was an opportunity for the therapist to *address parental beliefs* about depressive symptoms and the level of Sophie's control over them. Sophie's father reflected that he was unaware his well-meaning comments may have been perceived as critical by Sophie; and he hadn't realized that she found it so hard to concentrate because of her low mood. The therapist helped the parents *identify new ways of responding* to Sophie, with an emphasis on a *calm and empathic* parenting style, *positive reinforcement* (particularly when Sophie showed approach-type behavior and engagement with family and activities, as opposed to withdrawal) and *lower and more realistic expectations*.

Family communication and conflict resolution

Communication and conflict difficulties arise in most families from time to time, but they are particularly important in the context of anxiety and depression in children and young people. Interpersonal conflicts within the home environment are often stressful and, as such, they present risk and function as maintaining factors, for depression in particular (Grant, Compas, Thurm, McMahon, and Gipson 2004; Joiner, Coine, and Blalock 1999). Families where there is a young person with depression have been found to experience more communication problems and greater levels of interpersonal conflict (e.g., Kaslow, Deering, and Racusin 1994; Rapee 1997), and young people with depression report more frequent perceptions of family conflict (Stein et al. 2000). In addition, conflict with parents is associated with suicidal behavior in young people (Kerfoot, Dyer, Harrington, Woodham, and Harrington 1996).

The interpersonal difficulties experienced by children and young people with depression (Gotlib and Hammen 1992; Sheeber, Davis, Lever, Hops, and Tildesley 2007) may be influenced by negative cognitive biases associated with depressed mood (Beck 1976). For example, young people with depression are more likely to make negative attributions about their parents' behaviors and to underreport parental happy and neutral affect, by comparison with young people who do not have depression (Ehrmantrout, Allen, Leve, Davis, and Sheeber 2011), so the former may be inclined to respond in a more hostile manner to their parents. These interactions may be exacerbated in the presence of parental psychopathology, in particular depressed mood (e.g., Goodman and Gotlib 1999), which is likely to influence both cognitive and behavioral parental responses. Taken together or in combination, these factors may create an environment that is vulnerable to a vicious cycle characterized by frequent family discord and depression in both young people and their parents.

Several empirically tested treatments for children and young people with depression include strategies aimed at *family communication and conflict resolution* (e.g., Brent and Poling 1997; Clarke, Lewinsohn, and Hops 1990; Curry et al. 2005). The main aim of the strategies is to help family members to communicate more effectively with each other in order to improve the relationship between parents and their children and to reduce the likelihood of interpersonal conflict. One of the most common conflict resolution strategies employed with families in treatment programs is family problem-solving skills training. In conflict resolution or family problem-solving skills training, those family members involved in the conflict are taught by the therapist to (i) identify the problem; (ii) generate potential solutions together; (iii) evaluate the predicted outcome for each of these solutions; (iv) choose the most appropriate course of action; and (v) evaluate the outcome (e.g., Curry et al. 2005; Rapee et al. 2006). Case 19.2b illustrates how therapists may use family problem-solving skills training (in combination with other CBT strategies and techniques) to address *family communication and conflict resolution*.

Parental intrusiveness and overprotection management

It is well established that there is a link between anxiety in children and young people and parental control (e.g., Wood, McLeod, Sigman, Hwang, and Chu 2003), in particular a lack of autonomy granting (McLeod, Wood, and Weisz 2007). In addition, experimental research has supported the hypothesis that a lack of autonomy granting leads to an increase in anxiety symptoms in children and young people (e.g., de Wilde and Rapee 2008; Thirlwall and Creswell 2010). With regard to low mood, psychological control – such as manifest in the induction of guilt and/or shame – has been linked to childhood depression (e.g., Barber 1996). Similarly, depressed children describe their parents as more controlling than do those without depression (e.g., Stark, Humphrey, Crook and Lewis 1990).

Case 19.2b   Reducing conflict and improving communication with Sophie and her family

The therapist encouraged Sophie and her parents to engage in several exercises aimed to teach them *effective problem-solving strategies* in order to reduce conflict and rehearse alternatives to avoidance in dealing with problems. They were encouraged to draw up *common problem lists*, generate solutions, evaluate them, and choose appropriate ones with *action plans*. It became apparent that Sophie and her parents had very different views about how to solve particular problems (e.g., how little quality time the family had together), and at first there was quite a bit of resentment and conflict about how to tackle these things together. This was an opportunity for the therapist to help the family with skills such as *active listening, negotiation and compromise, assertiveness and disclosure of feelings*, and *making contracts of agreement*. Making written contracts for how to manage common problems was particularly helpful when emotions escalated at home and the contract (hanging on the fridge in the kitchen) could be consulted to remind everyone of the agreed steps. The therapist also helped the family to *schedule pleasant family activities* in order to ensure that opportunities for positive time together were created and acted upon.

Reducing parental overprotectiveness and intrusiveness is thus seen as an important part of the treatment for children and young people with anxiety disorders, where these parental behaviors are evident in the family environment. Such reduction can be achieved by using a number of strategies, which ultimately aim to promote independence in the young person. Initially it is helpful for the therapist to identify the type of situations in which the parent is being intrusive or overprotective; and these situations may well be linked to areas in which the parent experiences anxiety (Creswell et al. 2012). For example, Figure 19.2 demonstrates the maintenance cycle that was developed for Case 19.1a, which then informed treatment interventions.

Consideration of what is appropriate for the young person's developmental level is also important. Supporting the parent in allowing the child to be more independent might involve providing the parent with alternative ways to support the young person, such as promoting the young person's use of particular CBT strategies, for instance problem solving or Socratic questioning. It may also involve contingency management, whereby the parent actively rewards the young person for independent activity. The reduction of parental provisions of reassurance is often a key part of promoting autonomy; instead, the therapist should enable parents to encourage their child to challenge their anxious thoughts and should give the young person clear positive messages about his/her ability to cope on his/her own. Some parents may find reducing their overprotectiveness extremely challenging. In our experience, empowering parents to feel confident about using alternative responses is often effective. However, at times parental emotions and expectations will need to be managed in the first instance, in order to allow them to change their behavioral responses to their child. Case 19.1c illustrates a therapist making use of *parental intrusiveness and overprotection management* in combination with other specific CBT techniques.

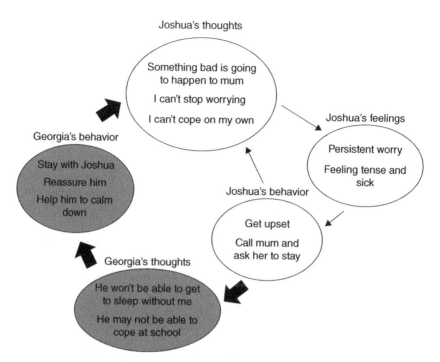

Joshua's thoughts

Something bad is going to happen to mum

I can't stop worrying

I can't cope on my own

Joshua's feelings

Persistent worry

Feeling tense and sick

Georgia's behavior

Stay with Joshua

Reassure him

Help him to calm down

Joshua's behavior

Get upset

Call mum and ask her to stay

Georgia's thoughts

He won't be able to get to sleep without me

He may not be able to cope at school

Figure 19.2 The maintenance cycle around bedtimes that was developed with Georgia, Joshua's mum.

Case 19.1c   Increasing Joshua's autonomy and independence

The therapist discussed with Joshua's mum, Georgia, what might be developmentally appropriate ways of dealing with the situations where Joshua becomes anxious (e.g., at the beginning of the school day and at bedtimes) and considered how to *encourage Joshua's independence* in managing them. Using a process of *graded exposure and associated contingency management*, Georgia gradually withdrew her support in the morning on arrival at school, until Joshua was able to play in the playground with his friends before entering the classroom on his own. By doing this, Joshua learnt that he was able to cope without Georgia when he arrived at school. She *also encouraged him to problem-solve the issues* that arose at school, with her support, and to *independently try out one of the solutions* that were generated. For example, Joshua agreed to talk to his teacher at the end of class if he had found the work difficult, rather than asking Georgia to talk to the teacher for him. Once again, this challenged his beliefs about not being able to cope without Georgia. The therapist and Georgia also reflected on Joshua's general levels of independence, and Georgia elected to *encourage him to be more independent in a number of other areas*, including his packing his own school bag each morning and having an alarm clock to allow him to get up independently in the morning. The combination of these strategies was successful in increasing not only Joshua's level of independence, but also his confidence and self-esteem, and it enabled him to develop a belief that he was able to cope independently in a variety of different situations.

Parental contingency management

Contingency management is used, with excellent outcomes, in the treatment of children and young people with a number of disorders (most commonly, oppositional defiant and conduct disorder) (e.g., Webster-Stratton 1984). It is also routinely included, with good effect, in anxiety-focused interventions for young people (e.g., Cartwright-Hatton, Laskey, Rust, and McNally 2010; Rapee et al. 2006). Contingency management is, however, not a key component in the treatment for children and young people with depression. Nevertheless, there is some research to suggest that, in families where a young person is depressed, the levels of praise are lower (Cole and Rehm 1986), and that, when the young person expresses positive emotions or behavior, parents may respond in a negative or withdrawn way, while responding more positively when the young person appears more depressed (e.g., Schwartz et al. 2012). This suggests that there may be a role for contingency management in the treatment of depression in young people.

Contingency management encourages parents to reinforce positive, adaptive behaviors and to ignore or negatively reinforce unhelpful or undesirable behaviors. In the first instance, it is important for the therapist to acknowledge that it is often a natural response to pay particular attention to the young person when (s)he is struggling (whether this attention is manifested in providing reassurance, stepping in to solve the problem, or expressing frustration) and less attention when the person is managing well. It is then essential that the therapist provides a clear rationale for positively reinforcing attempts to cope with challenges or to try out new responses.

Therapists can then encourage parents to keep records of their own responses to the young person's behaviors in order to gather a clear picture of possible reinforcers. This will include parental responses to the young person when (s)he is anxious or depressed (e.g., the parents' being aware of whether they are critical to a greater or smaller extent depending on their child's mood, or their being aware of providing excessive comforting and reassurance to the child), as well as parental responses when the young person is managing well (e.g., the parents' not noticing, ignoring, or responding in withdrawn, negative ways). The therapist would then work with the parents to identify whether they are giving excessive reassurance or attention to anxious behaviors and/or are being overly critical of their depressed child, then to replace these actions with Socratic questioning, helping the child to make use of his/her own problem-solving strategies. Parents can also be taught to respond positively to adaptive behaviors by giving specific and labeled praise or by using a structured reward system, and to actively ignore undesirable behaviors. Case 19.3a provides an example of how parental contingency management (in combination with other CBT strategies and techniques) might be used by a therapist who is seeing a young boy with anxiety and his parents.

Parent modeling of adaptive behavior

Experimental and prospective longitudinal research has shown that children's responses to potentially fear-provoking stimuli are influenced by their observation of how adults behave (e.g., De Rosnay, Cooper, Tsigaras, and Murray 2006; Gerull and Rapee 2002; Murray, Cooper, Creswell, Schofield, and Sack 2007; Murray et al. 2008).

Case 19.3a   Background and contingency management with George's parents

George was a 6-year-old boy who experienced social anxiety. George's parents, Katherine and Mark, came to the clinic with George for the initial assessment. Mark reported that George had always been shy and found new situations difficult. George would become anxious as soon as he had to interact with anyone who was unfamiliar and would typically hide behind his mum or dad and refuse to speak or make eye contact. He worried a lot about being told off at school, and so he would never put his hand up to answer a question or speak in front of more than one or two other children.

Mark described how both he and Katherine would normally give George repeated reassurance that everything would be okay when he was faced with an anxiety-provoking situation, but he also reported feeling frustrated by George's anxious behavior; he would become cross with him. For example, he recently took George to a friend's birthday party, where George refused to join in and clung to his dad. Mark reassured him that everything would be fine but felt increasingly cross and frustrated that George would still not join in. After a while he found himself telling George that no one would want to be his friend if he didn't play with them and they would think he was a baby; but this appeared to make George even more reluctant to participate and left Mark feeling guilty.

The therapist worked with George's parents and they first *mapped out the cycle of parent and child cognitions and behaviors* that occurred between them in challenging situations such as the party. Through doing this, the therapist assisted George's parents to identify the need to respond to George in a manner that would be less likely to reinforce his anxious thoughts and behaviors. On this basis, the therapist and parents agreed that Mark and Katherine would *set up a reward system* for George's participation in social activities, such as parties, *in conjunction with a graded exposure hierarchy plan*. In addition, they *specifically praised George's attempts to join in* with other children, and they *endeavored to keep their own emotions in check*. On the occasions when George would not join in, they would *ignore his clinging behavior and repeated requests for reassurance*. Instead they would calmly remind him of what he had agreed to do and of the associated reward and then would *ignore all subsequent anxious behavior*.

Given that parents of children and young people with anxiety disorders are at an increased risk of an anxiety disorder themselves, it follows that young people with anxiety disorders are more likely to see their parents express anxiety than those young people without anxiety. Similarly, children and young people who are depressed may be more likely than those who do not have depression to have seen their parents withdraw and disengage as a result of their own low mood (Goodman and Gotlib 1999). The aim of parent modeling of adaptive behavior (Sburlati et al. 2011) is to encourage the parent to use strategies that are helpful and adaptive and to discourage behaviors that are unhelpful, such as avoidance or withdrawal. This is especially

Case 19.3b Modeling brave behavior to George

As the therapist talked with Katherine and Mark, George's parents, it became clear that Katherine experienced a great deal of anxiety in social situations, and this was also evident from her responses to a self-report measure of anxiety that she completed. Katherine described how she had experienced similar difficulties as a child and continued to find some social situations stressful. She reported that, where possible, she would try to avoid putting herself in unfamiliar or difficult situations and described how she was struggling with the renovations that were being carried out to their home, as it meant having workmen in the house that she had to speak to. Where possible, she would try to get Mark to speak to them, especially if she thought this may involve conflict, for instance when asking them to change something they had done. In social situations like parties, she described how she would try to keep busy and find jobs to do in the kitchen, so that she did not end up having to talk to someone she did not know very well.

One of the therapist's goals for the first session was to establish a *collaborative relationship* where Katherine and Mark felt able to openly discuss what was happening, without feeling that they were being blamed for George's difficulties. They then discussed *different factors that contributed toward the development of anxiety*, before considering which were the factors that Katherine and Mark had control over – for instance how they parented George, or what he might learn from their responses in anxious situations. The therapist described how children learn a lot by watching how their parents behave, so that, if *parents can behave in ways that promote coping and do not avoid anxious situations*, this is really helpful. She encouraged Katherine to use a *"Botox Face"* or adopt an *"Oscar-Winning Performance"* (see Cartwright-Hatton et al. 2010) for situations that she would find anxiety provoking, so that she could appear calm, even if she did not feel so underneath.

useful within the context of treatment for child anxiety. Case 19.3b highlights how a therapist assisted George's parents, Katharine and Mark, to model adaptive behavior.

Competence in Treating Anxiety Disorders and Depression

The application of the specific CBT techniques from the modifying the family environment category of Sburlati and colleagues' (2011) model is different for anxiety and for depressive disorders. In consequence, the therapist treating children and young people with anxiety disorders and/or depression ought to become proficient at identifying when these techniques are necessary (which is done on the basis of the disorder presentation or case formulation) and what is the most effective way of implementing them. The following section briefly highlights how, with the help of established, empirically supported treatments, a clinician can make use of the modifying the family environment techniques in the treatment of anxiety disorders and depression.

Anxiety disorders

It is yet to be established that the addition of family components in treatment provides benefit above and beyond individual CBT for anxiety disorders in children and young people (Creswell and Cartwright-Hatton 2007). Comparisons between studies are, however, difficult to make when different treatment studies include such a wide range of interventions for targeting the family environment. Many empirically supported treatments for anxiety disorders in children and young people make use of (i) *parent emotion management,* aimed at lowering the parent's own level of anxiety; (ii) *parent expectations management,* designed to increase unnecessarily low parental expectations; (iii) *parent intrusiveness and overprotection management,* designed to diminish parental overprotection; (iv) *parental contingency management,* undertaken in order to assist parents to praise and reward non-anxious behaviors; and (v) *parent modeling of adaptive behavior,* aimed at encouraging parents to model non-anxious behaviors (e.g., Cartwright-Hatton et al. 2010; Rapee et al. 2006). The modifying the family environment technique that is used less often when treating anxiety in children and young people is (vi) *family communication and conflict resolution,* but this is commonly included in empirically supported treatments for children and young people with depression. A number of anxiety disorder treatment manuals are available for anxiety disorders in children and young people; some of them are transdiagnostic, others are disorder-specific.

Transdiagnostic treatment packages
Probably the most commonly used manualized treatments are *Coping Cat* (8–13 years) (Howard, Chu, Krain, Marrs-Garcia, and Kendall 2000) and *Cool Kids* (7–16 years) (Rapee et al. 2006), and derivatives of these programs have successfully been employed with adolescents (e.g., the CAT Project, 14–17 years; see Kendall, Choudhury, Hudson, and Webb 2002) and with younger children (e.g., *From Timid to Tiger,* for children up to 10 years of age, a program delivered solely via parents; see Cartwright-Hatton et al. 2010).

   The most commonly used strategies in these treatment protocols are management of parental intrusiveness and over-involvement, parent contingency management, and parental modeling of adaptive behavior. For example, in *From Timid to Tiger* there is considerable focus on contingency management through the use of praise designed to build the young person's confidence, through rewards designed to help with motivation, through the setting of limits, and through withdrawal of attention from anxious behavior. Unhelpful parental cognitions – such as the idea that worry is dangerous for the young person – and behaviors – such as modeling anxiety – are also identified and addressed. In *Cool Kids, BRAVE,* and *Overcoming* contingency management, parental over-involvement, and parental modeling of adaptive behavior are all addressed in the parent sessions. Parents are asked to record their responses to their child in order to increase their awareness of their responses and to attempt to alter them where necessary. In *Cool Kids* and *Overcoming, parent emotion management* is also included. In particular, parents are encouraged to engage in their own exposure tasks if they are anxious, which provides them with an opportunity not only to tackle their own fears, but to model adaptive, brave behavior to their child.

Disorder-specific treatment packages

Social phobia   Children and young people with social phobia are commonly treated using a transdiagnostic approach; however, there are also treatments that are disorder-specific and have established excellent outcomes (e.g., Beidel, Turner, and Morris 1998; Spence, Donovan and Brechman-Toussaint 2000). Both of these particular programs place a great deal of emphasis on the young person's acquisition and development of social skills, and parents are involved to varying degrees to support the newly acquired skills. Beidel and colleagues' *social effectiveness therapy* for children and young people involves the parents, with the aim of enabling them to support the young person in completing exposure tasks successfully between sessions, and it positively reinforces the young person's brave behavior. In the treatment devised by Spence and colleagues, for one of the groups of children and young people having CBT, the authors included a parent component where parents were taught to regularly model, prompt, and reinforce their child's developing social skills, in an attempt to generalize them to new environments. The addition of the parent component was associated with a 50 percent improvement in the number of children and young people who became free of social phobia after treatment.

Specific phobia   While it is likely that parental factors are relevant in the development and maintenance of the child's phobia, Öst and Ollendick's (2001) single-session phobia treatment does not require parents to be involved beyond being consulted in case the child is unable to respond to certain instructions, bringing the child to treatment, and taking the child to designated locations for the homework or practice to take place. Recent developments of this approach have, however, augmented the standard treatment with a parental component, which primarily involves psycho-education to parents about phobias and their causes and observation of the child's treatment, with a commentary designed to highlight the steps that the child is working through. During this process the various components and the importance of the reinforcement of child exposure and of continual rehearsal beyond the treatment session are emphasized (Ollendick 2013).

Panic disorder   Parents of children and young people with panic disorder are known to have elevated rates of panic disorder themselves (Last and Strauss 1989), so including parents in the treatment may be of clear benefit in this context. Similar techniques to those seen in transdiagnostic anxiety treatments are included in Pincus, Ehrenreich and Mattis' (2008) panic control treatment for adolescents (PCT-A). In this program parents can be included in a portion of the treatment sessions, in order to ensure that they can help reinforce the concepts that the young person learns in therapy. Therapists are encouraged to engage parents as co-therapists and coaches, rather than seeing them as clients in their own right and potentially getting embroiled in larger family issues. Pincus and colleagues describe how parents are often worried that their child may be in significant distress during a panic attack and therefore may inadvertently reinforce the young person's avoidance of places or situations that could trigger panic symptoms. Therefore parents are given educational handouts and are involved in sessions; the idea is to enable them to better understand their parenting styles and how they inadvertently maintain their child's anxiety. Parents are also instructed in how to encourage more helpful ways of responding, for instance by being compassionate but encouraging the child to push through the anxiety, downplaying the physical feelings and building up the young person's exposure to anxiety-provoking situations in a realistic and manageable way. The importance of consistency between parents is addressed, and parents are taught contingency-management techniques in order to positively reinforce brave behaviors.

Obsessive–compulsive disorder   There is some evidence to suggest that family factors are relevant for understanding obsessive–compulsive disorder (OCD) in childhood. In particular, Barrett, Shortt, and Healy (2002) found that parents of young people with OCD were less confident about their child's abilities and independence skills than parents of young people with other anxiety disorders and less likely to use positive problem-solving techniques. Furthermore, Derisley, Libby, Clarke, and Reynolds (2005) found that parents of young people with OCD tended to cope with problems by avoiding them. It is not clear, however, whether these cognitions and behaviors have a maintaining role (rather than, say, simply being a response to the OCD), and hence whether targeting them in treatment would improve outcomes. Empirically supported treatment approaches for OCD in children and young people (March and Mulle 1998; Waite and Williams 2009) consider the role of parents largely in relation to maintaining the young person's OCD through participation in safety behaviors (e.g., by providing reassurance, carrying out rituals for the child, or enabling avoidance).

Waite, Gallop and Atkinson (2009) suggest a flexible approach to parental involvement – an approach based on the wishes of the young person and the individual case conceptualization. In contrast, March and Mulle's (1998) approach is more structured and involves parent sessions at specific time points in treatment. Both treatment approaches involve the therapist assessing potential family maintaining factors and providing psycho-education about how the parents' behavior can inadvertently keep the young person's problem alive. Parent contingency management is used to enable parents to reinforce their child's brave behavior and to make them deal effectively with situations where the young person becomes anxious.

When OCD takes up so much time and is such a large part of family life, it is not surprising that parents can start to see the OCD as part of their child. It is therefore important that attention is paid to the positive elements of the young person's life and that goals are planned that involve dreams and hopes for the future and that do not relate to OCD (Waite et al. 2009). With this in mind, March and Mulle (1998) encourage families to plan ceremonies and notifications, so that the young person is positively reinforced when (s)he is practicing exposure and response prevention or engages in activities unrelated to the OCD.

Post-traumatic stress disorder   Various factors relating to the family environment appear to be connected to the development and maintenance of post-traumatic stress symptoms in children and young people. In particular, parental depression predicts the development of post-traumatic stress symptoms in children and young people following exposure to a traumatic event (e.g., Smith, Perrin, Yule, and Rabe-Hesketh 2001; Wolmer, Laor, Gershon, Mayes, and Cohen 2000), and this association is mediated by parental endorsement of worry as a coping strategy (Meiser-Stedman, Yule, Dalgleish, Smith, and Glucksman 2006). Furthermore, a number of authors have suggested that parental support is the most critical factor influencing the young person's adjustment after the trauma, particularly in the case of sexual abuse (e.g., Conte and Schuerman 1987; Everson, Hunter, Runyon, Edelsohn, and Coulter 1989). Parental involvement in therapy may therefore be extremely important for enabling parents to manage their own distress, as well as to provide appropriate support for the young person. In their empirically supported treatment for sexual abuse in children and young people, Deblinger and Heflin (1996) recommend individual sessions with the non-offending parent in order to provide support and information and to develop skills. The approach includes an educational component with information about sexual abuse and involves parents being taught coping skills, so that they are able to deal with their own thoughts and emotions effectively, for example by moving from thinking "I am a bad mother for not protecting my son from being abused" to "The secretive nature of sexual abuse makes it difficult for anyone, even parents, to pick it up. It is not possible to supervise my son every minute of the day." Parents are also helped to confront and cope with discussions about the young person's abuse, and they are trained in how to talk to their child about the experience. In addition, they are taught behavior management strategies in order to deal with behaviors such as angry outbursts, anxiety, or sexualized behaviors and to encourage more adaptive ones.

Depression

Despite the fact that many clinicians agree about the usefulness, and at times necessity, of family involvement in treatments for children and young people with depression, the extent to which the effectiveness of treatments for adolescent depression is enhanced by the inclusion of family components is not clear at present. To date, very few studies have specifically evaluated the possible advantages of interventions that include strategies aimed at modifying the family environment for children and young people with depression. Where they have, a trend toward better outcomes where parents are involved in treatment has been observed; but differences in outcomes are not statistically significant (e.g., Clarke, Rhode, Lewinsohn, Hops, and Seeley 1999; Lewinsohn, Clarke, Hops, and Andrews 1990). Despite this, the evidence for associations between family factors and depression in children and young people would suggest that families should be taken into consideration in some way when treating the child or young person.

Empirically supported treatments vary in the amount of family and parent involvement and often apply a formulation-led, modular approach in determining the degree of use of family strategies for individual clients (e.g., Brent and Poling 1997; Clarke et al. 1990; Curry et al. 2005). This degree will depend on individual family functioning, on the quality of relationships, and on whether the parents are able and willing to participate in treatment. Empirically supported treatments for depression in children and young people typically make use of (i) *family communication and conflict resolution* – to improve negative communication, increase positive communication, improve conflict resolution, and ultimately enhance the quality of the parent–adolescent relationship; (ii) *parent expectations management* – aimed at lowering unnecessarily high parental expectations of the child or young person with depression; and (iii) *parental contingency management* – to provide children and young people with positive reinforcement and to reduce negative reinforcement or punishment of the young person with depression (e.g., Brent and Poling 1997; Clarke et al. 1990; Curry et al. 2005). Unlike anxiety treatments, depression treatments typically make less use of (iv) *parent modeling of adaptive behavior*, (v) *parental intrusiveness and overprotection management*; and (vi) *parent emotion management* from the modifying the family environment category. However, if parental depression is identified, parents are encouraged to seek their own treatment, and referrals are arranged accordingly. Some treatment programs stress that parental psychopathology must be addressed, and treatment for parents is seen as a necessary component of the overall intervention (e.g., Brent and Poling 1997).

Competence in Working with Different Ages and Presenting Problems

The age of the child or young person ought to be considered by therapists when planning the degree of parent involvement in treatment. Research suggests that parental involvement may lead to better outcomes for younger children (e.g., Barrett et al. 1996), which means that the specific CBT techniques from the modifying the family environment category of Sburlati and colleagues' (2011) model may be more useful with younger children than with adolescents. In fact some interventions for very young children, from age 4 to 8 (Waters, Ford, Wharton, and Cobham 2009) or 4 to 9 (Cartwright-Hatton et al. 2010), do not include the child in the treatment at all; rather the therapist engages only with the parents. Recently, parent-led CBT has been implemented as a low-intensity intervention in which parents are guided through a self-help book to overcome their child's difficulties with anxiety. This approach has been effective both in the UK (Thirlwall et al. 2013) and in rural Australian settings (Lyneham and Rapee 2006). It is notable, however, that, when it comes to parent-led CBT like this, Creswell and colleagues (2010) found that poorer outcomes were associated with higher levels of anxiety in parents, and Waters and colleagues (2009) found that more families dropped out of treatment when the young person was not included in the treatment sessions. These considerations clearly need to be taken into account by therapists when they make decisions about how and when to include families in treatment in order to optimize outcomes for children and young people.

It is worth noting, however, that factors other than the child's age contribute to whether parental involvement in treatment is going to be advantageous. For instance, parent involvement in treatment enhances outcomes when the child is school-refusing (Heyne et al. 2002), when the child is anxious about separating from caregivers (e.g., Choate, Pincus, Eyberg, and Barlow 2005), or when parents experience high levels of anxiety themselves (e.g., Cobham et al. 1998). Thus, when implementing treatment with younger children, with children who refuse school, and with children who suffer from separation anxiety and/or live in the context of parental anxiety, therapists ought to involve parents in the treatment.

The degree of parental involvement varies across treatments packages. While some treatment protocols involve parents in a structured number of sessions (e.g., Curry et al. 2005; Spence et al. 2000; Spence et al. 2011), the majority are flexible in how parents should be involved. When treatment approaches have been evaluated through randomized control trials, the nature of the family's involvement in therapy has not typically been the main focus of study. Where family involvement in CBT is the main focus of study, the variation in the nature and amount of family involvement across trials is such that it becomes difficult to draw any clear conclusions about who should be involved and how.

Common Obstacles to Competent Practice and Methods to Overcome Them

There are many factors that can make it difficult to modify the family environment. To begin with, parents can often feel that it is their fault that the young person is experiencing difficulties with anxiety or depression, and this can lead to feelings of guilt and shame. They may feel that they are not a good enough parent, feel stigmatized to be seen by a mental health service, and feel judged by other people – family, friends, other parents, and professionals (e.g., Hinshaw 2005). Where there are two parents in a family, it is not uncommon that they will have different and conflicting perspectives on how to deal with the young person's anxiety or low mood, and this can make it difficult for them to use a consistent approach. Where parents are separated or divorced, they may not be willing or able to discuss and agree on a way forward. There may be other family members, such as step-parents or grandparents, who are also very involved in the child's life but see the problem differently or are unwilling to change the way they deal with things. Teachers at school may also be handling things in a way that inadvertently perpetuates the problem. Families can be in the midst of having to cope with other stressful life events – redundancy, ill health, relationship breakdown, bereavement, financial concerns, or mental health difficulties (Goodman and Gotlib 1999) – and this makes it difficult for parents to find the energy or time to attend sessions or to support the child to develop and practice new strategies and skills outside sessions. Parents may understand the need to support and encourage their child to expose him-/herself to situations (s)he has been regularly avoiding because of anxiety or low mood, but they may struggle to successfully implement strategies due to difficulties in tolerating the child's negative emotions (Tiwari et al. 2008). Finally, there may be some elements of the young person's difficulties that are not unpleasant, or may even be beneficial for family members, and therefore become positively reinforced (Choate et al. 2005); for example, having the young person sleeping in the same bed may at times be pleasant for a parent, especially if there is a lack of physical contact at other times, if the parent lacks other intimate relationships, or if this happens in the context of marital difficulties.

When families are involved in treatment, it is important that the therapist provides the parents with a clear, understandable rationale for their inclusion. Where difficulties are encountered, the therapist needs to attend to them as early as possible. From the beginning, it is crucial that the therapist fosters a collaborative relationship with the family; therapist and family should function as a team in order to make sense of the problem and try out new ways of dealing with it. By adopting a validating, empathic, and curious stance, the therapist can identify any negative or unhelpful thoughts and beliefs held by parents and any parental behaviors that may be maintaining the problem and need to be addressed in therapy. However, it is also critical to identify and reinforce what parents are doing that works well, in often very difficult circumstances. When parents feel that they are to blame for the young person's difficulties, it can be helpful if the therapist provides psycho-education about the many factors that contribute to the development and maintenance of anxiety or depression in young people (Hinshaw 2005) and if (s)he makes use of Socratic questioning and open discussion to explore matters further. For families where there are conflicting perspectives about how to manage the young person's anxiety or depression, it may be necessary to find goals that everyone can agree on.

For example, in the case of school refusal, where one parent believes that the child should not have to attend school and should be home-tutored while the other parent believes that attending school is essential for getting a good education, it may be possible to identify a goal based on a shared wish for the young person to receive an education that enables him/her to get the necessary qualifications as well as to have opportunities to develop and maintain social relationships. The therapist may need to engage other family members in order to explore their beliefs, provide psycho-education, and encourage them to behave in ways that promote the young person's adaptive behavior. The therapist may need to closely attend to parental mental health difficulties by routinely assessing parental anxiety and depression, being proactive in discussing the impact of difficulties on the child, and facilitating and encouraging parents to seek help for themselves. Where parents struggle to implement strategies due to their difficulty in tolerating the child's distress, they may need support in order to develop a more adaptive view of their child – a view that allows them to recognize the child's ability to cope with potential challenges, with appropriate support (e.g., Duncan, Coatsworth, and Greenberg 2009). Finally, where there is evidence that parents may find some elements of the young person's difficulties beneficial, the therapist will need to explore this further through Socratic questioning and problem solving, in order to discover with the parents how they can achieve the same feeling in a more adaptive way (e.g., by having quality time with the young person at other times, or by developing their own social network and interests, separate from the child's).

Summary

Factors relating to the family environment play a role in the development and maintenance of anxiety and depressive disorders in children and young people. This is recognized in many empirically supported treatments through the inclusion of specific interventions targeting parental cognitions and behaviors. In this chapter we have illustrated how, in a range of anxiety disorders and depression, clinicians can teach parents strategies for managing their own anxiety or low mood as it relates to their child, how they can identify and modify unrealistically high parental expectations, intervene to improve family communication and conflict resolution, or encourage parents to grant more autonomy, reinforce their child's more adaptive behaviors and model adaptive behaviors.

While these strategies target particular parental processes that appear to be associated with anxiety or depression in children and young people, it is yet to be established that the addition of family components in treatment provides benefit above and beyond individual CBT (Creswell and Cartwright-Hatton 2007). Further specification of the family processes that maintain emotional disorders in children and young people (such as parental psychopathology and parental behaviors) are likely to lead to more clearly defined family interventions. Factors such as symptom severity, comorbidity, specific diagnoses (of the young person and, where relevant, of the parent(s)) may be important to consider in order to clarify at whom family-based interventions should be targeted.

References

Asarnow, Joan R., Michael J. Goldstein, Martha Tompson, and Donald Guthrie. 1993. "One-Year Outcomes of Depressive Disorders in Child Psychiatric Inpatients: Evaluation of the Prognostic Power of a Brief Measure of Expressed Emotion." *Journal of Child Psychology and Psychiatry and Allied Disciplines*, 34: 129–37. DOI: 10.1111/j.1469-7610.1993.tb00975.x

Barber, Brian K. 1996. "Parental Psychological Control: Revisiting a Neglected Construct." *Child Development*, 67 (6): 3296–319. DOI: 10.1111/j.1467-8624.1996.tb01915.x

Barrett, Paula M., Alison Shortt, and Lara Healy. 2002. "Do Parent and Child Behaviors Differentiate Families Whose Children Have Obsessive–Compulsive Disorder from Other Clinic and Non-Clinic Families?" *Journal of Child Psychology and Psychiatry*, 43: 597–607. DOI: 10.1111/1469-7610.00049

Barrett, Paula M., Ronald M. Rapee, Mark R. Dadds, and Sharon M. Ryan. 1996. "Family Enhancement of Cognitive Style in Anxious and Aggressive Children." *Journal of Abnormal Child Psychology*, 24: 187–203. DOI: 10.1007/BF01441484

Beck, Aaron T. 1976. *Cognitive Therapy and the Emotional Disorders*. New York: International Universities Press.

Beidel, Deborah C., Samuel M. Turner, and Tracy L. Morris. 1998. *SET-C: Social Effectiveness Therapy for Children and Adolescents*. Unpublished manuscript.

Birmaher, Boris. 2011. "Remission of a Mother's Depression Is Associated with Her Child's Mental Health." *American Journal of Psychiatry*, 168: 563–5. DOI: 10.1176/appi.ajp.2011.11020305

Brent, David A., and Kimberly Poling. 1997. *Cognitive Therapy Treatment Manual for Depressed and Suicidal Youth*. Pittsburgh, CA: University of Pittsburgh, Services for Teens at Risk.

Cartwright-Hatton, Sam, Ben Laskey, Stewart Rust, and Deborah McNally. 2010. *From Timid to Tiger: A Treatment Manual for Parenting the Anxious Child*. Chichester, England: Wiley-Blackwell.

Choate, Molly, L., Donna B. Pincus, Sheila M. Eyberg, and David H. Barlow. 2005. "Parent–Child Interaction Therapy for Treatment of Separation Anxiety Disorder in Young Children: A Pilot Study." *Cognitive and Behavioral Practice*, 12: 126–35.

Clarke, Gregory N., Peter M. Lewinsohn, and Hyman Hops. 1990. *Leader's Manual for Adolescent Groups: Coping with Depression Course*. Portland, OR: Kaiser Permanente Center for Health Research.

Clarke, Gregory N., Paul Rhode, Peter M. Lewinsohn, Hyman Hops, and John R. Seeley. 1999. "Cognitive–Behavioral Treatment of Adolescent Depression: Efficacy of Acute Group Treatment and Booster Sessions." *Journal of the American Academy of Child and Adolescent Psychiatry*, 38: 272–9.

Cobham, Vanessa E., Susan H. Spence, and Mark R. Dadds. 1998. "The Role of Parental Anxiety in the Treatment of Childhood Anxiety." *Journal of Consulting and Clinical Psychology*, 66: 893–905. DOI: 10.1037/0022-006X.66.6.893

Cole, David A., and Lynn P. Rehm. 1986. "Family Interaction Patterns and Childhood Depression." *Journal of Abnormal Child Psychology*, 14: 297–314. DOI: 10.1007/BF00915448

Conte, Jon R., and John R. Schuerman. 1987. "Factors Associated with an Increased Impact of Child Sexual Abuse." *Child Abuse and Neglect*, 11: 201–11. DOI: 10.1016/0145-2134

Cooper, Peter J., Catherine Gallop, Lucy Willetts, and Cathy Creswell. 2008. "Treatment Response in Child Anxiety Is Differentially Related to the Form of Maternal Anxiety Disorder." *Behavioural and Cognitive Psychotherapy*, 36: 41–8.

Cooper, Peter J., Vanessa Fearn, Lucy Willetts, Hannah Seabrook, and Monika Parkinson. 2006. "Affective Disorder in the Parents of a Clinic Sample of Children with Anxiety Disorders." *Journal of Affective Disorders*, 93: 205–12.

Creswell, Cathy, and Sam Cartwright-Hatton. 2007. "Family Treatment of Child Anxiety: Outcomes, Limitations and Future direction." *Clinical Child and Family Psychology*, 10: 232–52. DOI: 10.1007/s10567-007-0019-3

Creswell, Cathy, Frances Hentges, Monika Parkinson, Paul Sheffield, Lucy Willetts, and Peter Cooper. 2010. "Feasibility of Guided Cognitive Behaviour Therapy (CBT) Self-Help for Childhood Anxiety Disorders in Primary Care." *Mental Health in Family Medicine*, 7: 49–57.

Creswell, Cathy, Adela Apetroaia, Lynne Murray, and Peter Cooper. 2012. "Cognitive, Affective, and Behavioral Characteristics of Mothers with Anxiety Disorders in the Context of Child Anxiety Disorder." *Journal of Abnormal Psychology*, 121: 26–38. DOI: 10.1037/a0029516

Creswell, Cathy, Lynne Murray, Stacey James, and Peter Cooper. 2011. "Parenting and Child Anxiety." In Wendy K. Silverman and Andy P. Field (Eds.), *Anxiety Disorders in Children and Adolescents* (pp. 299–322). Cambridge: Cambridge University Press.

Curry, John F., Karen C. Wells, David A. Brent, Gregory N. Clarke, Paul Rohde, Anne Marie Albano, … John S. March. 2005. *Treatment for Adolescents with Depression Study (TADS) Cognitive Behavior Therapy Manual: Introduction, Rationale, and Adolescent Sessions.* Durham, NC: Duke University Medical Center, The TADS Team.

De Rosnay, Marc, Peter J. Cooper, Nicholas Tsigaras, and Lynne Murray. 2006. "Transmission of Social Anxiety from Mother to Infant: An Experimental Study Using a Social Referencing Paradigm." *Behavior Research and Therapy*, 44: 1165–75. DOI: 10.1016/j.brat.2005.09.003

de Wilde, Alice, and Ronald M. Rapee. 2008. "Do Controlling Maternal Behaviours Increase State Anxiety in Children's Responses to a Social Threat? A Pilot Study." *Journal of Behavior Therapy and Experimental Psychiatry*, 39: 526–37. DOI: 10.1016/j.jbtep.2007.10.011

Deblinger, Esther, and Anne Hope Heflin. 1996. *Treating Sexually Abused Children and Their Nonoffending Parents.* Thousand Oaks, CA: Sage.

Derisley, Jo, Sarah Libby, Sarah Clarke, and Shirley Reynolds. 2005. "Mental Health, Coping and Family-Functioning in Parents of Young People with Obsessive–Compulsive Disorder and with Anxiety Disorders." *British Journal of Clinical Psychology*, 44: 439–44. DOI: 10.1348/014466505X29152

Duncan, Larissa J., J. Douglas Coatsworth, and Mark T. Greenberg. 2009. "Pilot Study to Gauge Acceptability of a Mindfulness-Based, Family-Focused Preventive Intervention." *Journal of Primary Prevention*, 30: 605–18. DOI: 10.1007/s10935-009-0185-9

Ehrmantrout, Nikki, Nicholas B. Allen, Craig Leve, Betsy Davis, and Lisa Sheeber. 2011. "Adolescent Recognition of Parental Affect: Influence of Depressive Symptoms. *Journal of Abnormal Psychology*, 120: 628–34. DOI: 10.1037/a0022500

Eley, Thalia C., Jennifer L. Hudson, Cathy Creswell, Maria Tropeano, Kathryn J. Lester, Peter Cooper, ... David A. Collier. 2011. "Therapygenetics: The 5HT-TLPR and Response to Psychological Therapy." *Molecular Psychiatry*, 17: 236–7. DOI: 10.1038/mp.2011.132

Everson, Mark D., Wanda M. Hunter, Desmond K. Runyon, Gail A. Edelsohn, and Martha L. Coulter. 1989. "Maternal Support following Disclosure of Incest." *American Journal of Orthopsychiatry*, 59 (2): 197–207. DOI: 10.1111/j.1939-0025.1989.tb01651.x

Gerull, Friederike C., and Ronald M. Rapee. 2002. "Mother Knows Best: Effects of Maternal Modelling on the Acquisition of Fear and Avoidance Behaviour in Toddlers." *Behaviour Research and Therapy*, 40: 279–87. DOI: 10.1016/S0005-7967(01)00013-4

Goodman, Sherryl H., and Ian H. Gotlib. 1999. "Risk for Psychopathology in the Children of Depressed Mothers: A Developmental Model for Understanding Mechanisms of Transmission." *Psychological Review*, 106: 458–90. DOI: 10.1037/0033-295X.106.3.458

Gotlib, Ian H., and Constance L. Hammen. 1992. *Psychological Aspects of Depression: Toward a Cognitive–Interpersonal Integration*. Chichester, Englans: Wiley.

Grant, Kathryn E., Bruce E. Compas, Audrey E. Thurm, Susan D. McMahon, and Polly Y. Gipson. 2004. "Stressors and Child and Adolescent Psychopathology: Measurement Issues and Prospective Effects." *Journal of Clinical Child and Adolescent Psychology*, 33: 412–25. DOI: 10.1207/s15374424jccp3302_23

Greenberger, Ellen, Chuansheng S. Chen, Steven R. Tally, and Qi Dong. 2000. "Family, Peer, and Individual Correlates of Depressive Symptomatology among US and Chinese Adolescents." *Journal of Consulting and Clinical Psychology*, 68 (2): 209–19. DOI: 10.1037//0022-006X.68.2.209

Hammen, Constance L., David Gordon, Dorli Burge, Adrian Cheri, Carol Jaenicke, and Donald Hiroto. 1987. "Maternal Affective Disorders, Illness, and Stress: Risk for Children's Psychopathology." *The American Journal of Psychiatry*, 144: 736–41.

Heyne, David, Neville J. King, Bruce J. Tonge, Stephanie Rollings, Dawn Young, Melinda Pritchard, and Thomas H. Ollendick. 2002. "Evaluation of Child Therapy and Caregiver Training in the Treatment of School Refusal." *Journal of the American Academy of Child and Adolescent Psychiatry*, 41 (6): 687–95.

Hinshaw, Stephen P. 2005. The Stigmatization of Mental Illness in Children and Parents: Developmental Issues, Family Concerns, and Research Needs. *Journal of Child Psychology and Psychiatry*, 46 (7): 714–34. DOI: 10.1111/j.1469-7610.2005.01456.x

Hollander, Eric. 1997. "Obsessive–Compulsive Disorder: The Hidden Epidemic." *Journal of Clinical Psychiatry*, 58 (suppl. 12): 3–6.

Howard, Bonnie, Brian C. Chu, Amy L. Krain, Abbe L. Marrs-Garcia, and Philip C. Kendall. 2000. *Cognitive–Behavioral Family Therapy for Anxious Children: Therapist Manual* (2nd ed.). Ardmore, PA: Workbook.

Hudson, Jennifer L., and Ronald M. Rapee. 2004. "From Anxious Temperament to Disorder: An Etiological Model of Generalized Anxiety Disorder." In Richard G. Heimberg, Cynthia L. Turk, and Douglas S. Mennin (Eds.), *Generalized Anxiety Disorder: Advances in Research and Practice* (pp. 51–74). New York: Guilford Press.

Joiner, Thomas, James C. Coyne, and Janice Blalock. 1999. "On the Interpersonal Nature of Depression: Overview and Synthesis." In Thomas Joiner and James C. Coyne (Eds.),

The Interactional Nature of Depression: Advances in Interpersonal Approaches (pp. 3–19). Washington, DC: American Psychological Association.

Kaslow, Nadine J., Catherine Gray Deering, and Gary R. Racusin. 1994. "Depressed Children and Their Families." *Clinical Psychology Review*, 14: 39–59. DOI: 10.1016/0272-7358(94)90047-7

Kendall, Phillip C., Muniya Choudhury, Jennifer Hudson, and Alicia Webb. 2002. *The C.A.T. Project Workbook for the Cognitive–Behavioral Treatment of Anxious Adolescents (Ages 14–17)*. Ardmore, PA: Workbook.

Kerfoot, Michael, Elizabeth Dyer, Val Harrington, Adrine Woodham, and Richard Harrington. 1996. "Correlates and Short-Term Course of Self-Poisoning in Adolescents." *British Journal of Psychiatry*, 168: 38–42. DOI: 10.1192/bjp.168.1.38

Last, Cynthia G., and Cyd C. Strauss. 1989. "Panic Disorder in Children and Adolescents." *Journal of Anxiety Disorders*, 3: 87–95. DOI: 10.1016/0887-6185

Last, Cynthia G., Michel Hersen, Alan Kazdin, Helen Orvaschel, and Sean Perrin. 1991. "Anxiety Disorders in Children and Their Families." *Archives of General Psychiatry*, 48: 928–39. DOI: 10.1001/archpsyc.1991.01810340060008

Lewinsohn, Peter M., Gregory N. Clarke, Hyman Hops, and Judy Andrews. 1990. "Cognitive–Behavioral Treatment for Depressed Adolescents." *Behavior Therapy*, 21: 385–401. DOI: 10.1016/S0005-7894(05)80353-3

Lyneham, Heidi J., and Ronald M. Rapee. 2006. "Evaluation of Therapist-Supported Parent-Implemented CBT for Anxiety Disorders in Rural Children." *Behaviour Research and Therapy*, 44: 1287–300. DOI: 10/1016/j.brat.2005.09.009

March, John S., and Karen Mulle. 1998. *OCD in Children and Adolescents: A Cognitive–Behavioral Treatment Manual*. New York: Guilford Press.

McLeod, Bryce D., Jeffrey J. Wood, and John R. Weisz. 2007. "Examining the Association between Parenting and Childhood Anxiety: A Meta-Analysis." *Clinical Psychology Review*, 27: 155–72. DOI: 10.1016/j/cpr.2006.09.002

Meiser-Stedman, Richard A., William Yule, Tim Dalgleish, Patrick Smith, and Edward Glucksman. 2006. "The Role of the Family in Child and Adolescent Posttraumatic Stress following Attendance at an Emergency Department." *Journal of Pediatric Psychology*, 31: 397–402. DOI: 10.1093/jpepsy/jsj005

Murray, Lynne, Peter J. Cooper, Cathy Creswell, Elizabeth Schofield, and Caroline Sack. 2007. "The Effects of Maternal Social Phobia on Mother–Infant Interactions and Infant Social Responsiveness." *Journal of Child Psychology and Psychiatry*, 48: 45–52. DOI: 10.1111/j.1469-7610.2006.01657.x

Murray, Lynne, Marc DeRosnay, Joanna Pearson, Caroline Bergeron, Elizabeth Schofield, Melanie Royal-Lawson, and Peter J. Cooper. 2008. "Intergenerational Transmission of Maternal Social Anxiety: The Role of the Social Referencing Process." *Child Development*, 79: 1049–64. DOI: 10.1111/j.1467-8624.2008.01175.x

Öst, Lars-Göran, and Thomas H. Ollendick. 2001. *Manual for One-Session Treatment of Specific Phobias*. Unpublished manuscript.

Ollendick, Thomas H. (2013). *Guidelines for Parent Therapist Competency in One-Session Treatment*. Unpublished manuscript.

Pincus, Donna B., Jill T. Ehrenreich, and Sara G. Mattis. 2008. *Mastery of Anxiety and Panic for Adolescents: Riding the Wave Therapist Guide (Treatments That Work)*. New York: Oxford University Press.

Pineda, Ashley Q., David A. Cole, and Alanna E. Bruce. 2007. "Mother–Adolescent Interactions and Adolescent Depressive Symptoms: A Sequential Analysis." *Journal of Social and Personal Relationships*, 24: 5–19. DOI: 10.1177/0265407507072564

Rapee, Ronald M. 1997. "Potential Role of Childrearing Practices in the Development of Anxiety and Depression." *Clinical Psychology Review*, 17: 47–67. DOI: 10.1016/S0272-7358(96)00040-2

Rapee, Ronald M., Heidi J. Lyneham, Carolyn A. Schniering, Viviana Wuthrich, Maree A. Abbot, Jennifer L. Hudson, and Ann Wignall. 2006. *The Cool Kids "Chilled" Adolescent Anxiety Program Therapist Manual.* Sydney, Australia: Centre for Emotional Health, Macquarie University.

Sburlati, Elizabeth S., Carolyn A. Schniering, Heidi J. Lyneham, and Ronald M. Rapee. 2011. "A Model of Therapist Competencies for the Empirically Supported Cognitive Behavioral Treatment of Child and Adolescent Anxiety and Depressive Disorders." *Clinical Child and Family Psychology Review*, 14: 89–109. DOI: 10.1007/s10567-011-0083-6

Schwartz, Orli S., Paul Dudgeon, Lisa B. Sheeber, Marie B. H. Yap, Julian G. Simmons, and Nicholas B. Allen. 2012. "Parental Behaviors During Family Interactions Predict Changes in Depression and Anxiety Symptoms During Adolescence." *Journal of Abnormal Child Psychology*, 40: 59–71. DOI 10.1007/s10802-011-9542-2

Sheeber, Lisa B., Betsy Davis, Craig Lever, Hyman Hops, and Eilzabeth Tildesley. 2007. "Adolescents' Relationships with Their Mothers and Fathers: Associations with Depressive Disorder and Subdiagnostic Symptomatology." *Journal of Abnormal Psychology*, 116: 144–54. DOI: 10.1037/0021-843X.116.1.144

Smith, Patrick, Sean Perrin, Willian Yule, and Sophia Rabe-Hesketh. 2001. "War Exposure and Maternal Reactions in the Psychological Adjustment of Children from Bosnia-Hercegovina." *Journal of Child Psychology and Psychiatry and Allied Disciplines*, 42: 395–404.

Southam-Gerow, Michael A., Philip C. Kendall, and V. Robin Weersing. 2001. "Examining Outcome Variability: Correlates of Treatment Response in a Child and Adolescent Anxiety Clinic." *Journal of Clinical Child and Adolescent Psychology*, 30: 422–36. DOI: 10.1207/S15374424JCCP3003_13

Spence, Susan H., Caroline Donovan, and Margaret Brechman-Toussaint. 2000. "The Treatment of Childhood Social Phobia: The Effectiveness of a Social Skills Training-Based, Cognitive–Behavioural Intervention, with and without Parental Involvement." *Journal of Child Psychology and Psychiatry*, 41: 713–26. DOI: 10.1111/1469-7610.00659

Spence, Susan H., Caroline L. Donovan, Sonja March, Amanda Gamble, Renee E. Anderson, Samantha Prosser, and Justin Kenardy. 2011. "A Randomized Controlled Trial of Online versus Clinic-Based CBT for Adolescent Anxiety." *Journal of Consulting and Clinical Psychology*, 79: 629–42. DOI: 10.1037/a0024512

Stark, Kevin D., Laura Lynn Humphrey, Kim Crook, and Kay Lewis. 1990. "Perceived Family Environments of Depressed and Anxious Children: Child's and Maternal Figure's Perspectives." *Journal of Abnormal Psychology*, 18, 527–47. DOI: 10.1007/BF00911106

Stein, Daniel, Douglas E. Williamson, Boris Birmaher, David A. Brent, Joan Kaufman, Ronald E. Dahl, James M. Perel, and Neal D. Ryan. 2000. "Parent–Child Bonding and Family Functioning in Depressed Children and Children at High Risk and Low Risk for Future Depression." *Journal of the American Academy of Child and Adolescent Psychiatry*, 39: 1387–95. DOI: 10.1097/00004583-200011000-00013

Stobie, Blake, Tracey Taylor, Alexandra Quigley, Sandra Ewing, and Paul M. Salkovskis. 2007. "'Contents May Vary': A Pilot Study of Treatment Histories of OCD Patients." *Cognitive and Behavioural Psychotherapy*, 35: 273–82: DOI: 10.1017/S135246580700358X

Thirlwall, Kerstin, and Cathy Creswell. 2010. "The Impact of Maternal Control on Children's Anxious Cognitions, Behaviour and Affect: An Experimental Study." *Behaviour Research and Therapy*, 48: D1041–46. DOI: 10.1016/j.brat.2010.05.030

Thirlwall, Kerstin, Peter J. Cooper, Jessica Karalus, Merryn Voysey, Lucy Willetts, and Cathy Creswell. 2013. "Treatment of Child Anxiety Disorders via Guided Parent-Delivered Cognitive-Behavioural Therapy: Randomised Controlled Trial." *The British Journal of Psychiatry.* DOI: 10.1192/bjp.bp.113.126698

Tiwari, Shilpee, Jennifer C. Podell, Erin D. Martin, Matt P. Mychailyszyn, Jami M. Furr, and Philip C. Kendall. 2008. "Experiential Avoidance in the Parenting of Anxious Youth: Theory, Research and Future Directions." *Cognition and Emotion*, 22 (3): 480–96. DOI: 10.1080/02699930801886599

Waite, Polly, and Tim Williams (Eds.). 2009. *CBT with Children, Adolescents and Families: Cognitive Behavioral Approaches and Interventions for Obsessive Compulsive Disorder.* London: Taylor Francis.

Waite, Polly, Catherine Gallop, and Linda Atkinson. 2009. "Planning and Carrying Out Treatment." In Polly Waite and Tim Williams (Eds.), *CBT with Children, Adolescents and Families: Cognitive Behavioral Approaches and Interventions for Obsessive Compulsive Disorder* (pp. 51–76). London: Taylor Francis.

Waters, Allison M., Louise A. Ford, Trisha A. Wharton, and Vanessa E. Cobham. 2009. "Cognitive–Behavioural Therapy for Young Children with Anxiety Disorders: Comparison of a Child + Parent Condition versus a Parent Only Condition. *Behaviour Research and Therapy*, 47: 654–62. DOI: 10.1016/j.brat.2009.04.008

Webster-Stratton, Carolyn. 1984. "Randomized Trial of Two Parent-Training Programs for Families with Conduct-Disordered Children." *Journal of Consulting and Clinical Psychology*, 52: 666–70. DOI: 10.1037/0022-006X.52.4.666

Weissman, Myrna M., Daniel J. Pilowsky, Priya J. Wickramaratne, Ardesheer Talati, Stephen R. Wisniewski, Maurizio Fava, … A. John Rush. 2006. "Remissions in Maternal Depression and Child Psychopathology: A STAR*D-Child Report." *The Journal of the American Medical Association*, 295: 1389–1398. DOI: 10.1001/jama.295.12.1389

Wickramaratne, Priya, Marc J. Gameroff, Daniel J. Pilowsky, Carroll W. Hughes, Judy Garber, Erin Malloy, … Myrna M. Weissman. 2011. "Children of Depressed Mothers 1 Year after Remission of Maternal Depression: Findings from the STAR*D-Child Study." *The American Journal of Psychiatry*, 168: 593–602. DOI: 10.1176/appi.ajp.2010.10010032

Wolmer, Leo, Nathaniel Laor, Avner Gershon, Linda C. Mayes, and Donald Cohen. 2000. "The Mother–Child Dyad Facing Trauma: A Developmental Outlook." *The Journal of Nervous and Mental Disease*, 188: 409–15.

Wood, Jeffrey J., Bryce D. McLeod, Marian Sigman, Wei-Chin Hwang, and Brian C. Chu. 2003. "Parenting and Childhood Anxiety: Theory, Empirical Findings, and Future Directions." *Journal of Child Psychology and Psychiatry*, 44: 134–51.

Index

absenteeism 89, 147
  see also school refusal
ACTION program 15
ADIS-C/P 87
affective bond 65, 71
age-appropriate activities 30, 70
age-appropriate rewards 69, 70
aggression 100, 221, 234, 266, 269
  in family 56
agoraphobia 240
American Psychological Association
    (APA) 39
anhedonia 50
anxiety disorders
  and avoidant coping style 104
  and cognitive restructuring 173
  and conditioning 105–6
  and emotional liability 104–5
  and emotion regulation 231–2
  and environmental factors 105–7
  and family environment 105, 276–7,
    288–91
  and internal factors 104–5
  and life events 106–7
  and negative thoughts 187, 189
  and parenting styles 105, 108, 289
  and positive imagery 182–3
  and problem solving skills 250–1

  and self-talk 185
  and social skills training 267–8
  comorbidity 85–6, 89, 172
  competence in treating 7, 41–2, 67–8,
    144–7, 172–3, 182–3, 185, 187, 189,
    213–16, 231–2, 236, 239, 242, 250–3,
    267–9, 287–92
  exposure therapy 194–207
  integrated model of 107–8
  see also generalized anxiety disorder (GAD)
applied tension (AT) 237–40
arousal 108, 225, 227
"assertive imagery" technique 265
assertiveness skills 264–5
assertiveness training 144
assessment
  consideration of different diagnosis 85–6
  developmental factors 86–7, 90
  during treatment 122–3
  evidence-based (EBA) 80–2
  integration of data 84–5
  key features of competencies 80
  multi-informant 84
  multi-method 83–4
  multi-systemic 87–8
  obstacles to 89–90
  of self-harm risk 88–9
  of suicide risk 88–9

Evidence-Based CBT for Anxiety and Depression in Children and Adolescents: A Competencies-Based Approach,
First Edition. Edited by Elizabeth S. Sburlati, Heidi J. Lyneham, Carolyn A. Schniering, and Ronald M. Rapee.
© 2014 John Wiley & Sons, Ltd. Published 2014 by John Wiley & Sons, Ltd.